# METHYLATION - FROM DNA, RNA AND HISTONES TO DISEASES AND TREATMENT

Edited by **Anica Dricu**

**Methylation - From DNA, RNA and Histones to Diseases and Treatment**
http://dx.doi.org/10.5772/2932
Edited by Anica Dricu

**Contributors**

Anica Dricu, Dmitri Nikitin, Attila Kertesz-Farkas2, Alexander Solonin, Marina Mokrishcheva, Hirokazu Suzuki, Robert Peter Mason, Mark Brown, Xian Wang, Hongchuan Jin, Elena Kubareva, Alexandra Ryazanova, Liudmila Abrosimova, Tatiana Oretskaya, Zvonko Magic, Gordana Supic, Nebojsa Jovic, Mirjana Brankovic-Magic, Jianrong Li, Rita Castro, Byron Baron

**Published by InTech**

Janeza Trdine 9, 51000 Rijeka, Croatia



**Publishing Process Manager** Iva Simcic
**Technical Editor** InTech DTP team
**Cover** InTech Design team

Additional hard copies can be obtained from orders@intechopen.com

Methylation - From DNA, RNA and Histones to Diseases and Treatment , Edited by Anica Dricu
p. cm.
ISBN 978-953-51-0881-8

For EU product safety concerns:
IN TECH d.o.o., Prolaz Marije Krucifikse Kozulić 3, 51000 Rijeka, Croatia,
info@intechopen.com or visit our website at intechopen.com.

# Meet the editor

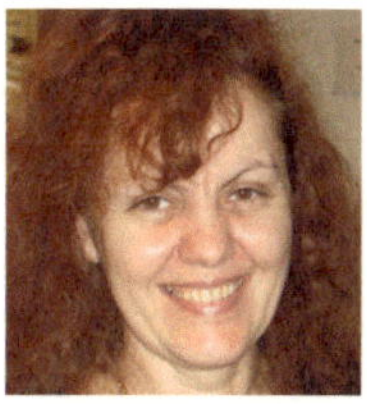

Prof. Anica Dricu was awarded his PhD in Experimental Pathology by the University of Medicine „ Karolinska Institute" , Stockholm, in 1997. She became Docent in Molecular Oncology at the University of Medicine „Karolinska Institute", Stockholm, in 2007. Dr. Anica Dricu was appointed Professor at the University of Medicine and Pharmacy Craiova, in 2009. As a faculty member at the University of Medicine and Pharmacy Craiova, Prof. Anica Dricu is involved in teaching medical students, residents, clinical fellows, graduate and undergraduate students. In addition to her research and teaching activities, Prof. Dricu is actively involved in service at national and institutional levels; she is currently, director of the Doctoral School and head of the Division of Biochemistry at the University of Medicine and Pharmacy Craiova and she also serves as a member of the National Council for Titles, Diplomas and Certificates. She is a editorial member of several medical journal. Her special interests include: stem cell research, experimental pathology, molecular oncology, medical biochemistry.

# Contents

# Preface

There is a widespread interest in the today scientific literature for methylation field, which started to be published in the early 60's and continues to be a future line of research. This book represents a comprehensively reviewed literature on the importance of methylation processes in human health and disease. The book, covers the basic mechanism of DNA and protein methylation, along with the role of mRNA cap methylation in viral replication, gene expression and viral pathogenesis. Human health risks from metals methylation in the natural environment has been well describe in the literature. As a consequence, the formation processes, the biotic and abiotic degradation and the accumulation of the methylated metals and metalloids in the aquatic environment is reviwed in the book.

DNA methylation is a well-characterized process, allowing cells to control gene expression, while the study of histone methylation is more recent. The enzymes responsible for histone methylation (histone methyltransferases and histone demethylases) are important for transcriptional regulation in both normal and abnormal states, representing an important target for drug discovery. The interconection between DNA methylation and other regulatory molecules such as: enzymes, transcription factors, proteins and growth factors is discussed, providing key information about the mechanisms that trigger cell proliferation, differentiation, aging and malignant transformation. This textbook strongly point out the importance of methylated DNA as a biological marker of cancer an also gives the reader insights into the recently emerged treatment modalities targeting methylation mechanism, in various diseases including cancer.

The textbook addresses the following topics: Gene expression and methylation, DNA-methyltransferases: structure and function in eukaryotic and prokaryotic system; Protein arginine methylation in mammals; Cancer research through study of methylation cell processes; Bacteria, viruses and metals methylation: risk and benefit for human health.

The book aims at the advanced undergraduate and graduate biomedical students and researchers working in the epigenetic area, providing readers with both classical and relevant recent discoveries that have been made in the research field of methylation and also pointing out pathways where questions remain.


**Prof. Anica Dricu**
University of Medicine and Pharmacy
Faculty of Medicine
Craiova, Romania

Section 1

# Gene Expression and Methylation

Chapter 1

# Breaking the Silence: The Interplay Between Transcription Factors and DNA Methylation

Byron Baron

Additional information is available at the end of the chapter

http://dx.doi.org/10.5772/55021

## 1. Introduction

DNA methylation is best known for its role in gene silencing through a methyl group ($CH_3$) being added to the 5' carbon of cytosine bases (giving 5-methylcytosine) in the promoters of genes leading to supression of transcription [1]. However this is far from the whole story.

*De novo* methylation, which involves the addition of a methyl group to unmodified DNA, is described as an epigenetic change because it is a chemical modification to DNA not a change brought about by a DNA mutation. Unlike mutations, methylation changes are potentially reversible. Epigenetic changes also include changes to DNA-associated molecules such as histone modifications, chromatin-remodelling complexes and other small non-coding RNAs including miRNAs and siRNAs [2]. These changes have key roles in imprinting (gene-expression dependent on parental origin), X chromosome inactivation and heterochromatin formation among others [3-5].

DNA methylation leading to silencing is a very important survival mechanism used on repetitive sequences in the human genome, which come from DNA and RNA viruses or from mRNA and tRNA molecules that are able to replicate independently of the host genome. Such elements need to be controlled from spreading throughout the genome, by being silenced through CpG methylation, as they cause genetic instability and activation of oncogenes [6-10]. Such elements can be categorised into three groups: SINEs (Small Interspersed Nuclear Elements), LINEs (Long Interspersed Nuclear Elements) and LTRs (Long Terminal Repeats) [6,11-13]. Repetitive sequences are recognised by Lymphoid-Specific Helicase (LSH) also known as the 'heterochromatin guardian' [14,15], which additionally acts on single-copy genes [16].

DNA methylation generally occurs when a cytosine is adjacent 5′ to a guanine, called a CpG dinucleotide. Such dinucleotides are spread all over the genome and over 70% of CpGs are methylated. Clusters of CpGs, called CpG Islands (CGI), consist of stretches of 200–4000bp that are 60 to 70% G/C rich, found in TATAless promoters and/or first exons of genes [17-19].

In the human genome almost 50% of transcription start sites (TSS) [20], and about 70% of all genes contain CGIs [21,22]. CGIs present in the promoters or first exons of ubiquitously expressed housekeeping and tightly regulated developmental genes are usually hypomethylated, irrispective of transcription activity [1,19,21,23-29] and become silenced when they are hypermethylated [20]. On the contrary, promoters of some tissue-specific genes, with low CpG density, are commonly methylated without loss of transcription activity [21,26,30].

Many active promoters were shown to contain a low percentage of methylation (4 - 7%) indicating that supression through DNA hypermethylation is density-dependent [21]. The opposite was shown for the cAMP-responsive element (CRE)-binding sites, which are found in the promoters of numerous tissue-specific genes, including hormone-coding and viral genes [31]. Methylation of the CpG at the centre of the CRE sequence inhibits transcription, by inhibiting transcription factor binding, indicating that methylation at specific CpG sites can contribute to the regulation of gene expression [32].

Low-density gene body methylation has been observed in actively transcribed genes and is implicated in reducing 'transcriptional noise' – the inappropriate gene transcription from alternative start sites or in cells where it is meant to be silenced [33]. Moreover it is thought to inhibit antisense transcription, to direct RNA splicing and to have a role in replication timing [34-37]. Methylation is thought to play a role in transcriptional elongation, termination and splicing regulation due to higher CpG methylation in exons compared to introns [38,39] and the transacription start and termination regions lacking methylation [40,41].

CpG dinucleotides are not the only sequences that can be methylated, although non-CpG methylation was thought to be infrequent until the methylome of embryonic stem (ES) cells revealed that such non-CpG methylation, generally occuring in a CHG and CHH context, constitues 25% of total methylated sites in the genome [40]. Non-CpG methylation was also reported in some genes from mouse ES cells [42,43]. The distribution of such non-CG methylation was high in gene bodies and low in promoters and regulatory sequences with almost complete loss during differentiation [40].

DNA methyltransferases (DNMTs) are enzymes that catalyse the addition of methyl groups to cytosine residues in DNA. Mammals have three important DNMTs: DNMT1 is responsible for the maintenance of existing methylation patterns following DNA replication, while DNMT3a and DNMT3b are *de novo* methyltransferases [1,44-46]. As a result of DNA replication, fully methylated DNA becomes hemi-methylated and DNMT1 binds hemi-methylated DNA to add a methyl group to the 5′ carbon of cytosines [2].

Overall, most DNA methylation changes can be observed invariantly in all tissues [47]. However, the small portion of tissue-specific methylation has a profound effect on cellular activity including cell differentiation, disease and cancer [48-53].

DNA methylation shows different effects on gene expression, brought about by an interplay of several different mechanisms, which can be grouped into three categories [2,54]: i. effects on direct transcription factor binding at CpG dinucleotides; ii. binding of specific methylation-recognition factors (such as MeCP1 and MeCP2) to methylated DNA; iii. changes in chromatin structure.

## 2. Methylation in development and aging

Key stages in development make use of methylation to switch on/off and regulate gene expression. DNA methylation was shown to be essential for embryonic development through homozygous deletion of the mouse Mtase gene which leads to embryonic lethality [52]. Germline cells show 4% less methylation in CGI promoters, including almost all CGI promoters of germline-specific genes, compared to somatic cells [21].

Immediately after fertilisation but before the first cell division, the paternal DNA undergoes active demethylation throughout the genome [55-58]. After the first cell cycle, the maternal DNA undergoes passive demethylation as a result of a lack of methylation maintenance after mitosis [56,59], and this genome-wide demethylation continues, except for the imprinted genes, until the formation of the blastocyst [60,61].

After implantation, the genome (except for CGIs) undergoes *de novo* methylation [54]. Active demethylation subsequently occurs during early embryogenesis [62] with tissue-specific genes undergoing demethylation in their respective tissues, creating a methylation pattern which is maintained in the adult, giving each cell type a unique epigenome. [54].

Somatic cells go through the process of aging as they divide and replicate. Aging is characterised by a genome-wide loss and a regional gain of DNA methylation [63]. CGI promoters present an increase in DNA methylation in normal tissues of older individuals at several sites throughout the genome [64,65]. This causes genomic instability and deregulation of tissue-specific and imprinted genes as well as silencing of tumour suppressor genes (controlling cell cycle, apoptosis or DNA repair) through hypermethylation of promoter CGIs [5,66].

The age-related change in methylation was shown in a genome-wide CGI methylation study comparing small intestine (and other tissues) from 3-month-old and 35-month-old mice, which presented linear age-related increased methylation in 21% and decreased methylation in 13% of tested CGIs with strong tissue-specificity [67]. Furthermore, human intestinal age-related aberrant methylation was shown to share similarities to mouse [67]. Although the majority of CGIs methylated in tumours are also methylated in a selection of normal tissues during aging, particular tumours exhibit methylation in specific promoters and are thus said to display a CpG island methylator phenotype (CIMP) [65].

Aging appears to exhibit common methylation features with carcinogenesis and in fact these processes share a large number of hypermethylated genes such as ER, IGF2, N33 and MyoD in colon cancer, NKX2-5 in prostate cancer and several Polycomb-group protein target genes, which suggests they probably have common epigenetic mechanisms driving them [68-70].

## 3. Methylation in carcinogenesis

DNA methylation can either affects key genes which act as a driving force in cancer formation or else be a downstream effect of cancer progression [71,72]. According to the widely accepted 'two-hit' hypothesis of carcinogenesis [73], loss of function of both alleles for a given gene, such as a tumour suppressor gene, is required for malignant transformation. The first hit is typically in the form of a mutation while the second hit tends to be due to aberrant methylation leading to gene suppression. While in familial cancers only one allele needs to be aberrantly methylated to result in carcinogenesis [74,75], both alleles have to be silenced by methylation in non-familial cancers [76,77]. Interestingly, cancer cells appear to use DNMT3b in addition to DNMT1 to maintain hypermethylation [78,79].

Hypermethylation and suppression of promoter CGIs through d*e novo* methylation is well-documented for numerous cancer, affecting mostly general but occasionally tumour-specific genes [3,4,66,80,81]. A study of over 1000 CGIs from almost 100 human primary tumours deduced that on average 600 CGIs out of an estimated 45,000 spread throughout the genome were aberrantly methylated in cancers. It was shown that while some CGI methylation patterns were common to all test tumours, others were highly specific to a specific tumour-type, implying that the methylation of certain groups of CGIs may have implications in the formation, malignancy and progression of specific tumour types [82].

CGI shores (the 2kb region at the boundary of CGIs) are methylated in a tissue-specific manner to regulate gene expression but become hypermethylated in cancer [83-85]. Methylation boundaries flanking the CGIs in the E-cad and VHL tumour suppressor genes were found to be over-ridden by *de novo* methylation, resulting in transcription supression and consequentially oncogenesis [86]. On the other hand, the location and function of non-CG methylation in cancer is still mostly unknown [87-88].

Aberrant methylation has been linked to cancer cell energetics. Most cancer cells exhibit the Warburg effect i.e. produce energy mainly through a high level of glycolysis followed by lactic acid fermentation in the cytosol even under aerobic conditions, rather than through a low level of glycolysis followed by oxidative phosphorylation in the mitochondria as is the case in normal cells [89].

In one study it was found that fructose-1,6-bisphosphatase-1 (FBP1), which reduces glycolysis, is down-regulated by the NF-κB pathway partly through hypermethylation of the FBP1 promoter [90]. It was proposed that NF-κB could interact with co-repressors such as Histone deacetylases 1 and 2 (HDAC1 and HDAC2) to suppress gene expression [91,92] and subsequently the HDACs could interact with DNMT1, which gives hypermethylation of the promoter resulting in gene silencing [93-96].

In another study it was proposed that environmental toxins bring about oxidative-stress which affects genome-wide methylation by activating the Ten-Eleven Translocation (TET) proteins (which convert methylcytosine to 5-hydroxymethylcytosine) and chromatin modifying proteins which interfere with oxidative phoshphorylation [97].

## 4. Effect of CpG methylation on transcription factor binding

The methylation of CpGs in transcription factor binding sites in general leads to transcription suppression and gene silencing by directly inhibiting the binding of specific transcription factors. Transcription factors that have CpGs in their recognition sequences and are thus methylation-sensitive include AP-2 [98-100], Ah receptor [101], CREB/ATF [32,100,102], E2F [103], EBP-80 [104], ETS factors [105], MLTF [106], MTF-1 [107], c-Myc, c-Myn [108-109], GABP [110], NF-κB [111-100], HiNF-P [112] and MSPF [113].

There are also some transcription factors that are not sensitive to methylation e.g. Sp1, CTF and YY1 [100]. Thus methylation does not hinder binding of gene-specific transcription factors, but rather prevents the binding of ubiquitous factors, and subsequently transcription, in cells where the gene should not be expressed [102].

A model of CpG *de novo* methylation through over-expression of DNMT1 revealed that despite the overall increase in CGI methylation, there was a differential response of specific sites. The vast majority of CGIs were resistant to *de novo* methylation, while seven novel sequence patterns proved to be particularly susceptible to aberrant methylation [114]. This essentially means that the sequence in itself plays a role in the methylation state of CGIs. The result of this study implies that specific CGI patterns have an intrinsic susceptibility to aberrant methylation, which means that the genes regulated by promoters containing such CGIs are more susceptible to *de novo* methylation and could lead to various cancers depending on the genes involved [114].

Various studies have identified three main groups of transcription factors as being important in human cancer: steroid receptors (e.g. oestrogen receptors in breast cancer and androgen receptors in prostate cancer), resident nuclear factors (always in the nucleus e.g. c-JUN) [115,116] and latent cytoplasmic factors (translocated from the cytopasm to the nucleus after activation e.g. STAT proteins) [115].

Resident nuclear proteins are proteins ubiquitously present in the nucleus irrespective of cell type which include bZip proteins e.g. c-JUN, c-FOS, ATFs, CREBs and CREMs, the cEBP family, the ETS proteins and the MAD-box family [117]. The different families vary greatly in overall structure and interaction profiles but have the common functional feature of promoting transcription by co-operating with other transcription factors through tandem recognition sequences in promoters as well as by interacting with co-activator proteins [116,118-124]. Resident nuclear transcription factors drive carcinogenesis by direct over-expression or as highly active fusion proteins e.g. MYC acting with MAX [125-127]. The two families of resident nuclear transcription factors that are most prominent in human cancers are the ETS family proteins and proteins composing the AP-1 transcription complexes. ETS family proteins are of particular interest because they promote transcription of a wide range of genes by providing a DNA-binding domain through fusion with other proteins or by mutation [123,128,129].

Latent cytoplasmic proteins are found in the cytoplasm of cells and rely on protein–protein interaction at the cell surface to produce a cascade which activates them as they are directed to the nucleus where they affect transcription by binding to activation sites in the promoters of inducible genes and interacting with transcription initiation factors. They can be activated either directly by tyrosine or serine kinases at the cell surface or by complex processes which include kinases along the pathway [117]. STATs (signal transducers and activators of transcription) are activated by JAK (a tyrosine kinase family) which is activated by various receptors [130,131].

## 5. Protection mechanisms against methylation

It has been generally accepted that methylation-resistant CGIs are associated with broad expression or housekeeping genes while the majority of methylation-prone CGIs are associated with tissue-specific and thus restricted-expression genes [132]. Exceptions to this pattern have also been found, including WNT10B, NPTXR and POP3. Thus the hypothesis that active transcription has an indirect protective effect against aberrant methylation of CGIs [1,133] has been repeatedly proven to be valid though not absolute [114].

A number of mechanisms have been put forward to explain the relationship between aberrant *de novo* methylation and cancer. One hypothesis proposed that an initial random methylation event is selected for as proliferation progresses [80]. Another hypothesis proposed the recruitment of DNA methyltransferases to methylation-sensitive sequences by cis-acting factors [134,135], histone methyltransferases such as G9a [136,137], or EZH2 [138]. Yet another hypothesis proposed the loss of chromatin boundaries or the absence of 'protective' transcription factors, leading to the spread of DNA methylation in CGIs [139].

The most recent hypothesis proposes the protective character of co-operative binding of transcription factors in maintaining CGIs unmethylated [140]. CGIs showed an unexpected resistance to *de novo* methylation when DNMT1 was over-expressed. The general pattern that emerged was that most *de novo* methylated CGIs were characterised by an absence of in-tandem transcription factor binding sites and an absence of bound transcription factors. Thus protection from *de novo* methylation requires the presence of tandem transcription factor binding sites that are stably co-bound by at least one general transcription factor, with the second factor being either a general or a tissue–specific transcription factor. Among the most prominent transcription factors found to be linked with aberrant methylation were GABP, SP1, NFY, NRF1 and YY1 [140].

This study re-confirmed that methylation-resistant CGIs were bound by combinations of ubiquitous transcription factors which regulated genes of basic cellular functions, while methylation-prone CGIs were mostly associated with development, differentiation and cell communication, which are frequently regulated by tissue–specific transcription factors [140].

## 6. Specificity protein 1 (Sp1)

Sp1 is an Sp/KLF (Krüppel-like factor) family member containing a zinc-finger DNA-binding domain [141]. Many KLF proteins regulate cellular proliferation and differentiation

[142-145], and play a role in malignancy e.g. Sp1 has been shown to be the key factor in epithelial carcinomas [146,147].

Multiple Sp1 binding sites are found in the CGI-promoters of housekeeping genes [148,149] as well as CGIs downstream of the TSS [150]. Sp1 sites in gene promoters have been shown to protect CGIs from *de novo* methylation and maintain expression of downstream genes [151,153] e.g. Sp1-binding site protect the APRT gene from *de novo* methylation in humans and mice [154,155]. However, Sp1 binding is not methylation-sensitive [151,156,157] and resistance to *de novo* methylation by DNMT1 is not correlated to the frequency of Sp1 sites in CGIs [114].

Sp1 co-operates with the GABP complex to activate genes which include the folate receptor b [158], CD18 [159], utrophin [141,160], heparanase-1 [161], the pem pd homeobox gene [162], the mouse thymidylate synthase promoter [163] and mouse DNA polymerase alpha primase with E2F [164,165].

## 7. GA-Binding Protein (GABP)

GABP is a transcription factor composed of two distinct subunits: GABPα and GABPβ. GABPα, also known as Nuclear Respiratory Factor 2 (NRF-2) or Adenovirus E4 Transcription Factor 1 (E4TF1-60), is a member of the E26 Transformation-Specific (ETS) family of proteins [166-169]. However unlike other ETS factors GABPα forms an obligate heteromeric protein complex with GABPβ [170-172]. Together they generally form a heterotetramer consisting of 2α and 2β subunits [173,174] and the presence of sites for GABP binding containing 2 tandem ETS consensus motifs has been reported [175]. On the other hand, single GABP binding sites tend to combine with another site that recognises a different transcription factor e.g. NRF-1, Sp1 or YY1 [175]. GABP is able to recruit co-activators such as PCG1 and p300/CBP that create a chromatin environment favouring transcription [176,177].

GABPα (like all other ETS factors) binds to purine-rich sequences containing a 5′- GGAA/T-3′ core by means of a highly conserved DNA-binding domain made up of an 85 amino acid sequence rich in tryptophan which forms a winged-helix-turn-helix structure, characteristic of the ETS protein family near its carboxy terminal [166,167,170,172,178-181]. The domain through which GABPα binds to the ankyrin repeats of GABPβ is found just downstream of the DNA-binding domain [167,168]. GABPα also has another two domains, the helical bundle pointed (PNT) domain found in its mid-region, which consists of five α-helices [182,183] and the On-SighT (OST) domain near the amino-terminus (residues 35–121), which folds as a 5-stranded β-sheet crossed by a distorted helix and contains two predominant clusters of negatively-charged residues, which might be used to interact with positively-charged proteins [184].

The role of GABP is very versatile and its ability to co-operate with other transcription factors gives it a key role in transcription regulation. GABP and PU.1 compete for binding to the promoter of the b2-integrin gene, yet co-operate to increase gene transcription [185]. GABP also acts as a repressor of mouse ribosomal protein gene transcription [186], apparently by interfering with the formation of the transcriptional initiation complex [187].

GABP is a methylation-sensitive transcription factor [110] and its modulation is best seen in the transactivation of the *Cyp*2d-9 promoter for the male-specific steroid 16a-hydroxylase in mouse liver where GABP does not bind to the promoter when the CpG site at -97 is methylated [187]. Interestingly, CpG sites located at -93 and -85, outside of the GABP recognition sequence in the Thyroid Stimulating Hormone Receptor (TSHR) gene promoter when methylated, affect the binding of GABP to the promoter, leading to a reduction in basal transcription [187].

## 8. Therapeutic applications

As more such data is accumulated, it presents methylation as a very interesting and promising tumour-specific therapeutic target especially since the lack of methylation of CGIs in normal cells makes it a safe therapy. Demethylation is known to reactivate the expression of many genes silenced in cultured tumour cells [82]. While high doses of DNMT inhibitors can inhibit DNA synthesis and eventually lead to cell death by cytotoxicity, administration of low doses of these drugs over a prolonged period has a therapeutic effect [188-191]. In fact, the United States Food and Drug Administration has approved the DNMT inhibitors, 5-azacytidine and its derivative 5-aza-2′-deoxycytidine (decitabine), for therapy of patients with solid tumours, myelodysplastic syndrome (which can lead to the development of acute leukemia) and myelogenous leukemia [192].

5-azacitidine acts by becoming phosphorylated and being incorporated into RNA, where it suppresses RNA synthesis and produces a cytotoxic effect [3,193]. It is converted by ribonucleotide reductase to 5-aza-2'-deoxycytidine diphosphate and subsequently phosphorylated. The triphosphate form is then incorporated into DNA in place of cytosine. The substitution of the 5' nitrogen atom in place of the carbon, traps the DNMTs on the substituted DNA strand and methylation is inhibited [194].

Several more stable analogues such as arabinofuranosyl-5-azacytosine [195], pseudo-isocytidine [196], 5-fluorocytidine [196], pyrimidone [197] and dihydro-5-azacytidine [198] have been tested, and others are undergoing clinical trials [199,200].

Targetting overactive transcription factors is another interesting tumour-specific therapeutic strategy. Many human cancers appear to have a small number of specific overactive transcription factors which are valid candidate targets to at least control further malignancy and metastasis. Such tumour-specific transcription factors are ideal targets because they are less numerous and more significant than other possible protein targets in the transcription activation pathway.

However it is not a simple task to target transcription factors in a controlled manner particularly if attempting to inhibit the interaction of DNA-binding proteins with their recognition sequences [201,202]. Inhibition of a DNA-binding transcription factor can alternatively be done in one of two ways: lowering the overall level of intracellular transcription factor through siRNA or directing methylation to the recognition sequence of the DNA-binding protein. Both options are extremely difficult to carry out *in vivo* even if their *in vitro* counterpart has proven to be successful.

## 9. Conclusion

Research into DNA methylation, particularly at CGIs has come a long way and it is now known that gene silencing, albeit essential, is not the only purpose of methylation processes. In particular, the interactions of transcription factors with promoters have been shown to modulate the function of genes through their methylation-sensitivity and may thus be regarded as viable targets for therapeutics. Unfortunately the biochemical mechanisms and principles required to successfully inhibit protein–protein interactions require further study and clarification [203-206]. Additionally, delivery systems for such cellular treatments also need further study and improvement. However as more focus is put on molecular medicine and with the shift towards personalised medicine, there will surely be significant advances in protein-targetting treatments.

## Author details

Byron Baron[1,2]

Address all correspondence to: angenlabs@gmail.com

1 Department of Anatomy and Cell Biology, Faculty of Medicine and Surgery, University of Malta, Msida, Malta

2 Department of Biochemistry and Functional Proteomics, Yamaguchi University Graduate School of Medicine, Ube-shi, Yamaguchi-ken, Japan

## References

[1] Bird A. DNA methylation patterns and epigenetic memory. Genes Dev. 2002: 16, 6–21

[2] Chatterjee R, Vinson C. CpG methylation recruits sequence specific transcription factors essential for tissue specific gene expression. Biochim. Biophys. Acta 2012: 1819, 763–770.

[3] Robertson KD, Jones PA. DNA methylation: past, present and future directions. Carcinogenesis 2000: 21, 461–467.

[4] Esteller M. CpG island hypermethylation and tumour suppressor genes: a booming present, a brighter future. Oncogene 2002: 21, 5427–5440.

[5] Berdasco M, Esteller M. Aberrant epigenetic landscape in cancer: how cellular identity goes awry, Dev. Cell 2010: 19, 698-711.

[6] Yoder JA, Walsh CP, Bestor TH. Cytosine methylation and the ecology of intragenomic parasites. Trends Genet. 1997: 13, 335–340.

[7] amada Y, Jackson-Grusby L, Linhart H, Meissner A, Eden A, Lin H, Jaenisch R. Opposing effects of DNA hypomethylation on intestinal and liver carcinogenesis. Proc. Natl. Acad. Sci. USA 2005: 102, 13580–13585.

[8] hoi IS, Estécio MR, Nagano Y, Kim do H, White JA, Yao JC, Issa JP, Rashid A. Hypomethylation of LINE-1 and Alu in welldifferentiated neuroendocrine tumours (pancreatic endocrine tumours and carcinoid tumours). Mod. Pathol. 2007: 20, 802–810.

[9] stécio MR, Yan PS, Ibrahim AE, Tellez CS, Shen L, Huang TH, Issa JP. High-throughput methylation profiling by MCA coupled to CpG island microarray. Genome Res. 2007: 17, 1529–1536.

[10] Wolff EM, Byun H-M, Han HF, Sharma S, Nichols PW, Siegmund KD, Yang AS, Jones PA, Liang G. Hypomethylation of a LINE-1 Promoter Activates an Alternate Transcript of the MET Oncogene in Bladders with Cancer. PLoS Genet. 2010: 6 (4), e1000917.

[11] Lander ES, Linton LM, Birren B, Nusbaum C, Zody MC, Baldwin J, Devon K et al. (2001) Initial sequencing and analysis of the human genome. Nature 2001: 409, 860–921.

[12] Venter JC, Adams MD, Myers EW, Li PW, Mural RJ, Sutton GG, Smith HO et al. The sequence of the human genome. Science 2001: 291, 1304–1351.

[13] Li Y, Zhu J, Tian G, Li N, Li Q, Ye M, Zheng H, Yu J, Wu H, Sun J, Zhang H, Chen Q, Luo R, Chen M, He Y, Jin X, Zhang Q, Yu C, Zhou G, Huang Y, Cao H, Zhou X, Guo S, Hu X, Li X, Kristiansen K, Bolund L, Xu J, Wang W, Yang H, Wang J, Li R, Beck S, Zhang X. The DNA methylome of human peripheral blood mononuclear cells, PLoS Biol. 2010: 8 (11), e1000533.

[14] Huang J, Fan T, Yan Q, Zhu H, Fox S, Issaq HJ, Best L, Gangi L, Munroe D, Muegge K. Lsh, an epigenetic guardian of repetitive elements. Nucleic Acids Res. 2004: 32 (17), 5019–5028.

[15] Yan Q, Cho E, Lockett S, Muegge K. Association of Lsh, a regulator of DNA methylation, with pericentromeric heterochromatin is dependent on intact heterochromatin. Mol. Cell. Biol. 2003: 23, 8416–8428.

[16] Xi S, Zhu H, Xu H, Schmidtmann A, Geiman TM, Muegge K. Lsh controls Hox gene silencing during development. Proc. Natl. Acad. Sci. USA 2007: 104, 14366–14371.

[17] Craig JM, Bickmore WA. The distribution of CpG islands in mammalian chromosomes. Nat. Genet. 1994: 7, 376–382.

[18] Gardiner-Garden M, Frommer M. CpG islands in vertebrate genomes. J. Mol. Biol. 1987: 196, 261–282.

[19] Illingworth RS, Bird AP. CpG islands—'a rough guide'. FEBS Lett. 2009: 583, 1713–1720.

[20] Deaton AM, Bird A. CpG islands and the regulation of transcription. Genes Dev. 2011: 25, 1010–1022.

[21] Weber M, Hellmann I, Stadler MB, Ramos L, Paabo S, Rebhan M, Schubeler D. Distribution, silencing potential and evolutionary impact of promoter DNA methylation in the human genome. Nat. Genet. 2007: 39, 457–466.

[22] Sharma S, Kelly TK, Jones PA. Epigenetics in cancer, Carcinogenesis 2010: 31 27-36.

[23] Takai D, Jones PA. Comprehensive analysis of CpG islands in human chromosomes 21 and 22, Proc. Natl. Acad. Sci. USA 2002: 99, 3740-3745.

[24] Gal-Yam EN, Egger G, Iniguez L, Holster H, Einarsson S, Zhang X, Lin JC, Liang G, Jones PA, Tanay A. Frequent switching of Polycomb repressive marks and DNA hypermethylation in the PC3 prostate cancer cell line, Proc. Natl. Acad. Sci. USA 2008: 105, 12979-12984.

[25] Saxonov S, Berg P, Brutlag DL. A genome-wide analysis of CpG dinucleotides in the human genome distinguishes two distinct classes of promoters, Proc. Natl. Acad. Sci. USA 2006: (103) 1412–1417.

[26] Eckhardt F, Lewin J, Cortese R, Rakyan VK, Attwood J, Burger M, Burton J, Cox TV, Davies R, Down TA, Haefliger C, Horton R, Howe K, Jackson DK, Kunde J, Koenig C, Liddle J, Niblett D, Otto T, Pettett R, Seemann S, Thompson C, West T, Rogers J, Olek A, Berlin K, Beck S. DNA methylation profiling of human chromosomes 6, 20 and 22. Nat. Genet. 2006: 38, 1378–1385.

[27] Fouse SD, Shen Y, Pellegrini M, Cole S, Meissner A, Van Neste L, Jaenisch R, Fan G. Promoter CpG methylation contributes to ES cell gene regulation in parallel with Oct4/Nanog, PcG complex, and histone H3 K4/K27 trimethylation, Cell Stem Cell 2008: (2) 160–169.

[28] Rollins RA, Haghighi F, Edwards JR, Das R, Zhang MQ, Ju J, Bestor TH. Large-scale structure of genomic methylation patterns. Genome Res. 2006: 16, 157–163.

[29] Bock C, Paulsen M, Tierling S, Mikeska T, Lengauer T, Walter J. CpG island methylation in human lymphocytes is highly correlated with DNA sequence, repeats, and predicted DNA structure. PLoS Genet 2006: 2 (3), e26.

[30] Rishi V, Bhattacharya P, Chatterjee R, Rozenberg J, Zhao J, Glass K, Fitzgerald P, Vinson C. CpG methylation of half-CRE sequences creates C/EBPalpha binding sites that activate some tissue-specific genes. Proc. Natl. Acad. Sci. USA 2010: 107, 20311–20316.

[31] Roesler WJ, Vandenbark GR, Hanson RW. Cyclic AMP and the induction of eukaryotic gene transcription. J. Biol. Chem. 1899: 263, 9063-9066.

[32] Iguchi-Ariga SM, Schaffner W. CpG methylation of the cAMP-responsive enhancer/ promoter sequence TGACGTCA abolishes specific factor binding as well as transcriptional activation. Genes Dev. 1989: 3, 612–619.

[33] Bird AP. Gene number, noise reduction and biological complexity. Trends Genet. 1995: 11, 94–100.

[34] Ball MP, Li JB, Gao Y, Lee J-H, LeProust EM, Park I-H, Xie B, Daley GQ, Church GM. Targeted and genome-scale strategies reveal genebody methylation signatures in human cells. Nat. Biotechnol. 2009: 27, 361–368.

[35] Maunakea AK, Nagarajan RP, Bilenky M, Ballinger TJ, D'Souza C, Fouse SD, Johnson BE, Hong C, Nielsen C, Zhao Y, Turecki G, Delaney A, Varhol R, Thiessen N, Shchors K, Heine VM, Rowitch DH, Xing X, Fiore C, Schillebeeckx M, Jones SJ, Haussler D, Marra MA, Hirst M, Wang T, Costello JF. Conserved role of intragenic DNA methylation in regulating alternative promoters. Nature 2010: 466, 253-257.

[36] Shenker N, Flanagan JM. Intragenic DNA methylation: implications of this epigenetic mechanism for cancer research. Br. J. Cancer 2012: 106, 248-253.

[37] Aran D, Toperoff G, Rosenberg M, Hellman A. Replication timing-related and gene body-specific methylation of active human genes. Hum. Mol. Genet. 2010: 20, 670-680.

[38] Choi JK. Contrasting chromatin organization of CpG islands and exons in the human genome. Genome Biol. 2010: 11, R70.

[39] Jeltsch A. Molecular biology. Phylogeny of methylomes. Science 2010: 328, 837–838.

[40] Lister R, Pelizzola M, Dowen RH, Hawkins DR, Hon G, Tonti-Filippini J, Nery JR, Lee L, Ye Z, Ngo Q-M, Edsall L, Antosiewicz-Bourget J, Stewart R, Ruotti V, Millar AH, Thomson JA, Ren B, Ecker JR. Human DNA methylomes at base resolution show widespread epigenomic differences. Nature 462, 315–322.

[41] Hodges E, Smith AD, Kendall J, Xuan Z, Ravi K, Rooks M, Zhang MQ, Ye K, Bhattacharjee A, Brizuela L, McCombie WR, Wigler M, Hannon GJ, Hicks JB. High definition profiling of mammalian DNA methylation by array capture and single molecule bisulfite sequencing, Genome Res. 2009: (19) 1593–1605.

[42] Haines TR, Rodenhiser DI, Ainsworth PJ. Allele-specific non- CpG methylation of the Nf1 gene during early mouse development. Dev. Biol. 2001: 240, 585–598.

[43] Ramsahoye BH, Biniszkiewicz D, Lyko F, Clark V, Bird AP, Jaenisch R. Non-CpG methylation is prevalent in embryonic stem cells and may be mediated by DNA methyltransferase 3a. Proc. Natl. Acad. Sci. USA 2000: 97, 5237–5242.

[44] Bestor TH. The DNA methyltransferases of mammals. Hum Mol Genet 2000 :9 2395–2402

[45] Okano M, Xie S. Li E. (1998) Cloning and characterization of a family of novel mammalian DNA (cytosine-5) methyltransferases. Nat Genet 1998: 19, 219–220

[46] Okano M, Bell DW, Haber DA, Li E. DNA methyltransferases Dnmt3a and Dnmt3b are essential for de novo methylation and mammalian development. Cell 1999: 99, 247–257

[47] Estécio M, Issa JP. Dissecting DNA hypermethylation in cancer. FEBS Letters 2011: 585, 2078–2086.

[48] Beard C, Li E, Jaenisch R. Loss of methylation activates Xist in somatic but not in embryonic cells. Genes Dev. 1995: 9, 2325–2334.

[49] Biniszkiewicz D, Gribnau J, Ramsahoye B, Gaudet F, Eggan K, Humpherys D, Mastrangelo M-A, Jun Z, Walter J, Jaenisch R. Dnmt1 overexpression causes genomic hypermethylation, loss of imprinting, and embryonic lethality. Mol. Cell. Biol. 2002: 22, 2124–2135.

[50] Ji H, Ehrlich LIR, Seita J, Murakami P, Doi A, Lindau P, Lee H, Aryee MJ, Irizarry RA, Kim K, Rossi DJ, Inlay MA, Serwold T, Karsunky H, Ho L, Daley GQ, Weissman IL, Feinberg AP. Comprehensive methylome map of lineage commitment from haematopoietic progenitors. Nature 2010: 467, 338–342.

[51] Jones PA, Taylor SM, Wilson V. DNA modification, differentiation, and transformation. J. Exp. Zool. 1983: 228, 287–295.

[52] Li E, Bestor TH, Jaenisch R. Targeted mutation of the DNA methyltransferase gene results in embryonic lethality. Cell 1992: 69, 915–926.

[53] Sanford JP, Clark HJ, Chapman VM. Rossant J. Differences in DNA methylation during oogenesis and spermatogenesis and their persistence during early embryogenesis in the mouse. Genes Dev. 1987: 1, 1039– 1046.

[54] Siegfried Z, Cedar H. DNA methylation: A molecular lock. Current Biol. 1997: 7, R305–R307.

[55] Reik W, Dean W, Walter J. Epigenetic reprogramming in mammalian development. Science 2001: 293, 1089–1093.

[56] Rougier N, Bourc'his D, Gomes DM, Niveleau A, Plachot M, Pàldi A, Viegas-Péquignot E. Chromosome methylation patterns during mammalian preimplantation development. Genes Dev. 1998: 12, 2108-2113.

[57] Mayer W, Niveleau A, Walter J, Fundele R, Haaf T. Demethylation of the zygotic paternal genome. Nature 2000: 403, 501–502.

[58] Oswald J, Engemann S, Lane N, Mayer W, Olek A, Fundele R, Dean W, Reik W, Walter J. Active demethylation of the paternal genome in the mouse zygote. Curr. Biol. 2000: 10, 475–478.

[59] Howlett SK, Reik W. Methylation levels of maternal and paternal genomes during preimplantation development. Development 1991: 113, 119-127.

[60] Carlson LL, Page AW, Bestor TH. Properties and localization of DNA methyltransferase in preimplantation mouse embryos: implications for genomic imprinting. Genes Dev. 1992: 6, 2536–2541.

[61] Cardoso MC, Leonhardt H. DNA methyltransferase is actively retained in the cytoplasm during early development. J. Cell Biol. 1999: 147, 25–32.

[62] Kafri T, Gao X, Razin A. Mechanistic aspects of genome-wide demethylation in the preimplantation mouse embryo. Proc Natl Acad Sci USA 1993: 90, 10558-10562.

[63] Dunn BK. Hypomethylation: one side of a larger picture. Ann. N. Y. Acad. Sci. 2003: 983, 28–42.

[64] Issa JP, Ottaviano YL, Celano P, Hamilton SR, Davidson NE, Baylin SB. Methylation of the oestrogen receptor CpG island links ageing and neoplasia in human colon. Nat. Genet. 1994: 7, 536–540.

[65] Toyota M, Ahuja N, Ohe-Toyota M, Herman JG, Baylin SB, Issa JP. CpG island methylator phenotype in colorectal cancer. Proc. Natl. Acad. Sci. USA 1999: 96, 8681–8686.

[66] Egger G, Liang G, Aparicio A, Jones PA. Epigenetics in human disease and prospects for epigenetic therapy, Nature 2004: 429, 457-463.

[67] Maegawa S, Hinkal G, Kim HS, Shen L, Zhang L, Zhang J, Zhang N, Liang S, Donehower LA, Issa JP. Widespread and tissue-specific age-related DNA methylation changes in mice. Genome Res. 2010: 20, 332–340.

[68] Ahuja N, Issa JP. Aging, methylation and cancer. Histol. Histopathol. 2000: 15, 835–842.

[69] Kwabi-Addo B, Wang S, Chung W, Jelinek J, Patierno SR, Wang BD, Andrawis R, Lee NH, Apprey V, Issa JP, Ittmann M. Identification of differentially methylated genes in normal prostate tissues from African American and Caucasian men. Clin. Cancer Res. 2010: 16, 3539–3547.

[70] Teschendorff AE, Menon U, Gentry-Maharaj A, Ramus SJ, Weisenberger DJ, Shen H, Campan M, Noushmehr H, Bell CG, Maxwell AP, Savage DA, Mueller-Holzner E, Marth C, Kocjan G, Gayther SA, Jones A, Beck S, Wagner W, Laird PW, Jacobs IJ, Widschwendter M. Age-dependent DNA methylation of genes that are suppressed in stem cells is a hallmark of cancer. Genome Res. 2010: 20, 440–446.

[71] Hosoya K, Yamashita S, Ando T, Nakajima T, Itoh F, Ushijima T. Adenomatous polyposis coli 1A is likely to be methylated as a passenger in human gastric carcinogenesis. Cancer Lett. 2009: 285, 182–189.

[72] Sawan C, Vaissiere T, Murr R, Herceg Z. Epigenetic drivers and genetic passengers on the road to cancer. Mutat. Res. 2008: 642, 1–13.

[73] Knudson AG. Two genetic hits (more or less) to cancer. Nat. Rev. Cancer 2001: 1, 157–162.

[74] Esteller M, Fraga MF, Guo M, Garcia-Foncillas J, Hedenfalk I, Godwin AK, Trojan J, Vaurs-Barrière C, Bignon YJ, Ramus S, Benitez J, Caldes T, Akiyama Y, Yuasa Y, Launonen V, Canal MJ, Rodriguez R, Capella G, Peinado MA, Borg A, Aaltonen LA, Ponder BA, Baylin SB, Herman JG. DNA methylation patterns in hereditary human cancers mimic sporadic tumorigenesis. Hum Mol Genet 2001: 10, 3001–3007

[75] Slavotinek AM, Stone EM, Mykytyn K, Heckenlively JR, Green JS, Heon E, Musarella MA, Parfrey PS, Sheffield VC, Biesecker LG. Methylation of the CDH1 promoter as the second genetic hit in hereditary diffuse gastric cancer. Nat Genet 2000: 26, 16–17

[76] Jones PA, Baylin SB. The fundamental role of epigenetic events in cancer. Nat Rev Genet 2002: 3, 415–428.

[77] Herman JG, Baylin SB. Gene silencing in cancer in association with promoter hypermethylation. N Engl J Med 2003: 349, 2042–2054.

[78] Rhee I, Jair KW, Yen RW, Lengauer C, Herman JG, Kinzler KW, Vogelstein B, Baylin SB, Schuebel KE. CpG methylation is maintained in human cancer cells lacking DNMT1. Nature 2000: 404, 1003–1007

[79] Rhee I, Bachman KE, Park BH, Jair KW, Yen RW, Schuebel KE, Cui H, Feinberg AP, Lengauer C, Kinzler KW, Baylin SB, Vogelstein B. DNMT1 and DNMT3b cooperate to silence genes in human cancer cells. Nature 2002: 416, 552–556

[80] Jones PA, Baylin SB. The epigenomics of cancer. Cell 2007: 128, 683– 692.

[81] Toyota M, Issa JP. Epigenetic changes in solid and hematopoietic tumours. Semin. Oncol. 2005: 32, 521–530.

[82] Costello JF, Frühwald MC, Smiraglia DJ, Rush LJ, Robertson GP, Gao X, Wright FA, Feramisco JD, Peltomäki P, Lang JC, Schuller DE, Yu L, Bloomfield CD, Caligiuri MA, Yates A, Nishikawa R, Su Huang HJ, Petrelli NJ, Zhang X, O'Dorisio MS, Held WA, Cavenee WK, Plass C.. Aberrant CpG-island methylation has non-random and tumour-type-specific patterns. Nat. Genet. 2000: 24, 132–138.

[83] Irizarry RA, Ladd-Acosta C, Wen B, Wu Z, Montano C, Onyango P, Cui H, Gabo K, Rongione M, Webster M, Ji H, Potash JB, Sabunciyan S, Feinberg AP. The human colon cancer methylome shows similar hypo- and hypermethylation at conserved tissue-specific CpG island shores, Nat. Genet. 2009: 41, 178-186.

[84] Feber A, Wilson GA, Zhang L, Presneau N, Idowu B, Down TA, Rakyan VK, Noon LA, Lloyd AC, Stupka E, Schiza V, Teschendorff AE, Schroth GP, Flanagan A, Beck S. Comparative methylome analysis of benign and malignant peripheral nerve sheath tumours, Genome Res. 2011: 21, 515-524.

[85] Ogoshi K, Hashimoto S, Nakatani Y, Qu W, Oshima K, Tokunaga K, Sugano S, Hattori M, Morishita S, Matsushima K. Genome-wide profiling of DNA methylation in human cancer cells, Genomics 2011: 98, 280-287.

[86] Mancini DN, Singh SM, Archer TK, Rodenhiser DI. Site-specific DNA methylation in the neurofibromatosis (NF1) promoter interferes with binding of CREB and SP1 transcription factors. Oncogene 1999: 18, 4108 – 4119.

[87] Prazeres H, Torres J, Rodrigues F, Pinto M, Pastoriza MC, Gomes D, Cameselle-Teijeiro J, Vidal A, Martins TC, Sobrinho-Simões M, Soares P. Chromosomal, epigenetic and microRNA-mediated inactivation of LRP1B, a modulator of the extracellular environment of thyroid cancer cells. Oncogene 2011: 30, 1302–1317.

[88] Woodcock DM, Linsenmeyer ME, Doherty JP, Warren WD. DNA methylation in the promoter region of the p16 (CDKN2/MTS-1/INK4A) gene in human breast tumours. Br. J. Cancer 1999: 79, 251–256.

[89] Kim JW, Dang CV. Cancer's molecular sweet tooth and the Warburg effect, Cancer Res. 2006: 66, 8927–8930.

[90] Liu X, Wang X, Zhang J, Lam EK, Shin VY, Cheng AS, Yu J, Chan FK, Sung JJ, Jin HC. Warburg effect revisited: an epigenetic link between glycolysis and gastric carcinogenesis, Oncogene 2010: (29) 442–450.

[91] Ashburner BP, Westerheide SD, Baldwin Jr. AS. The p65 (RelA) subunit of NFkappaB interacts with the histone deacetylase (HDAC) corepressors HDAC1 and HDAC2 to negatively regulate gene expression. Mol. Cell. Biol. 2001: 21, 7065–7077.

[92] Bhat KP, Pelloski CE, Zhang Y, Kim SH, deLaCruz C, Rehli M, Aldape KD. Selective repression of YKL-40 by NF-kappaB in glioma cell lines involves recruitment of histone deacetylase-1 and -2. FEBS Lett. 2008: 582, 3193–3200.

[93] Robertson KD, Ait-Si-Ali S, Yokochi T, Wade PA, Jones PL, Wolffe AP. DNMT1 forms a complex with Rb, E2F1 and HDAC1 and represses transcription from E2F-responsive promoters. Nat Genet 2000: 25, 338–342

[94] Rountree MR, Bachman KE, Baylin SB. DNMT1 binds HDAC2 and a new co-repressor, DMAP1, to form a complex at replication foci. Nat Genet 2000: 25, 269–277

[95] Fuks F, Burgers WA, Brehm A, Hughes-Davies L, Kouzarides T. DNA methyltransferase Dnmt1 associates with histone deacetylase activity. Nat Genet 2000: 24, 88–91

[96] Wang X, Jin H. The epigenetic basis of the Warburg effect. Epigenetics 2010: (5) 566–568.

[97] Chia N, Wang L, Lu X, Senut MC, Brenner C, Ruden DM. Hypothesis: environmental regulation of 5-hydroxymethylcytosine by oxidative stress, Epigenetics 2011: 6, 853–856.

[98] Comb M, Goodman HM. CpG methylation inhibits proenkephalin gene expression and binding of the transcription factor AP-2. Nucleic Acids Res. 1990: 18, 3975–3982.

[99] Hermann R, Hoeveler A, Doerfler W. Sequence-specific methylation in a downstream region of the late E2A promoter of adenovirus type 2 DNA prevents protein binding. J. Mol. Biol. 1989: 210, 411–415.

[100] Tate PH, Bird A. Effects of DNA methylation on DNA binding proteins and gene expression. Curr. Opin. Genet. Dev. 1993: 3, 226–231.

[101] Shen ES, Whitlock Jr JP. The potential role of DNA methylation in the response to 2,3,7,8-tetrachlorodibenzo-p-dioxin. J. Biol. Chem. 1989: 264, 17754–17758.

[102] Becker PB, Ruppert S, Schutz G. Genomic footprinting reveals cell type-specific DNA binding of ubiquitous factors. Cell 1987: 51, 435–443.

[103] Kovesdi I, Reichel R, Nevins JR. Role of an adenovirus E2 promoter binding factor in E1A-mediated coordinate gene control. Proc. Natl Acad. Sci. USA. 1987: 84, 2180–2184.

[104] Falzon M, Kuff EL. Binding of the transcription factor EBP 80 mediates the methylation response of an intracisternal A-particle long terminal repeat promoter. Mol. Cell Biol. 1991: 11, 117–125.

[105] Gaston K, Fried M. CpG methylation has differential effects on the binding of YY1 and ETS proteins to the bi-directional promoter of the Surf-1 and Surf-2 genes. Nucleic Acids Res. 1995: 23, 901–909.

[106] Watt F, Molloy PL. Cytosine methylation prevents binding to DNA of a HeLa cell transcription factor required for optimal expression of the adenovirus major late promoter. Genes Dev. 1988: 2, 1136–1143.

[107] Radtke F, Hug M, Georgiev O, Matsuo K, Schaffner W. Differential sensitivity of zinc finger transcription factors MTF-1, Sp1 and Krox-20 to CpG methylation of their binding sites. Biol. Chem. Hoppe-Seyler 1996: 377, 47–56.

[108] Prendergast GC, Lawe D, Ziff EB. Association of Myn, the murine homolog of Max, with c-Myc stimulates methylation-sensitive DNA binding and ras co-transformation. Cell 1991: 65, 395–407.

[109] Prendergast GC, Ziff EB. Methylation-sensitive sequencespecific DNA binding by the c-Myc basic region. Science 1991: 251, 186–189.

[110] Yokomori N, Moore R, Negishi M. Sexually dimorphic DNA demethylation in the promoter of the Slp (sex-limited protein) gene in mouse liver. Proc. Natl Acad. Sci. USA 1995: 92, 1302–1306.

[111] Bednarik DP, Duckett C, Kim SU, Perez VL, Griffis K, Guenthner PC, Folks TM. DNA CpG methylation inhibits binding of NF-kappa B proteins to the HIV-1 long terminal repeat cognate DNA motifs. New. Biol. 1991: 3, 969–976.

[112] van Wijnen AJ, van den Ent FM, Lian JB, Stein JL, Stein GS. Overlapping and CpG methylation-sensitive protein–DNA interactions at the histone H4 transcriptional cell cycle domain: distinctions between two human H4 gene promoters. Mol. Cell Biol. 1992: 12, 3273–3287.

[113] List HJ, Patzel V, Zeidler U, Schopen A, Ruhl G, Stollwerk J, Klock G. Methylation sensitivity of the enhancer from the human papillomavirus type 16. J. Biol. Chem. 1994: 269, 11902–11911.

[114] Feltus FA, Lee EK, Costello JF, Plass C, Vertino PM. Predicting aberrant CpG island methylation. Proc. Natl. Acad. Sci. USA 2003: 100, 12253– 12258.

[115] Brivanlou AH, Darnell Jr JE. Signal transduction and the control of gene expression. Science 2002: 295, 813–818.

[116] Blume-Jensen P, Hunter T. Oncogenic kinase signalling. Nature 2001: 411, 355–365.

[117] Darnell Jr. JE Transcription factors as targets for cancer therapy. Nat Rev Cancer. 2002: 2(10), 740-749.

[118] Dérijard B, Hibi M, Wu IH, Barrett T, Su B, Deng T, Karin M, Davis RJ. JNK1: a protein kinase stimulated by UV light and Ha-Ras that binds and phosphorylates the c-Jun activation domain. Cell 1994: 76, 1025–1037.

[119] Vogt P.K. Jun, the oncoprotein. Oncogene 2001: 20, 2365–2377.

[120] Zhang X, Wrzeszczynaska MH, Horvath CM, Darnell Jr JE. Interacting regions in Stat3 and c-Jun that participate in cooperative transcriptional activation. Mol. Cell. Biol. 1999: 19, 7138–7146.

[121] Hartl M, Vogt PK. A rearranged junD transforms chicken embryo fibroblasts. Cell Growth Differ. 1992: 3, 909–918.

[122] Vandel L, Montreau N, Vial E, Pfarr CM, Binetruy B, Castellazzi M. Stepwise transformation of rat embryo fibroblasts: c-Jun, JunB, or JunD can cooperate with Ras for focus formation, but a c-Jun-containing heterodimer is required for immortalization. Mol. Cell. Biol. 1996: 16, 1881–1888.

[123] Davidson B, Reich R, Goldberg I, Gotlieb WH, Kopolovic J, Berner A, Ben-Baruch G, Bryne M, Nesland JM. Ets-1 messenger RNA expression is a novel marker of poor survival in ovarian carcinoma. Clin. Cancer Res. 2001: 7, 551–557.

[124] Shaywitz AJ, Greenberg ME. CREB: a stimulus-induced transcription factor activated by a diverse array of extracellular signals. Annu. Rev. Biochem. 1999: 68, 821–861.

[125] Nesbit CE, Tersak JM, Prochownik EV. MYC oncogenes and human neoplastic disease. Oncogene 1999, 18, 3004–3016.

[126] Grandori C, Cowley SM, James LP, Eisenman RN. The Myc/Max/Mad network and the transcriptional control of cell behavior. Annu. Rev. Cell Dev. Biol. 2000: 16, 653–699.

[127] Eisenman RN. Deconstructing Myc. Genes Dev. 2001: 15, 2023–2030.

[128] Gilliland DG. The diverse role of the ETS family of transcription factors in cancer. Clin. Cancer Res. 2001: 7, 451–453.

[129] Denhardt DT. Oncogene-initiated aberrant signaling engenders the metastatic phenotype: synergistic transcription factor interactions are targets for cancer therapy. Crit. Rev. Oncog. 1996: 7, 261–291.

[130] Stark GR, Kerr IM, Williams BR, Silverman RH, Schreiber RD. How cells respond to interferons. Annu. Rev. Biochem. 1998: 67, 227–264.

[131] Levy D, Darnell Jr. JE. STATs: transcriptional control and biological impact. Nature Rev. Mol. Cell Biol. 2002: 3, 651–662.

[132] Bakin AV, Curran T. Role of DNA 5-Methylcytosine Transferase in Cell Transformation by fos. Science 1999: 283, 387–390.

[133] Clark SJ, Melki J. DNA methylation and gene silencing in cancer: which is the guilty party? Oncogene 2002: 21, 5380–5387.

[134] Métivier R, Gallais R, Tiffoche C, Le Péron C, Jurkowska RZ, Carmouche RP, Ibberson D, Barath P, Demay F, Reid G, Benes V, Jeltsch A, Gannon F, Salbert G. Cyclical DNA methylation of a transcriptionally active promoter. Nature 2008: 452, 45–50.

[135] Suzuki M, Yamada T, Kihara-Negishi F, Sakurai T, Hara E, Tenen DG, Hozumi N, Oikawa T. Site-specific DNA methylation by a complex of PU.1 and Dnmt3a/b. Oncogene 2006: 25, 2477–2488.

[136] Feldman N, Gerson A, Fang J, Li E, Zhang Y, Shinkai Y, Cedar H, Bergman Y. G9a-mediated irreversible epigenetic inactivation of Oct-3/4 during early embryogenesis. Nat Cell Biol 2006: 8, 188–94.

[137] Tachibana M, Matsumura Y, Fukuda M, Kimura H, Shinkai Y. G9a/GLP complexes independently mediate H3K9 and DNA methylation to silence transcription. EMBO J 2008: 27, 2681–2690.

[138] Viré E, Brenner C, Deplus R, Blanchon L, Fraga M, Didelot C, Morey L, Van Eynde A, Bernard D, Vanderwinden JM, Bollen M, Esteller M, Di Croce L, de Launoit Y, Fuks F. The Polycomb group protein EZH2 directly controls DNA methylation. Nature 2006: 439, 871–874.

[139] Turker MS. Gene silencing in mammalian cells and the spread of DNA methylation. Oncogene 2002: 21, 5388–5393.

[140] Gebhard C, Benner C, Ehrich M, Schwarzfischer L, Schilling E, Klug M, Dietmaier W, Thiede C, Holler E, Andreesen R, Rehli M. General Transcription Factor Binding at CpG Islands in Normal Cells Correlates with Resistance to De novo DNA Methylation in Cancer Cells. Cancer Res. 2010: 70 (4), 1398-1407.

[141] Galvagni F, Capo S, Oliviero S. Sp1 and Sp3 physically interact and cooperate with GABP for the activation of the utrophin promoter. J. Mol. Biol., 2001: 306, 985–996.

[142] Marin M, Karism A, Visser P, Grosveld F, Philipsen S. Transcription factor Sp1 is essential for early embryonic development but dispensable for cell growth and differentiation. Cell, 1997: 89, 619-628.

[143] Black AR, Black JD, Azizkhan-Clifford J. Sp1 and kruppel-like factor family of transcription factors in cell growth regulation and cancer. J. Cell Physiol., 2001: 188, 143-160.

[144] Black AR, Jensen D, Lin SY, Azizkhan JC. Growth/cell cycle regulation of Sp1 phosphorylation. J. Biol. Chem. 1999: 274, 1207-1215.

[145] Adam PJ, Regan CP, Hautmann MB, Owens GK. Positive- and negative acting kruppel-like transcription factors bind a transforming growth factor beta control element required for expression of the smooth muscle cell differentiation marker SM22alpha in vivo. J. Biol. Chem. 2000: 275, 37798-37806.

[146] Foster KW, Ren S, Louro ID, Lobo-Ruppert SM, McKie-Bell P, Grizzle WE, Hayes MR, Broker TR, Chow LT, Ruppert JM. Oncogene expression cloning by retroviral transduction of adenovirus E1Aimmortalized rat kidney RK3E cells: transformation of a host with epithelial features by c-MYC and the zinc finger protein GKLF. Cell Growth Differ. 1999: 10, 423-434.

[147] Kumar AP, Butler AP. Enhanced Sp1 DNA-binding activity in murine keratinocyte cell lines and epidermal tumors. Cancer Lett. 1999: 137, 159-165.

[148] Bird AP. CpG-rich islands and the function of DNA methylation, Nature 1986: 321, 209–213.

[149] Bird AP. CpG islands as gene markers in the vertebrate nucleus. Trends Genet. 1987: 3, 324-347.

[150] Graff JR, Herman JG, Myöhänen S, Baylin SB, Vertino PM. Mapping Patterns of CpG Island Methylation in Normal and Neoplastic Cells Implicates Both Upstream and Downstream Regions inde NovoMethylation. J Bio Chem 1997: 272, 22322-22329.

[151] Höller M, Westin G, Jiricny J, Schaffner W. Spl transcription factor binds DNA and activates transcription even when the binding site is CpG methylated. Genes Dev. 1988: 2, 1127-1135.

[152] Turker MS. The establishment and maintenance of DNA methylation patterns in mouse somatic cells. Semin. Cancer Biol 1999: 9, 329–337.

[153] Straussman R, Nejman D, Roberts D, Steinfeld I, Blum B, Benvenisty N, Simon I, Yakhini Z, Cedar H. Developmental programming of CpG island methylation profiles in the human genome, Nat. Struct. Mol. Biol. 2009: (16), 564–571.

[154] Brandeis M, Frank D, Keshet I, Siegfried Z, Mendelsohn M, Names A, Temper V, Razin A, Cedar H. Sp1 elements protect a CpG island from de novo methylation. Nature 1994: 371, 435–438.

[155] Macleod D, Charlton J, Mullins J, Bird AP. Sp1 sites in the mouse aprt gene promoter are required to prevent methylation of the CpG island. Genes Dev 1994: 8, 2282–2292.

[156] Ben-Hattar J, Jiricny J. Methylation of single CpGs within the second distal promoter element of the HSV-1 tk gene downregulates its transcription in vivo. Gene 1988: 65, 219-227.

[157] Harrington MA, Jones PA, Imagawa M, Karin M. Cytosine methylation does not affect binding of transcription factor Spl. Proc. Natl. Acad. Sci. 1988: 85, 2066-2070.

[158] Sadasivan E, Cedeno MM, Rothenberg SP. Characterization of the gene encoding a folate-binding protein expressed in human placenta. Identification of promoter activity in a G-rich SP1 site linked with the tandemly repeated GGAAG motif for the ets encoded GA-binding protein. J. Biol. Chem. 1994: 269, 4725–4735.

[159] Rosmarin AG, Luo M, Caprio DG, Shang J, Simkevich CP. Sp1 cooperates with the ets transcription factor, GABP, to activate the CD18 (β2 leukocyte integrin) promoter. J. Biol. Chem. 1998: 273, 13097–13103.

[160] Gyrd-Hansen M, Krag TO, Rosmarin AG, Khurana TS. Sp1 and the ets-related transcription factor complex GABP $\alpha/\beta$ functionally cooperate to activate the utrophin promoter. J. Neurol. Sci. 2002: 197, 27–35.

[161] Jiang P, Kumar A, Parrillo JE, Dempsey LA, Platt JL, Prinz RA, Xu X. Cloning and characterization of the human heparanase-1 (HPR1) gene promoter: role of GA-binding protein and Sp1 in regulating HPR1 basal promoter activity. J. Biol. Chem. 2002: 277, 8989–8998.

[162] Rao MK, Maiti S, Ananthaswamy HN, Wilkinson MF. A highly active homeobox gene promoter regulated by Ets and Sp1 family members in normal granulosa cells and diverse tumor cell types. J. Biol. Chem. 2002: 277, 26036– 26045.

[163] Rudge TL, Johnson LF. Synergistic activation of the TATA-less mouse thymidylate synthase promoter by the Ets transcription factor GABP and Sp1. Exp. Cell Res. 2002: 274, 45– 55.

[164] Nishikawa N, Izumi M, Yokoi M, Miyazawa H, Hanaoka F. E2F regulates growth-dependent transcription of genes encoding both catalytic and regulatory subunits of mouse primase. Genes Cells 2001: 6, 57–70.

[165] Izumi M, Yokoi M, Nishikawa NS, Miyazawa H, Sugino A, Yamagishi M, Yamaguchi M, Matsukage A, Yatagai F, Hanaoka F. Transcription of the catalytic 180-kDa subunit gene of mouse DNA polymerase $\alpha$ is controlled by E2F, an Ets-related transcription factor, and Sp1. Biochim. Biophys. Acta 2002: 1492, 341–352.

[166] Watanabe H, Wada T, Handa H. Transcription factor E4TF1 contains two subunits with different functions. EMBO J. 1990: 9, 841– 847.

[167] Thompson CC, Brown TA, McKnight SL. Convergence of Ets and notch-related structural motifs in a heteromeric DNA binding complex. Science 1991: 253, 762– 768.

[168] Brown TA, McKnight SL. Specificities of protein–protein and protein-DNA interaction of GABPα and two newly defined ets-related proteins. Genes Dev. 1992: 6, 2502–2512.

[169] Flory E, Hoffmeyer A, Smola U, Rapp UR, Bruder JT. Raf-1 kinase targets GA-binding protein in transcriptional regulation of the human immunodeficiency virus type 1 promoter. J. Virol. 1996: 70, 2260– 2268.

[170] Sharrocks AD, Brown AL, Ling Y, Yates PR. The ETS-domain transcription factor family. Int. J. Biochem. Cell Biol. 1997: 29, 1371– 1387.

[171] Oikawa T, Yamada T. Molecular biology of the Ets family of transcription factors. Gene, 2003: 303, 11–34.

[172] Sharrocks AD. The ETS-domain transcription factor family. Nat. Rev. Mol. Cell Biol. 2001: 2, 827–837.

[173] Sawa C, Goto M, Suzuki F, Watanabe H, Sawada J, Handa H. Functional domains of transcription factor hGABP β1/E4TF1-53 required for nuclear localization and transcription activation. Nucleic Acids Res. 1996: 24, 4954–4961.

[174] Rosmarin AG, Resendes KK, Yang ZF, McMillan JN, Fleming SL. GA-binding protein transcription factor: A review of GABP as an integrator of intracellular signaling and protein-protein interactions. Blood Cells Mol. Diseases 2004: 32, 143–154.

[175] Valouev A, Johnson DS, Sundquist A, Medina C, Anton E, Batzoglou S, Myers RM, Sidow A. Genome-wide analysis of transcription factor binding sites based on ChIP-Seq data. Nature Methods 2008: 5, 829 - 834.

[176] Izumi H, Ohta R, Nagatani G, Ise T, Nakayama Y, Nomoto M, Kohno K. p300/CBP-associated factor (P/CAF) interacts with nuclear respiratory factor-1 to regulate the UDP-N-acetyl-α-D-galactosamine: polypeptide N-acetylgalactosaminyltransferase-3 gene. Biochem J 2003: 373, 713–722.

[177] Wu Z, Puigserver P, Andersson U, Zhang C, Adelmant G, Mootha V, Troy A, Cinti S, Lowell B, Scarpulla RC, Spiegelman BM. Mechanisms controlling mitochondrial biogenesis and respiration through the thermogenic coactivator PGC-1. Cell 1999: 98, 115–124.

[178] LaMarco K, Thompson CC, Byers BP, Walton EM, McKnight SL. Identification of Ets- and notch-related subunits in GA binding protein. Science 1991: 253, 789– 792.

[179] Wasylyk B, Hahn SL, Giovane A. The Ets family of transcription factors. Eur. J. Biochem. 1993: 211, 7–18.

[180] Gugneja S, Virbasius JV, Scarpulla RC. Four structurally distinct, non-DNA-binding subunits of human nuclear respiratory factor 2 share a conserved transcriptional activation domain. Mol. Cell. Biol. 1995: 15, 102–111.

[181] Batchelor AH, Piper DE, De la Brousse FC, McKnight SL, Wolberger C. The structure of GABPα/β: an ETS domain - ankyrin repeat heterodimer bound to DNA. Science 1998: 279, 1037–1041.

[182] Slupsky CM, Gentile LN, Donaldson LW, Mackereth CD, Seidel JJ, Graves BJ, McIntosh LP. Proc. Natl. Acad. Sci. USA 1998: 95, 12129-12134.

[183] Mackereth CD, Scharpf M, Gentile LN, MacIntosh SE, Slupsky CM, McIntosh LP. Diversity in structure and function of the Ets family PNT domains. J. Mol. Biol. 2004: 342, 1249–1264.

[184] Kang HS, Nelson ML, Mackereth CD, Scharpf M, Graves BJ, McIntosh LP. Identification and Structural Characterization of a CBP/p300- Binding Domain from the ETS Family Transcription Factor GABPα. J Mol. Biol. 2008: 377 (3), 636–646.

[185] Rosmarin AG, Caprio DG, Kirsch DG, Handa H, Simkevich CP. GABP and PU.1 compete for binding, yet cooperate to increase CD18 (β2 leukocyte integrin) transcription. J. Biol. Chem. 1995: 270, 23627– 23633.

[186] Genuario RR, Perry RP. The GA-binding Protein Can Serve as Both an Activator and Repressor of ribosomal protein Gene Transcription. J. Biol. Chem. 1996: 271 (8), 4388–4395.

[187] Yokomori N, Tawata M, Saito T, Shimura H, Onaya T. Regulation of the Rat Thyrotropin Receptor Gene by the Methylation- Sensitive Transcription Factor GA-Binding Protein. Mol. Endo. 1998: 12 (8), 1241-1249

[188] Issa JP, Kantarjian HM. Targeting DNA methylation, Clin. Cancer Res. 2009: (15) 3938–3946.

[189] Fenaux P, Mufti GJ, Hellstrom-Lindberg E, Santini V, Finelli C, Giagounidis A, Schoch R, Gattermann N, Sanz G, List A, Gore SD, Seymour JF, Bennett JM, Byrd J, Backstrom J, Zimmerman L, McKenzie D, Beach C, Silverman LR. Efficacy of azacitidine compared with that of conventional care regimens in the treatment of higher-risk myelodysplastic syndromes: a randomised, open-label, phase III study, Lancet Oncol. 2009: (10) 223–232.

[190] Vigil CE, Martin-Santos T, Garcia-Manero G. Safety and efficacy of azacitidine in myelodysplastic syndromes, Drug Des. Devel. Ther. 2010: (4) 221–229.

[191] Garcia JS, Jain N, Godley LA. An update on the safety and efficacy of decitabine in the treatment of myelodysplastic syndromes, Onco Targets Ther. 2010: (3) 1–13.

[192] Von Hoff DD, Slavik M, Muggia FM. 5-Azacytidine: A new anticancer drug with effectiveness in acute myelogenous leukemia. Ann. Int. Med. 1976: 85, 237–245.

[193] Glover AB, Leyland-Jones B. Biochemistry of azacitidine: a review. Cancer Treat Rep. 1987: 71, 959–964.

[194] Juttermann R, Li E, Jaenisch R. Toxicity of 5-aza-2'-deoxycytidine to mammalian cells is mediated primarily by covalent trapping of DNA methyltransferase rather than DNA demethylation. Proc. Natl. Acad. Sci. USA 1994: 91, 11797–11801.

[195] Wallace RE, Lindh D, Durr FE. Arabinofuranosyl-5- azacytosine: activity against human tumors in athymic mice. Cancer Chemother. Pharmacol. 1989: 25, 117–123.

[196] Jones PA, Taylor SM. Cellular differentiation, cytidine analogs and DNA methylation. Cell 1980: 20, 85–93.

[197] Taylor C, Ford K, Connolly BA, Hornby DP. Determination of the order of substrate addition to MspI DNA methyl-transferase using a novel mechanism-based inhibitor. Biochem. J. 1993: 291, 493–504.

[198] Beisler JA, Abbasi MM, Driscoll JS. Dihydro-5-azacytidine hydrochloride, a biologically active and chemically stable analog of 5- azacytidine. Cancer Treat. Rep. 1976: 60, 1671–1674.

[199] Rodriguez-Paredes M, Esteller M. Cancer epigenetics reaches mainstream oncology. Nat. Med. 2011: 17, 330–339.

[200] Baylin SB, Jones PA. A decade of exploring the cancer epigenome — biological and translational implications, Nat. Rev. Cancer 2011: 11, 726–734.

[201] Gibbs JB. Mechanism-based target identification and drug discovery in cancer. Science 2000: 287, 1969–1973.

[202] Fitzgerald K, Harrington A, Leder P. Ras pathway signals are required for notch-mediated oncogenesis. Oncogene 2000: 19, 4191–4198.

[203] Park HS, Lin Q, Hamilton AD. Supramolecular chemistry and self-assembly special feature: modulation of protein–protein interactions by synthetic receptors. Design of molecules that disrupt serine protease-proteinaceous inhibitor interaction. Proc. Natl Acad. Sci. USA 2002: 99, 5105–5109.

[204] Ohkanda J, Knowles DB, Blaskovich MA, Sebti SM, Hamilton AD. Inhibitors of protein farnesyltransferase as novel anticancer agents. Curr. Top. Med. Chem. 2002: 2, 303–323.

[205] Peczuh MW, Hamilton AD. Peptide and protein recognition by designed molecules. Chem. Rev. 2000: 100, 2479–2494.

[206] Cochran AG. Antagonists of protein–protein interactions. Chem. Biol. 2000: 7, R85–R94.

Section 2

# DNA-Methyltransferases: Structure and Function in Eukaryotic and Prokaryotic System

Chapter 2

# Diverse Domains of (Cytosine-5)-DNA Methyltransferases: Structural and Functional Characterization

A. Yu. Ryazanova, L. A. Abrosimova,
T. S. Oretskaya and E. A. Kubareva

Additional information is available at the end of the chapter

http://dx.doi.org/10.5772/52046

## 1. Introduction

(Cytosine-5)-DNA methyltransferases (C5-DNA MTases) are enzymes which catalyze methyl group transfer from *S*-adenosyl-*L*-methionine (AdoMet) to C5 atom of cytosine residue in DNA. As a result, AdoMet is converted into *S*-adenosyl-*L*-homocysteine (AdoHcy). The recognition sites of C5-DNA MTases are usually short palindromic sequences (2–6 bp) in double-stranded DNA. One or both DNA strands can be methylated. The introduced methyl group is localized in the major groove of the DNA double helix and thus does not disrupt Watson–Crick interactions [1].

In prokaryotes, DNA methylation underlies several important processes, *e.g.* host and foreign DNA distinction as well as maternal and daughter strand discrimination that is vital for correction of replication errors in the newly synthesized DNA strand. DNA methylation is also responsible for DNA replication control and its interconnection with cell cycle [1]. The majority of the known DNA MTases are components of restriction–modification (R–M) systems which protect bacterial cells from bacteriophage infection. A typical R–M system consists of a MTase which modifies certain DNA sequences and a restriction endonuclease (RE) which hydrolyses DNA if these sequences remain unmethylated [2].

In eukaryotes, DNA methylation has diverse functions such as control of gene expression, regulation of genome imprinting, X-chromosome inactivation, genome defense from endogenous retroviruses and transposons, participation in development of immune system and in brain functioning. Anomalous methylation patterns in humans are associated with psychoses, immune system diseases and different cancers [3].

Different C5-DNA MTases share high similarity both in the primary and in the tertiary structure that enables their easy identification by bioinformatic tools. At the moment (July 2012), the Pfam database (http://pfam.sanger.ac.uk/) contains 5065 protein sequences that possess the characteristic domain of C5-DNA MTases (PF00145). Among this moiety, 3072 sequences (61%) contain the only domain PF00145 while the others have a duplication of this domain and/or other additional domains. The diversity of such domains fused in a single polypeptide with the C5-DNA MTase domain is rather wide (Table 1): there are MTases, RE, transcription factors, chromatin-associated domains *etc.*

To date, the structural characteristics of the catalytic domain from different MTases, the details of the catalytic mechanism and the biological functions of C5-DNA MTases from different organisms are summarized in a variety of reviews (for example, see [1, 4-8]). Therefore, these aspects are discussed here rather briefly. The present review is focused on the additional activities of C5-DNA MTases, on the structure and functions of the domains which are additional to the catalytic one. The data about C5-DNA MTases have not yet been summarized from this point of view.

## 2. The methyltransferase domain in prokaryotic and eukaryotic (cytosine-5)-DNA methyltransferases

The most studied enzyme among the prokaryotic C5-DNA MTases is MTase HhaI (M.HhaI) from *Haemophilus haemolyticus*. It methylates the inner cytosine residue in the sequence 5′-GCGC-3′/3′-CGCG-5′ (italicised). M.HhaI consists of only the MTase domain (Figure 1). The structural organization and catalytic mechanism of C5-DNA MTases were extensively studied using this enzyme as a model.

The catalytic domain of C5-DNA MTases consists of two subdomains, a large one and a small one, separated by a DNA-binding cleft. The tertiary structure of the large (catalytic) subdomain has a common structural core – a β-sheet that consists of 7 β-strands and is flanked by 3 α-helices from each side. Six of seven β-strands have a parallel orientation, while the $7^{th}$ β-strand is located between the $5^{th}$ and the $6^{th}$ β-strands in an antiparallel orientation (Figure 1, b). Thus, the large subdomain consists of 2 parts: the first one (β1–β3) forms the AdoMet binding site while the second one (β4–β7) forms the binding site for the target cytosine. The small subdomain contains a TRD region (target recognition domain) that has a unique sequence in each MTase and is responsible for the substrate specificity. The small subdomains of C5-DNA MTases vary substantially in size and spatial structure [1].

http://dx.doi.org/10.5772/52046

| Domain name and number | Domain description |
|---|---|
| **Methyltransferase domains** | |
| **DNA_methylase (PF00145)** | C5-cytosine-specific DNA methyltransferase |
| Eco57I (PF07669) | Eco57I restriction–modification methyltransferase |
| Methyltransf_26 (PF13659) | Methyltransferase domain |
| MethyltransfD12 (PF02086) | D12 class N6-adenine-specific DNA methyltransferase |
| N6_Mtase (PF02384) | N6-DNA methyltransferase |
| N6_N4_Mtase (PF01555) | DNA methyltransferase |
| Cons_hypoth95 (PF03602) | Conserved hypothetical protein 95 |
| EcoRI_methylase (PF13651) | Adenine-specific methyltransferase EcoRI |
| Dam (PF05869) | DNA N6-adenine-methyltransferase (Dam) |
| **Endonuclease domains** | |
| RE_Eco47II (PF09553) | Eco47II restriction endonuclease |
| RE_HaeII (PF09554) | HaeII restriction endonuclease |
| RE_HaeIII (PF09556) | HaeIII restriction endonuclease |
| RE_HpaII (PF09561) | HpaII restriction endonuclease |
| HNH_3(PF13392) | HNH endonuclease |
| Vsr (PF03852) | DNA mismatch endonuclease Vsr |
| DUF559 (PF04480) | Domain of unknown function |
| BsuBI_PstI_RE (PF06616) | BsuBI/PstI restriction endonuclease C-terminus |
| TaqI_C (PF12950) | TaqI-like C-terminal specificity domain |
| **Transcription regulators** | |
| HTH_3 (PF01381) | Helix–turn–helix (HTH) |
| HTH_17 (PF12728) | HTH |
| HTH_19 (PF12844) | HTH |
| HTH_23 (PF13384) | Homeodomain-like domain |
| HTH_26 (PF13443) | Cro/C1-type HTH DNA-binding domain |
| HTH_31 (PF13560) | HTH |
| MerR (PF00376) | MerR family regulatory protein |
| MerR_1 (PF13411) | MerR HTH family regulatory protein |
| DUF1870 (PF08965) | Domain of unknown function |
| PHD (PF00628) | PHD-finger (plant homeo domain) |
| **Domains of other DNA-operating enzymes** | |
| SNF2_N (PF00176) | SNF2 family N-terminal domain |

| | |
|---|---|
| Helicase_C (PF00271) | Helicase conserved C-terminal domain |
| Terminase_6 (PF03237) | Terminase-like family |
| RVT_1 (PF00078) | Reverse transcriptase (RNA-dependent DNA polymerase) |
| MutH (PF02976) | DNA mismatch repair enzyme MutH |
| DEDD_Tnp_IS110 (PF01548) | Transposase |
| DYW_deaminase (PF14432) | DYW family of nucleic acid deaminases |
| DNA_pol3_beta_2 (PF02767) | DNA polymerase III beta subunit, central domain |
| DNA_pol3_beta_3 (PF02768) | DNA polymerase III beta subunit, C-terminal domain |
| HhH-GPD (PF00730) | HhH-GPD superfamily base excision DNA repair protein |
| Transposase_20 (PF02371) | Transposase IS116/IS110/IS902 family |
| **Chromatin-associated domains** | |
| Chromo (PF00385) | CHRromatin Organisation MOdifier |
| PWWP (PF00855) | PWWP domain (conserved Pro-Trp-Trp-Pro motif) |
| BAH (PF01426) | BAH domain (bromo-adjacent homology) |
| DMAP_binding (PF06464) | DMAP1-binding domain |
| DNMT1-RFD (PF12047) | Cytosine specific DNA methyltransferase replication foci domain |
| zf-CXXC (PF02008) | CXXC zinc finger domain |
| RCC1_2 (PF13540) | Regulator of chromosome condensation (RCC1) repeat |
| **Others** | |
| Pkinase_Tyr (PF07714) | Protein tyrosine kinase |
| YTH (PF04146) | YT521-B-like domain |
| PPR (PF01535) | PPR repeat (pentatricopeptide repeat) |
| AOX (PF01786) | Alternative oxidase |
| Cullin (PF00888) | Cullin family |
| Cyt-b5 (PF00173) | Cytochrome b5-like heme/steroid binding domain |
| PALP (PF00291) | Pyridoxal-phosphate dependent enzyme |
| CH (PF00307) | Calponin homology (CH) domain |
| Dabb (PF07876) | Stress responsive A/B barrel domain |
| Hint_2 (PF13403) | Hint domain |
| DUF1152 (PF06626) | Domain of unknown function |
| DUF3444 (PF11926) | Domain of unknown function |

**Table 1.** Domains existing in a single polypeptide chain with the C5-DNA MTase domain (PF00145) according to the Pfam database.

http://dx.doi.org/10.5772/52046

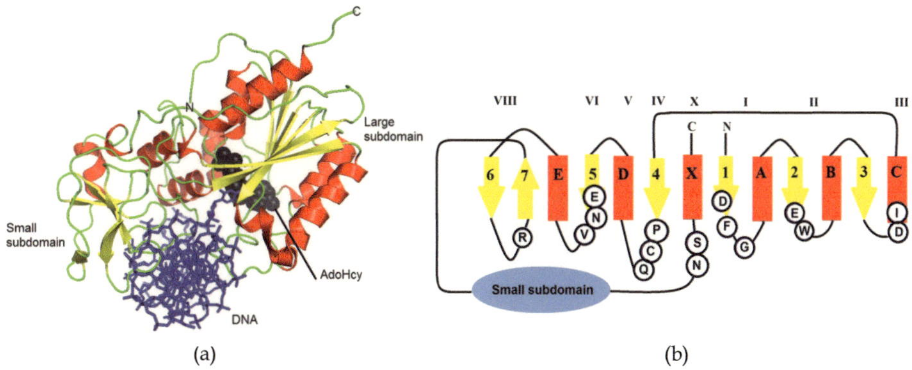


**Figure 1.** *a)* Secondary and tertiary structure typical for the C5-DNA MTase domain (M.HhaI in complex with DNA and AdoHcy, PDB code: 3mht). α-Helices are depicted in pink, β-strands are in yellow, DNA is in blue. AdoHcy is in black, spacefill representation. (*b*) The structural core and the order of the conservative motifs in the large subdomain of C5-DNA MTases. α-Helices are depicted as boxes, β-strands – as arrows. The conservative motifs are numbered using Roman numerals.

Mammalian DNA MTase Dnmt1 is responsible for maintenance methylation. Its main recognition site is monomethylated 5′-CG-3′/3′-GC-5′ DNA fragment. The structures of M.HhaI and Dnmt1 in their complexes with DNA were compared [9]. Their catalytic subdomains are rather similar (the root mean square deviation of $C_\alpha$ atoms is 2.0 Å over 218 aligned residues). However, the TRD primary and tertiary structures differ significantly between Dnmt1 and M.HhaI. The larger part of the Dnmt1 TRD is structurally isolated and stabilized by $Zn^{2+}$ ion, the latter one being coordinated by three Cys and one His residues. A β-hairpin in the C-terminal part of the Dnmt1 TRD forms hydrophobic contacts with the catalytic subdomain and the BAH1 domain (see section 4.1.5). The side chains of a few residues (presumably arginine) in the catalytic subdomain make contacts with the phosphate groups that flank unmethylated 5′-CG-3′/3′-GC-5′ sites. In the M.HhaI structure, the DNA is located in the cleft between the catalytic subdomain and the TRD, whereas the DNA in Dnmt1 complex is distant from the Dnmt1 catalytic center. This is likely to be connected with the fact that the activity of the Dnmt1 catalytic domain is regulated by the N-terminal part of the protein. An isolated Dnmt1 catalytic domain proved to be inactive [10-13].

## 3. The mechanism of DNA methylation

To catalyze the methylation reaction, a MTase binds DNA containing its recognition site and the cofactor AdoMet. Specific DNA–protein contacts are formed between the MTase and heterocyclic bases of the recognition site except the cytosine to be methylated. The target cytosine is methylated according to $S_N2$ mechanism. The whole methylation process can be divided into 3 steps: a cytosine flipping out of the DNA double helix, a formation of a covalent enzyme–substrate intermediate and a methyl group transfer to the cytosine residue [14-23] (Figure 2).

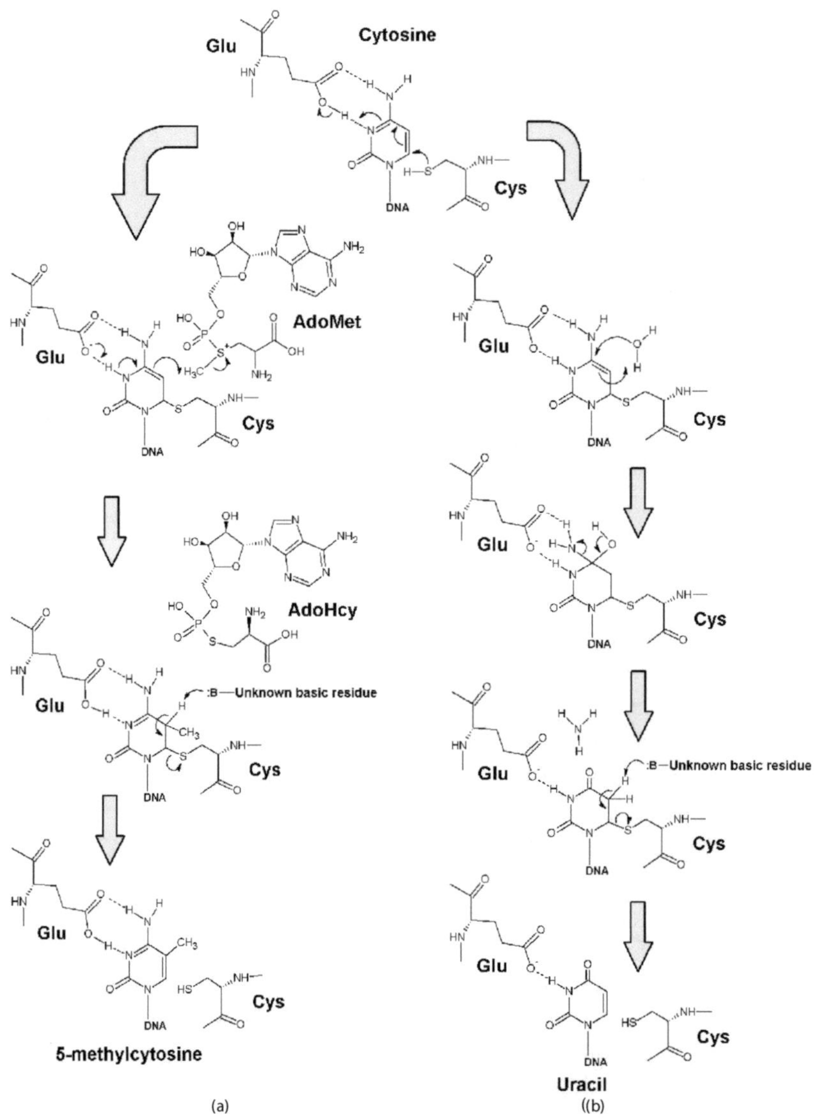


**Figure 2.** *a*) Mechanism of cytosine C5 atom methylation by a C5-DNA MTase. (*b*) Mechanism of cytosine deamination as a possible side reaction of the methylation process.

The target nucleotide flipping can occur spontaneously or with the help of an enzyme [20]. The catalytic loop (residues 81–100 in M.HhaI) shifts substantially towards the DNA almost simultaneously with the target cytosine flipping. As a result, the flipped out base occurs in close proximity with the cofactor molecule inside of a closed catalytic cavity [23-25].

A nucleophilic attack of M.HhaI Cys81 thiol group on the cytosine C6 atom results in a formation of M.HhaI–DNA conjugate. The Cys81 residue is a part of a conservative ProCys dipeptide of the protein (motif IV, Figure 2). The Glu119 residue from GluAsnVal tripeptide (motif

VI) protonates the cytosine N3 atom thus facilitating the nucleophilic attack by the thiol group. In the conjugate, the negative charge of the cytosine C5 atom causes its alkylation by the AdoMet methyl group. Proton elimination from the C5 atom of the methylated cytosine and β-elimination of the Cys residue result in a breakdown of the covalent DNA–protein complex and restore aromaticity of the modified cytosine base (Figure 2, a). The rate constant for methyl group transfer catalyzed by M.HhaI is about 0.14–0.26 $s^{-1}$ [17, 18]. The following release of the reaction products is a rate-limiting step of the M.HhaI catalytic cycle [17, 18].

C5-DNA MTases HhaI and HpaII catalyze the methylation reaction in a distributive manner, *i.e.* dissociate from the DNA substrate after every catalytic act [1, 18]. Each one of these MTases is a component of a R–M system where the cognate RE searches for its recognition sites *via* scanning DNA by a linear diffusion mechanism. The MTase distributivity provides for the corresponding RE a possibility to bind an unmodified site before the MTase and to cleave it. On the other hand, C5-DNA MTase SssI [26] has no cognate RE and is able to methylate several recognition sites located in one DNA substrate in a processive manner, *i.e.* without dissociation from DNA after each catalytic act.

The affinity of prokaryotic C5-DNA MTases to their DNA ligands in the presence of non-reactive cofactor analogs increases in the following manner: dimethylated DNA << unmethylated DNA < monomethylated DNA [1, 2, 27, 28]. A similar correlation is observed for the eukaryotic enzyme Dnmt1. The Dnmt1 affinity to monomethylated 5′-CG-3′/3′-GC-5′ sites is 2–200 times higher than to unmethylated ones depending on the experimental conditions [13, 29-35]. Dnmt1 modifies monomethylated sites processively (more than 50 sites per one binding act on average). Unmethylated sites (mainly 5′-CCGG-3′) are methylated by Dnmt1 in a distributive manner [36].

Mammalian C5-DNA MTases Dnmt3a and Dnmt3b methylate presumably unmodified sites in DNA and are responsible for *de novo* DNA methylation during embryonic development. Dinucleotides 5'-CG-3'/3′-GC-5′ are the main recognition sites of Dnmt3a and Dnmt3b. These enzymes are also able to modify dinucleotides 5′-CA-3′ but 10–100 times less efficiently [37]. The efficiency of methylation by Dnmt3a and Dnmt3b is also dependent on the sequences flanking the recognition site: 5′-RCGY-3′ is the most frequently methylated site whereas 5′-YCGR-3′ is methylated with a lower efficiency (R and Y are purine and pyrimidine nucleosides respectively). The difference in the methylation rate of these sites can exceed 500 times [38]. The primary structures of the Dnmt3a and Dnmt3b catalytic domains share identity of 84%. In contrast to Dnmt1, isolated catalytic domains of Dnmt3a and Dnmt3b retain their activity [12, 39]. Dnmt3a methylates DNA in a distributive manner while Dnmt3b modifies DNA processively since the DNA binding center of Dnmt3b is more positively charged than DNA binding center of Dnmt3a [37, 39]. Interestingly, a Cys residue substitution in the catalytic ProCys motif of an isolated Dnmt3a catalytic domain does not totally abolish the enzyme activity but merely decreases it 2–6 times. This Cys residue is shown to take part in the DNA–Dnmt3a conjugate formation. However, the Dnmt3a catalytic domain looses its activity completely after a substitution of a Glu residue in the GluAsnVal motif. The active center of Dnmt3a seems to have an unusual conformation and the Cys residue perhaps does not have its optimal orientation. Therefore, the nucleophilic attack onto the cytosine C6 atom can be performed by some other residue or hydroxyl ion. Post-translational modifications or interaction with other proteins are likely to be needed for the Dnmt3a activation [40].

Murine Dnmt3a is able to perform automethylation, a methyl group transfer to the Cys residue of its own catalytic center in the presence of AdoMet. This reaction is irreversible and rather slow but its can be activated by Dnmt3L. In the presence of a duplex containing 5′-CG-3′/3'-GC-5' sites Dnmt3a methylates the substrate DNA but not its own Cys residue. The automethylation seems to have a regulatory function that enables to inactivate excessive enzyme molecules in a cell. On the other hand, it can be just a side reaction which takes place in the absence of DNA [41].

A protein called Dnmt3L is also a member of Dnmt3 family. It is catalytically inactive but plays an important role as a stimulator of the Dnmt3a and Dnmt3b activity. A structure of a complex consisting of Dnmt3a and Dnmt3L C-terminal domain has been determined by X-ray crystallography (PDB-code 2qrv) [42]. The complex is a heterotetramer where the subunits are localized in the following order: Dnmt3L–Dnmt3a–Dnmt3a–Dnmt3L. Two active centers of Dnmt3a are localized nearby and probably can methylate two 5′-CG-3′/3′-GC-5′ sites simultaneously. These recognition sites should be separated by 8–10 bp (about one turn of DNA double helix). Twelve murine genes which undergo maternal imprinting contain 5′-CG-3′/3′-GC-5′ sites localized in such a manner. Moreover, highly methylated regions of human chromosome 21 possess 5′-CG-3′/3′-GC-5′ sites separated by 9, 18 and 27 bp more frequently in comparison to the unmethylated regions [43]. The effective methylation of these regions could be determined by the proper distribution of 5′-CG-3′/3′-GC-5′ sites. A substitution of Dnmt3a and Dnmt3L residues which do not take part in catalysis but are important for the interface formation (Dnmt3a–Dnmt3L or Dnmt3a–Dnmt3a interfaces) results in a suppression of Dnmt3a activity. This fact confirms the importance of the appropriate complex formation between Dnmt3a and Dnmt3L [42]. The orientation of the Dnmt3a–Dnmt3L complex relative to the substrate DNA is still unclear.

## 4. Additional functions of prokaryotic (cytosine-5)-DNA methyltransferases

### 4.1. DNA methyltransferases with multiple methyltransferase domains

Some C5-DNA MTases contain more than one MTase domain. The "additional" domain can belong to (cytosine-5)-DNA or (adenine-N6)-DNA MTases. Up to date, the Pfam database contains 5065 protein sequences that possess the characteristic domain of C5-DNA MTases (PF00145). Among them, 676 sequences (13%) contain two PF00145 domains and 42 sequences (1%) – even three PF00145 domains. Such structures might have arisen as fusions of two adjacent genes encoding different MTases. However, none of these proteins has been studied experimentally.

The ability of a single molecule to methylate both the cytosine C5 atom and the adenine N6 atom is typical for MTases that recognize asymmetric DNA sequences. This phenomenon was demonstrated for M.Alw26I from *Acinetobacter lwoffi* RFL26 (recognition site 5′-GTCTC-3′/3′-CAGAG-5′) and for M.Esp3I from *Hafnia alvei* RFL3 (recognition site 5′-CGTCTC-3′/3′-GCAGAG-5′) [44]. Each of these proteins contains the N6-DNA MTase domain in its N-terminal part and the C5-DNA MTase domain – in its C-terminal part [45]. The ability of each domain to methylate its recognition site in the absence of the second domain has not been investigated.

A gene coding for another enzyme consisting of two MTase domains has been constructed from two genes of *Helicobacter pylori* 26695 [46]. These genes are located in tandem orientation and code for DNA MTases M.HpyAVIB and M.HpyAVIA. One nucleotide insertion before the stop codon results in a formation of a fused gene. A similar mutation has been occurred naturally in *H. pylori* D27 strain [47]. M.HpyAVIB methylates the cytosine C5 atom and M.HpyAVIA methylates the adenine N6 atom in the sequence 5′-*C*CTC-3′/3′-GG*A*G-5′ (italicised). The obtained bifunctional protein contains the C5-DNA MTase domain and the N6-DNA MTase domain in its N-terminal and C-terminal parts, respectively. The both domains recognize in DNA the same sites as the initial proteins. The methylation kinetics and the properties of point mutants demonstrate that these domains function independently from each other. Each one of them contains its own catalytic and AdoMet binding motifs [46].

### 4.2. Deamination of cytosine and 5-methylcytosine

Prokaryotic C5-DNA MTases M.HpaII, M.HhaI, M.SssI, Dcm (from *E. coli*), M.EcoRII, and M.SsoII are shown to increase the rate of C → dU → T and $m^5C$ (5-methyl-2'-deoxycytidine) → T mutagenesis *in vitro* [48-55]. Some of them demonstrate the mutagenic activity (M.HpaII, M.EcoRII, and Dcm) also *in vivo* increasing the mutagenesis rate up to 50 times [50, 54, 56]. Interestingly, prokaryotic M.MspI does not stimulate cytosine deamination *in vitro* but its mutagenic effect is comparable with the effect of other C5-DNA MTases when M.MspI is expressed in *E. coli* cells [57]. Moreover, M.EcoRII is shown to catalyze 5-methylcytosine conversion into thymine [52].

The enzymatic catalysis of cytosine deamination is a side reaction of the methylation process. According to the standard mechanism (Figure 2), the cysteine thiol group performs a nucleophilic attack onto the cytosine C6 atom and at the same time the cytosine N3 atom gets protonated that altogether leads to the DNA–enzyme conjugate formation. As a result, the cytosine base aromaticity is disrupted and the C5 atom becomes negatively charged. However, the following step (the methyl group transfer to the C5 atom) becomes impossible in the absence of AdoMet. If water penetrates into the enzyme active center, hydroxylation of the cytosine C4 atom is likely to occur. These processes initiate the deamination reaction (Figure 2, b). Afterwards, the cytosine amino group is substituted with a carboxyl group and the base is converted into uracil [58, 59]. The presence of AdoMet or AdoHcy prevents water penetration into the active center and therefore inhibits deamination. A point mutant of M.HpaII incapable of AdoMet binding is a very effective catalyst of C → dU conversion [56].

The AdoMet analogs such as sinefungin and 5′-amino-5′-deoxyadenosine can increase the rate of enzymatic deamination even in the presence of AdoMet and AdoHcy [53]. They seem to trigger other reaction mechanisms which are not completely clarified yet. The supposed mechanisms include a water molecule direct attack onto the cytosine C4 atom. It becomes possible after the N3 atom protonation by a MTase which is a step of the methylation reaction. Two alternative mechanisms are suggested (Figure 3). According to the first one (mechanism 1), the hydroxyl group of 5′-amino-5′-deoxyadenosine activates a water molecule producing a hydroxyl ion which attacks the cytosine C4 atom (Figure 3). According to the mechanism 2, 5′-amino-5′-deoxyadenosine acts as an acid and protonates the cytosine N4 atom (Figure 3) thus facilitating the amino group elimination in the form of ammonium ion [59]. The mechanisms 1 and 2 are based on a water molecule direct attack onto the C4 atom and differ considerably from the others as they do not require a MTase interaction with the cytosine C6 atom. Therefore, a mutant form of a MTase which does not catalyze the methylation reaction should be able to catalyze these side reactions. Indeed, it has been shown experimentally for an M.EcoRII point mutant where catalytic Cys was substituted with Ala [59].

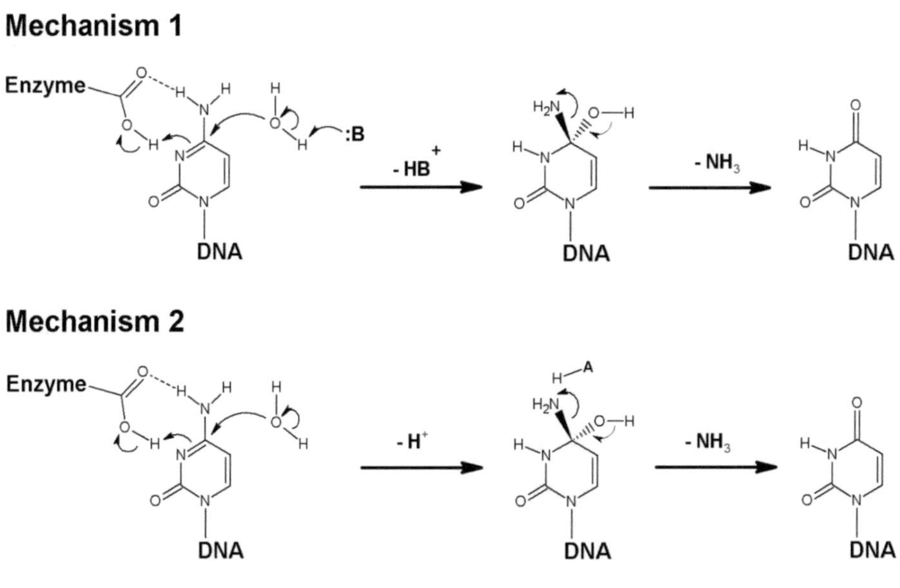


**Figure 3.** The supposed mechanisms of cytosine deamination catalyzed by an AdoMet analogue (sinefungin or 5′-amino-5′-deoxyadenosine). The AdoMet analogue might act as a base (mechanism 1) or as an acid (mechanism 2).

Both the methylation and the deamination reactions require flipping out of the cytosine residue. Thus, the longer cytosine base remains flipped out the faster these reactions go. The both reactions share a common intermediate – the enzyme–substrate conjugate (Figure 2). The usage of tritiated cytosine allows an estimation of tritium to hydrogen exchange rate at the cytosine C5 atom which can serve as a measure of the conjugate formation rate. In the absence of the cofactor, such an exchange catalyzed by murine Dnmt1 is slower than the one catalyzed by M.HhaI [60]. Thus, Dnmt1 forms the conjugate in the absence of AdoMet with a lower probability and therefore is less mutagenic than M.HhaI [60]. On the contrary, prokaryotic MTases catalyze effectively the deamination reaction in the absence of the cofactor [48, 53, 57].

The different rates of the covalent enzyme–substrate complex formation in the absence of the cofactor could reflect different physiological functions of prokaryotic and eukaryotic C5-DNA MTases. Limited nutrition decreases AdoMet amounts in prokaryotic cells. The mutations derived from the cytosine deamination might not be lethal for a bacterial cell and could help to prevent hydrolysis of cellular DNA by phage endonucleases. So, the ability of a C5-DNA MTase to catalyze deamination can turn out a physiological advantage for a bacterial cell [5]. On the contrary, mammalian cells are not likely to benefit from this kind of mutagenesis and therefore have developed mechanisms which provide low mutagenesis rate.

### 4.3. Topoisomerase activity

Two prokaryotic C5-DNA MTases are shown to have a topoisomerase activity, namely M.SssI from *Spiroplasma* MQI and M.MspI from *Moraxella species*. M.SssI is not a part of R–M system (there is no corresponding RE in *Spiroplasma* genome). As well as eukaryotic MTases, M.SssI modifies cytosine C5 atom in 5′-CG-3′/3′-GC-5′ sequences [61]. In the presence of 10 mM $Mg^{2+}$, M.SssI provides relaxation of negatively supercoiled plasmids which leads to accumulation of plasmids with different degree of supercoiling. The obtained set of plasmids is similar to the products of topoisomerase I from calf thymus. An ATP addition does not influence the topoisomerase activity of M.SssI. Since type II topoisomerases need ATP for the enzymatic activity, M.SssI can be regarded as a type I topoisomerase [62]. The MTase and the topoisomerase activities of M.SssI are functionally independent. The methylation process requires AdoMet, while the topoisomerase reaction demands $Mg^{2+}$ ions. The M.SssI conservative motifs IV and VIII share a certain similarity with topoisomerase sequences. In particular, the motif IV contains Tyr that is an important catalytic residue in topoisomerases. A more detailed analysis of M.SssI regions responsible for the topoisomerase activity has not been conducted.

Different speculations are proposed to explain why these two activities are combined in one M.SssI molecule. Firstly, the topoisomerase activity alters the supercoiling degree of plasmid DNA and thus could facilitate or complicate the cytosine flipping out of the DNA helix. Secondly, the methylation of 5′-CG-3'/3′-GC-5′ sites by M.SssI could change the DNA structure. For example, a negatively supercoiled DNA region with large amount of methylated 5′-CG-3′/3′-GC-5′ sites is likely to be converted into Z-form. For the B-form restoration, topoisomerase activity is necessary. Thirdly, the change in DNA topology perhaps influences the level of gene expression in *Spiroplasma*. Finally, the two different activities can be combined in one protein for the purpose of genome economy. *Spiroplasma* belongs to mycoplasmas – cellular organisms which have the smallest genome (from 600 to 1800 kbp). For a comparison, the T4 bacteriophage genome consists of 165 kbp and the *E. coli* genome – of 4600 kbp [62].

M.MspI is a part of MspI R–M system and methylates the first cytosine residue in the sequence 5′-CCGG-3′/3′-GGCC-5′ [63]. The unique property of this MTase is its ability to bend DNA at 142 ± 4° upon its binding to the methylation site. This was demonstrated using 127 bp DNA duplex and has not been shown for any other MTase [64]. Unlike M.SssI, M.MspI has an N-terminal part responsible for the topoisomerase activity. This part consists of 107 residues and is located before the conservative motif I. There are two regions of M.MspI that share similarity with topoisomerase sequences: the residues 32–98 and the conservative motif VIII. In contrast to M.SssI, there is no similarity between the M.MspI conservative motif IV and the topoisomerase sequences. A mutant form of M.MspI lacking the first 34 residues retains the ability to methylate DNA but loses its topoisomerase activity. Mutant proteins M.MspI(W34A) and M.MspI(Y74A) also do not have topoisomerase activity but are still able to methylate the DNA substrate [65]. Additionally, the M.MspI C-terminal part contains a region (245–287 a.a.) that shares similarity with DNA ligase I active center. This is in accordance with the fact that the topoisomerase I activity includes ligation of the DNA strands [65].

### 4.4. (Cytosine-5)-DNA methyltransferases as transcription factors

According to the Table 1, some C5-DNA MTases contain domains that can function as transcription factors. These domains are located in the N-terminal parts of the proteins and are followed by the MTase domains. The main structural element of these domains is a characteristic helix-turn-helix (HTH) motif that is also present in many transcription factors. To date, the Pfam database contains 68 sequences that include a domain with HTH motif followed by the C5-DNA MTase domain. Among them, 25 sequences belong to the HTH_3 family (PF01381). The ability to downregulate expression of its own gene was shown experimentally only for 7 DNA MTases (M.MspI, M.EcoRII, M.ScrFIA, M1.LlaJI, M.Eco47II, M.SsoII, and M.Ecl18kI) [66-68]. Among them, M.SsoII and M.Ecl18kI are the most remarkable ones as they not only suppress the transcription of their own genes but also stimulate the transcription of their cognate RE genes.

M.EcoRII from *E. coli* R245 strain methylates C5 atom of the second cytosine in the sequence 5′-CCWGG-3′/3′-GGWCC-5′ (W = A or T). *In vitro* experiments demonstrate that M.EcoRII can bind both its methylation site and the promoter region of its own gene. The enzyme's binding site has been determined by footprinting with DNase I: M.EcoRII protects 47 nucleotides in the "top" strand and 49 nucleotides in the "bottom" strand from DNase I hydrolysis [69]. Thus, the binding site of M.EcoRII is located upstream of the MTase gene coding region and overlaps with its –10 and –35 promoter elements. This localization of M.EcoRII prevents RNA polymerase binding to the promoter and results in a suppression of the MTase gene transcription. The M.EcoRII binding site in the promoter region contains an imperfect inverted repeat (with 2 nucleotide substitutions). The repeat consists of two 11 bp sequences spaced by 12 bp. This kind of symmetry supposes the MTase to bind the promoter region as a dimer though this protein is a monomer in solution. Investigation of M.EcoRII catalytically inactive forms shows that the efficiency of the MTase binding to the promoter region does not depend on its ability to methylate substrate. These facts demonstrate that M.EcoRII consists of two domains: a catalytic domain and a domain responsible for the interaction with the promoter region [70].

R–M system Eco47II from *E. coli* RFL47 strain contains a MTase that is also able to downregulate the expression of its own gene. M.Eco47II methylates the cytosine C5 atom in the sequence 5′-GGNCC-3′/3′-CCNGG-5′ (N = A, G, C, T). It remains unclear which one cytosine is modified. The M.Eco47II N-terminal part is predicted to contain an HTH motif and is demonstrated to be responsible for the transcription regulation but not for the MTase activity. Mutations introduced into the catalytic center of the enzyme result in suppression of the methylation activity but do not disrupt the regulatory function [68].

In the MspI R–M system, the *mspIM* and *mspIR* genes are transcribed divergently from the complementary DNA strands and their promoter regions (–35 elements) are separated by 6 bp. The regulatory site of M.MspI is located in the promoter region of the *mspIM* gene and contains a 12 bp inverted repeat. M.MspI protects from DNase I hydrolysis the region from –34 to +17 position in the "top" DNA strand and the region from –33 to +17 position in the "bottom" DNA strand (the numbers indicate the position relatively to the start point of the *mspIM* gene transcription). So, M.MspI interaction with the regulatory region prevents RNA polymerase binding to the promoter region and blocks transcription initiation from the *mspIM* gene. At the same time, M.MspI does not interact with the promoter region of the *mspIR* gene and does not interfere with the expression of RE MspI [71].

R–M system ScrFI from *Lactococcus lactis subsp. cremoris* also contains a C5-DNA MTase that regulates gene expression in its R–M system [66]. The RE gene (*scrFIR*) is flanked by two genes that code for MTases: *scrFIBM* and *scrFIAM*. The *scrFIAM* gene has its own promoter while the *scrFIBM* and *scrFIR* genes are transcribed together with a gene of unknown function – *orfX* (Figure 4). Both MTases from the ScrFI R–M system recognize and methylate the cytosine base in the sequence 5′-CCNGG-3′/3′-GGNCC-5′ (it remains unknown which one cytosine is methylated). The biological sense of existing of two MTase genes is not clear. The N-terminal part of M.ScrFIA is predicted to contain an HTH motif [72]. M.ScrFIA is also shown to bind to the regulatory region – a 15 bp inverted repeat located before the transcription start point for the *scrFIAM* gene. M.ScrFIA binds to this region and inhibits the expression of its own gene 72].

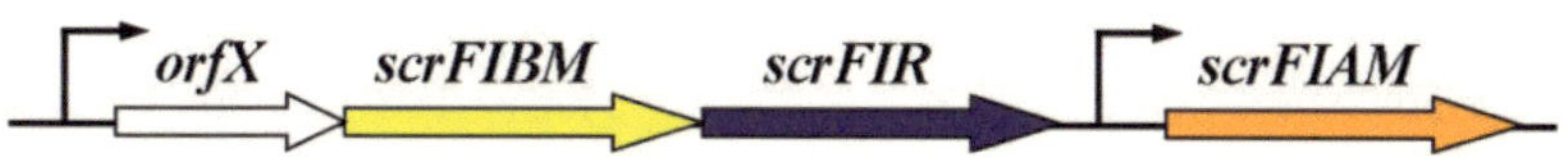


**Figure 4.** Genetic organization of the ScrFI R–M system. Thin arrows indicate the transcription initiation points.

R–M system LlaJI from *Lactococcus lactis* contains two C5-DNA MTases – M1.LlaJI and M2.LlaJI. These MTases have the same recognition site 5′-GACGC-3′/3′-CTGCG-5′ but methylate different cytosine bases (italicised) in the "top" and the "bottom" DNA strands respectively [73, 74]. Genes coding for these MTases and two RE compose one operon and are transcribed from the same promoter (Figure 5, a). The promoter region contains a 24 bp inverted repeat that is a regulatory site for the MTases. This palindrome sequence contains two methylation sites of the LlaJI MTases one of which overlaps with –35 promoter element (Figure 5, b). At first, M2.LlaJI modifies both sites that enables binding of M1.LlaJI and methylation of cytosine bases in the opposite strand. Interaction of M1.LlaJI with the unmethylated substrate has not been demonstrated [73]. M2.LlaJI acts only as a modifying enzyme while Ml.LlaJI has an additional capability of binding to the inverted repeat that contains –35 promoter element. The N-terminal part of Ml.LlaJI is predicted to contain an HTH motif. The M1.LlaJI binding to the inverted repeat results in suppression of gene transcription for the whole LlaJI operon. This mechanism seems to be unique since methylation usually decreases the binding efficiency of a repressor with its operator [74]. The complicated regulatory mechanism is likely to enable fine tuning of transcriptional level in LlaJI R–M system [74].

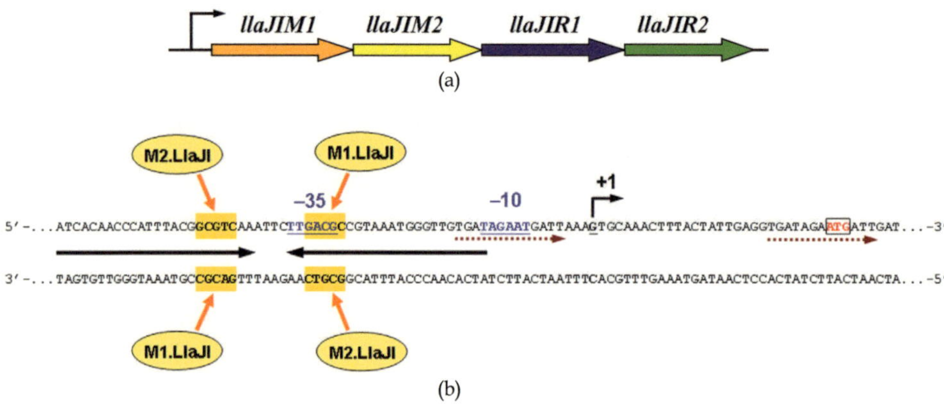


**Figure 5.** *a*) Genetic organization of the LlaJI R–M system. The thin arrow marks the transcription initiation point of the operon. (*b*) A fragment of the promoter region of the LlaJI R–M system. Two black arrows indicate the 24 bp inverted repeat. The methylation sites are highlighted with yellow. The transcription start point is marked by "+1", the promoter –10 and –35 elements are in blue. The start codon is in red.

Transcription regulation has been studied most thoroughly in the R–M systems SsoII from *Shigella sonnei* 47 and Ecl18kI from *Enterobacter cloacea* 18k. The nucleotide sequences of these systems share 99% identity. The sequences of the intergenic regions are completely identical while the proteins differ in 1 amino acid residue. We will refer to such R–M systems as to SsoII-like ones. The genes of the SsoII R–M system are located divergently and spaced by an intergenic region of 109 bp (Figure 6). To investigate the regulation mechanism of the system, two plasmids have been constructed, with both possible combinations of the intergenic region and a *lacZ* gene which encodes β-galactosidase. Thus, the expression of the *lacZ* gene is under control of a promoter of the *ssoIIM* gene (pACYC-SsoIIM) or the *ssoIIR* gene (pACYC-SsoIIR). The β-galactosidase expression level is found to be 540 times higher in the cells containing the pACYC-SsoIIM plasmid in comparison to the other plasmid. Therefore, the expression from the *ssoIIM* promoter is much higher than from the *ssoIIR* promoter. When transformed with an additional plasmid where the *ssoIIM* gene is under its own promoter, the cells containing pACYC-SsoIIM demonstrate a 20-fold decrease of the β-galactosidase expression while the cells containing pACYC-SsoIIR display an 8-fold increase of it [75]. Thus, M.SsoII is shown to downregulate the expression of its own gene and to stimulate the expression of the cognate RE gene. The transformation of the cells with a plasmid encoding a mutant M.SsoII without its first 72 residues does not influence the β-galactosidase expression level. The same effect is observed after the transformation with a plasmid encoding M.NlaX – a protein homologous to the M.SsoII domain responsible for methylation. On the contrary, a plasmid encoding a fusion of the M.SsoII first 72 residues with the full-length M.NlaX gives the same effect as the plasmid encoding the full-length M.SsoII [75]. These experiments demonstrate that the M.SsoII ability to regulate transcription in the SsoII R–M system is determined by its N-terminal part (72 residues). This part is predicted to contain an HTH motif.

M.SsoII is a typical C5-DNA MTase which modifies the second cytosine in the sequence 5′-CCNGG-3′/3′-GGNCC-5′. Moreover, M.SsoII interacts with the intergenic region of the SsoII R–M system protecting from DNase I hydrolysis 48 nucleotides in the top strand and 52 nucleotides in the bottom strand [75]. The intergenic region contains a 15 bp inverted repeat (regulatory site) [76]. Seven guanine bases interacting with M.SsoII are identified using protection footprinting; six of them are located inside the regulatory site symmetrically relative to the central A•T pair (Figure 7) [76]. Interference footprinting experiments with formic acid, hydrazine, dimethyl sulfate, and *N*-ethyl-*N*-nitrosourea show 6 guanine, 2 adenine, and 4 thymine residues as well as 6 phosphate groups interacting with M.SsoII. These nucleotides form two symmetrically located clusters: 5'-GGA-3' and 5'-TGT-3' in each DNA strand of the regulatory site (Figure 7) [77]. Such a symmetrical interaction with the both halves of the palindromic site is typical for many regulatory proteins which bind to the operator sequence in a dimeric form and contain an $\alpha$-helix that interacts with the DNA major groove recognizing the specific sequence. M.SsoII as a transcription factor is supposed to have the same mechanism of functioning.

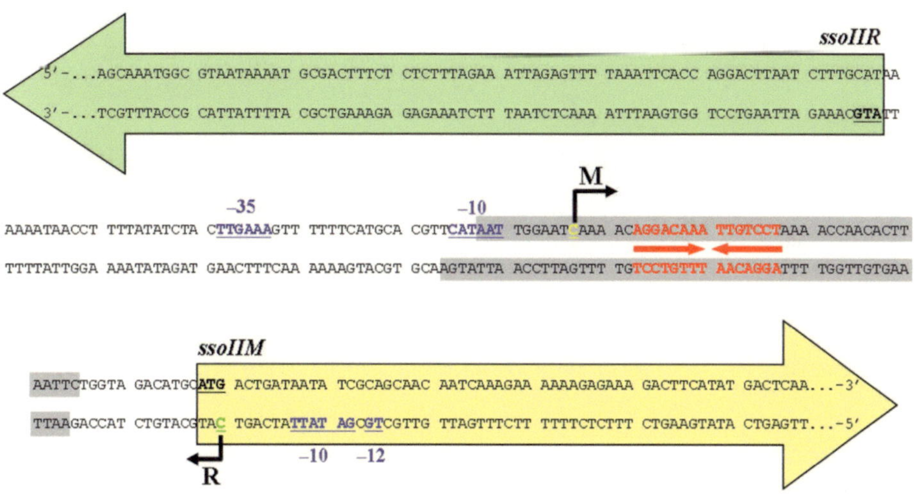


**Figure 6.** Genetic organization of the SsoII R–M system. The RE and MTase genes are depicted with green and yellow arrows respectively. The initiation codons are underlined. The region protected by M.SsoII from DNase I hydrolysis is highlighted with grey. The regulatory site is in red. The transcription initiation points of the RE and MTase genes are marked by black arrows, their promoter elements are in blue.

Arg35 or Arg38 substitution with Ala in M.Ecl18kI significantly impairs the protein binding to the regulatory site [79]. According to the computer simulation performed for M.SsoII, these residues belong to the second recognizing helix of the HTH motif [78]. Arg38 is supposed to form contacts with guanine bases of 5'-GGA-3' trinucleotide in one DNA strand while Arg35 can interact with thymine bases and DNA backbone of 5'-TGT-3' trinucleotide in the other strand (Figure 7). Amino acid substitutions in the M.Ecl18kI N-terminal part influence the ability of this protein to regulate transcription in the R–M system. However, there is no correlation between M.Ecl18kI affinity to the regulatory site and the amounts of the RNA transcripts [80]. Amino acid substitutions in the M.Ecl18kI N-terminal part increase the methylation activity of this enzyme in most of cases. There is also an inverse relationship: an M.SsoII point mutant which has Cys142 substituted with Ala is catalytically inactive but demonstrates an increased affinity to the regulatory site and effectively regulates transcription in the SsoII R–M system [79]. Thus, the interconnection between the two DNA binding sites is experimentally demonstrated for the SsoII-like DNA MTases. Moreover, it has been shown recently that M.SsoII binding to the regulatory site prevents its interaction with the methylation site. Thus, the two functions of the protein are mutually exclusive [67, 81].

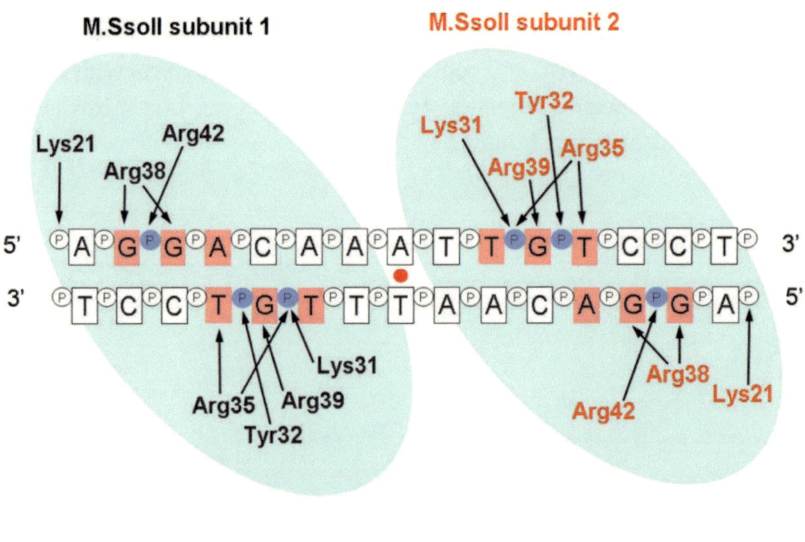


**Figure 7.** Scheme of the contacts formed between the two N-terminal domains of M.SsoII and the regulatory DNA site. The heterocyclic bases and the phosphate groups interacting with M.SsoII identified by footprinting are marked by red and blue respectively.

The transcription start point of the RE gene is located in the beginning of the MTase gene in the SsoII and Ecl18kI R–M systems (Figure 6) [67]. The transcription start point of the MTase gene is located inside the region protected by M.SsoII from DNase I hydrolysis, 5 bp away from the regulatory site. The suppression of the MTase gene transcription is based on the competitive binding of the MTase and RNA polymerase with the intergenic region of the SsoII (or Ecl18kI) R–M system. The MTase interaction with the regulatory site does not inter-

http://dx.doi.org/10.5772/52046

fere with RNA polymerase binding to the RE gene promoter. Thus, the RE gene is activated indirectly *via* averting of RNA polymerase binding with the MTase gene promoter [80].

# 5. Domains of eukaryotic DNA methyltransferases

All known eukaryotic DNA MTases methylate C5 atom of cytosine. Eukaryotic MTases are usually multidomain proteins (Figure 8).

## 5.1. Functional domains of mammalian Dnmt1

Murine and human Dnmt1 consist of 1620 and 1616 amino acid residues respectively. The primary structures of these proteins share 85% identity. Dnmt1 molecule contains the following domains and functionally important regions (listed starting from the N-end, Figure 8):

1. charge-rich domain or DMAP1-binding domain (DMAP1 is DNA methyltransferase associated protein, a transcription repressor);
2. PCNA-binding domain, PBD;
3. at least three functionally independent nuclear localization signals, NLS [82];
4. RFTS domain (replication foci targeting sequence), also called TS (targeting sequence), RFD (replication foci domain) or TRF (targeting to replication foci) domain;
5. cysteine-rich $Zn^{2+}$-binding domain, also called CXXC domain;
6. BAH1 and BAH2 (bromo-adjacent homology or bromo-associated homology) domains which are parts of the so-called PBHD domain (polybromo homology domain);
7. KG linker (consists of Lys and Gly residues) which connects N- and C-terminal parts of Dnmt1;
8. C-terminal catalytic domain.

The N-terminal part of Dnmt1 contains several domains that regulate the activity of the catalytic domain. Such a structural organization supposes that the Dnmt1 gene has arisen as fusion of a MTase gene with nonhomologous genes of other DNA-binding proteins [11, 83].

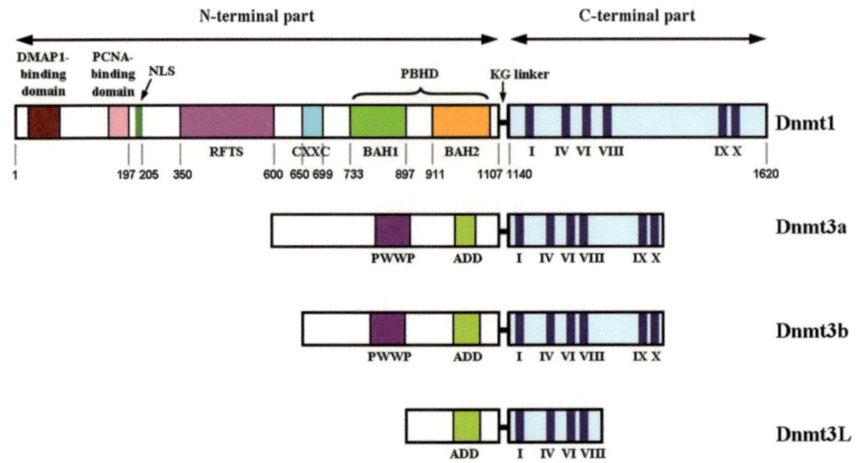


**Figure 8.** Domain architecture of mammalian C5-DNA MTases. The C-terminal domains are marked by a light blue filling. The other domains are signed. Roman numerals indicate the conservative motifs characteristic for C5-DNA MTases in the C-terminal domains. The borders of the Dnmt1 domains are shown according to [9].

Structures of two Dnmt1 complexes with DNA have been determined recently by X-ray crystallography: a fragment of murine Dnmt1 (residues 650–1602) with AdoHcy and a 19 bp DNA duplex containing two unmethylated 5′-CG-3′/3′-GC-5′ sites (PDB code: 3pt6) and a fragment of human Dnmt1 (residues 646–1600) with AdoHcy and the same duplex (PDB code: 3pta) [9]. The catalytic domain of Dnmt1 forms a core of the complex and makes contacts with the DNA on one side and with both BAH domains on the other side (Figure 9). AdoHcy molecule is located in the active center of the catalytic domain. The CXXC and BAH1 domains are located on different sides of the catalytic domain and are connected by a long CXXC–BAH1 linker. The BAH1 and BAH2 domains are located distantly from the bound DNA and are separated from each other by an $\alpha$-helical linker. The KG linker is disordered in the crystal. Different Dnmt1 domains are discussed further in this chapter.

It is worth to note that Dnmt1 targeting to replication foci is provided by three types of domains located in its N-terminal part: the PCNA binding domain, the RFTS domain, and the BAH domains [84-86]. Studying of Dnmt1 deletion mutants revealed 3 different DNA binding regions: the residues 1–343, the CXXC domain (residues 613–748), and the catalytic domain (residues 1124–1620) [13]. The catalytic domain binds preferentially monomethylated 5′-CG-3′/3′-GC-5′ sites while the fragment of residues 1–343 binds these sites independently of their methylation status [13]. The CXXC domain is shown to bind primarily dimethylated sites [13]. However, in the crystal structure the CXXC domain interacts with an unmethylated substrate [9].

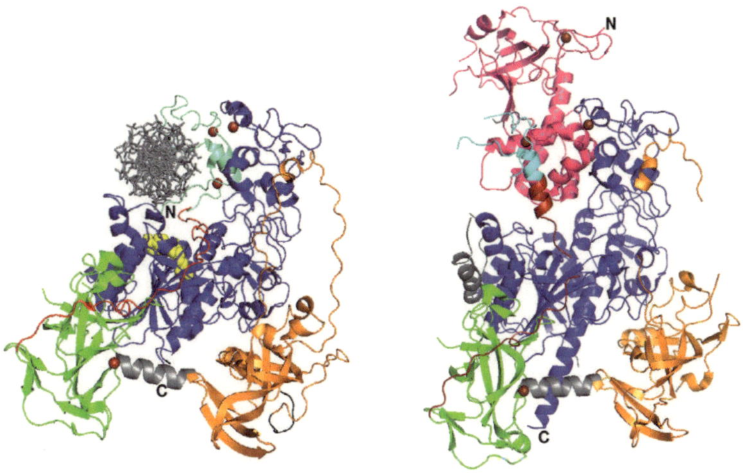


(a) (b)

**Figure 9.** Spatial structure of murine Dnmt1. (*a*) Dnmt1(650–1602) complexed with AdoHcy and a 19 bp DNA duplex containing two unmethylated 5′-CG-3′/3′-GC-5′ sites (PDB code: 3pt6). (*b*) Dnmt1(291–1620) in apo-form (PDB code: 3av4). The RFTS, CXXC, BAH1, BAH2, and MTase domains are colored in magenta, cyan, green, orange, and blue, respectively. $Zn^{2+}$ ions are in red and AdoHcy is in yellow, both in space-filling representation. DNA is in grey, in sticks representation. The autoinhibitory linker CXXC–BAH1 is colored in red. The borders of the domains are shown according to [9].

### *5.1.1. DMAP1-binding domain*

The first 120 residues of Dnmt1 can bind the transcription repressor DMAP1. This interaction provides DMAP1 presence in replication foci during the whole S phase of cell cycle. Moreover, Dnmt1 interacts directly with histone deacetylase 2 (HDAC2) during late S phase. Dnmt1, HDAC2, and DMAP1 form a complex *in vivo*. Since the direct interaction between HDAC2 and DMAP1 has not been demonstrated, Dnmt1 is likely to serve as a basis for this complex formation [88].

A special form of Dnmt1, Dnmt1o, is synthesized in oocytes. It lacks the first 118 residues that compose the DMAP1-binding domain. Dnmt1o is accumulated in oocyte cytoplasm and is transferred into nuclei of the 8-cell stage embryo where it is likely to be responsible for maintaining the methylation patterns of imprinted genes [82]. Dnmt1o is replaced by the regular Dnmt1 after implantation of the blastocyst. Homozygous mutant mice containing Dnmt1o in all somatic cells show a normal phenotype and have a normal level of genome methylation. This fact confirms the ability of Dnmt1o to perform all Dnmt1 functions. However, the Dnmt1o amounts and the corresponding enzymatic activity are much higher than the ones of Dnmt1. In heterozygous embryonic stem cells, the expression levels of Dnmt1o and Dnmt1 are the same. Though, in adult mice the Dnmt1o amount is 5 times higher than the Dnmt1 amount. So Dnmt1o seems to be more stable than Dnmt1 [89]. The DMAP1-binding domain is likely to decrease Dnmt1 stability *in vivo* and thus could be involved in Dnmt1 degradation.

*5.1.2. PCNA-binding domain*

The Dnmt1 residues 163–174 are responsible for binding of PCNA (proliferating cell nuclear antigen, also known as processivity factor for DNA polymerase δ). Dnmt1 relocates to DNA replication foci when the cell enters S phase [84, 90]. Its binding with PCNA is observed in the regions of newly synthesized DNA in intact cells. This binding does not influence the MTase activity of Dnmt1 [85].

In mammalian cells, newly replicated DNA is rapidly packaged into nucleosomes to which histone H1 is added further [91, 92]. Histone H1 has a high affinity to methylated DNA regardless its nucleotide sequence [93] and can suppress the Dnmt1 enzymatic activity [94]. Therefore, the maintenance methylation should be performed before DNA is packaged in nucleosomes. Dnmt1 binding with PCNA probably underlies a special mechanism required for coordination of these processes in a cell [85].

*5.1.3. RFTS domain*

Besides the presence in DNA replication foci during S phase (provided by the PCNA-binding domain) [84, 90], Dnmt1 is also associated with chromatin (mainly heterochromatin) from late S phase until early G1 phase [95]. This association is provided by the RFTS domain (replication foci targeting sequence) and does not depend on the methylation patterns specific for heterochromatin or on the histone binding proteins. Moreover, the association with chromatin does not depend on DNA replication, since it takes place in G2 phase and M phase *de novo* [95].

The RFTS domain inhibits the Dnmt1 binding with both free DNA and nucleosomal DNA. It functions as an intrinsic competitive inhibitor of Dnmt1 and can decrease its enzymatic activity up to 600 times [96]. The RFTS domain also inhibits the CXXC domain binding with nucleosomal DNA. The inhibition is observed for the isolated RFTS and CXXC domains as well as for the two domains in a single polypeptide chain. However, a deletion mutant containing both the CXXC domain and the catalytic domain is able to bind polynucleosomes in the presence of the isolated RFTS domain. Thus, the simultaneous presence of the two DNA binding domains seems to make the complex relatively resistant to exclusion of DNA by the RFTS domain [96].

The RFTS domain contains a $Zn^{2+}$-binding motif followed by a β-barrel and an $\alpha$-helical bundle (Figure 10). Hydrophobic interactions of the RFTS domains provide Dnmt1 dimerization, although its functional importance is still unknown [97]. In murine Dnmt1(291–1620), the negatively charged RFTS domain penetrates deeply into the positively charged DNA-binding center of the catalytic domain and forms several hydrogen bonds inside it. Such a structural organization could explain the mechanism of DNA displacement from the catalytic center by means of competition with the RFTS domain [87].

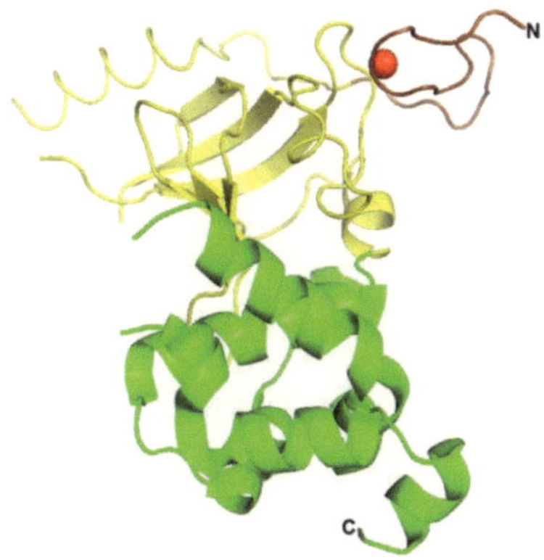


**Figure 10.** Spatial structure of the RFTS domain from human Dnmt1 (PDB code: 3epz). β-Barrel is colored in yellow, $Zn^{2+}$-binding motif – in brown, α-helical bundle – in green. $Zn^{2+}$ ion is shown as a red sphere.

*5.1.4. CXXC domain*

The cysteine-rich $Zn^{2+}$-binding domain contains several cysteine residues organized in CXXC motifs which provide a name to the domain. The CXXC domain of Dnmt1 is similar to cysteine-rich domains of other chromatin-associated proteins such as the MeCP2 protein, the CG binding protein (CGBP), the histone MTase MLL, and the histone demethylases JHDM1A and JHDM1B. This domain is shown to bind unmethylated 5′-CG-3′/3′-GC-5′ sites *in vitro* in the case of MBD1, MLL, CGBP, JHDM1B, and Dnmt1 proteins [3]. The CXXC domain of Dnmt1 is crescent-shaped and contains 8 conservative catalytically important Cys residues [98]. These residues are clustered in two groups and bind two $Zn^{2+}$ ions. In the structure of murine Dnmt1(650–1602) complexed with AdoHcy and 19 bp DNA (PDB code: 3pt6), all the specific contacts with DNA are formed by the CXXC domain which interacts with both major and minor grooves [9]. A loop region of the CXXC domain (Arg684-Ser685-Lys686-Gln687) penetrates into the major groove and forms contacts with heterocyclic bases and phosphate groups. The guanine bases of the 5′-CG-3′ dinucleotide are recognized by the side chains of Lys686 and Gln687, whereas the cytosine bases are recognized by the backbone interactions of Ser685 and Lys686. Salt bridges are formed between the Arg side chains and the DNA backbone.

The CXXC domain is known to bind specifically unmethylated 5′-CG-3′/3′-GC-5′ sites [98, 99]. The structural data confirm this type of specificity: a methyl group presence at the cytosine C5 atom would result in steric clashes between the DNA and the protein atoms [9]. The CXXC domain seems to bind newly synthesized unmethylated sites after DNA replication which would protect them from *de novo* methylation.

As mentioned above, Dnmt1 is a maintenance MTase that modifies mainly monomethylated sites. A deletion of the CXXC domain and the part of the CXXC–BAH1 linker results in a 7 times decrease of the Dnmt1 affinity to monomethylated DNA relatively to unmethylated one. The same effect is observed after a substitution of two residues (K686A/Q687A) in the CXXC domain that form contacts with the guanine bases in the recognition site [9].

Addition of dimethylated DNA stimulates murine Dnmt1 to methylate unmodified sites. Such an allosteric activation of Dnmt1 results in lowering its specificity [13, 29, 34, 100]. This effect depends on the presence of $Zn^{2+}$ ions and seems to be provided by the binding of the Dnmt1 residues 613–748 with dimethylated DNA [13]. This Dnmt1 region includes the CXXC domain. However, it remains unclear how the CXXC domain could bind dimethylated DNA.

### *5.1.5. BAH domains*

The BAH1 and BAH2 domains (bromo-adjacent homology) are the parts of the so-called PBHD domain (polybromo homology domain). This domain is present in some transcription regulators and is supposed to participate in protein–protein interactions that lead to gene repression. The BAH1 and BAH2 domains in Dnmt1 molecule are connected by an $\alpha$-helix and are arranged in a dumbbell shape (Figure 11). Three Cys and one His residues coordinate a $Zn^{2+}$ ion that keeps the BAH1 domain near the linker $\alpha$-helix. Despite low similarity of the primary structures, the both BAH domains have the same fold (Figure 11): the N-terminal subdomain consists of three antiparallel β-strands, the following subdomain consists of five antiparallel β-strands. Some smaller β-strands and loops which are located further are not homologous in different BAH domains.

Both BAH domains are physically associated with the MTase domain. Seven β-strands of the catalytic subdomain and two β-strands of the BAH1 domain form a common β-sheet. The BAH2 domain has a long loop (BAH2–TRD loop) which interacts with the TRD region of the MTase domain (Figure 11). Perhaps, this interaction prevents the TRD binding to DNA in the complex of murine Dnmt1(650–1602) with AdoHcy and 19 bp DNA duplex (PDB code: 3pt6) (Figure 9). The BAH1 and BAH2 domains have large solvent-accessible surfaces and thus could serve as platforms for interaction with other proteins.

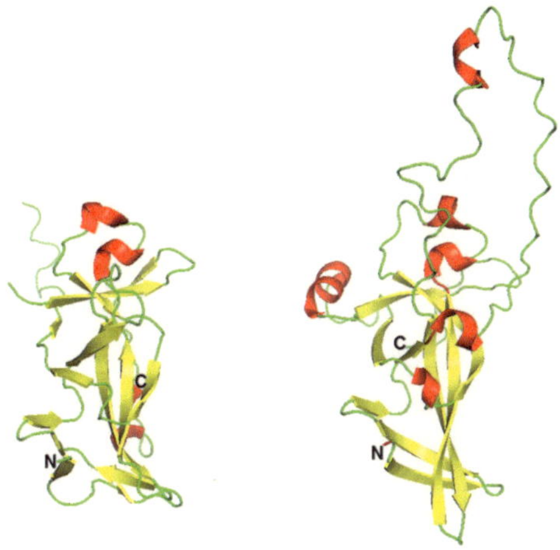


**Figure 11.** *a*) BAH1 and (*b*) BAH2 domains of murine Dnmt1 (PDB code: 3pt6) colored according to their secondary structure. α-Helices are in red, β-strands are in yellow.

The structure of Dnmt1(650–1602) complex with 19 bp DNA duplex and AdoHcy (PDB-код 3pt6) suggests an autoinhibition mechanism of Dnmt1: the CXXC domain binding with DNA results in DNA removal from the active center. The negatively charged CXXC–BAH1 linker is located between the DNA and the active center and thus prevents DNA entrance into the catalytic pocket (Figure 12). In addition, the BAH2–TRD loop fixes the TRD apart from DNA preventing its interaction with the major groove [9].

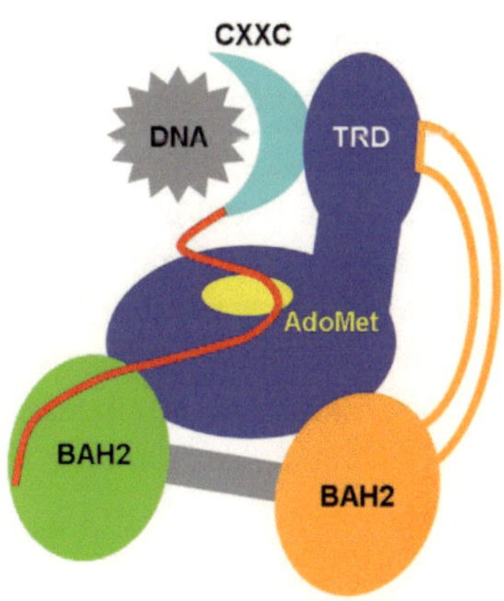


**Figure 12.** A model of the Dnmt1 autoinhibition mechanism in maintenance DNA methylation. The domains are colored as in Figure 9. The CXXC domain and the autoinhibitory linker (in red) close the active center of the enzyme. Additionally, the BAH2–TRD loop (in orange) keeps the TRD away from the DNA.

*5.1.6. KG linker*

The peptides containing the $(LysX)_nLys$ sequences (where X = Gly, Ala or Lys) can effectively bind to Z-DNA and stabilize it even at low NaCl concentrations (10–150 mM) and physiological pH. Such peptides can also induce B-DNA transition into Z-DNA. The efficacy of this process grows as the number of repeats ($n$) increases [101, 102]. The sequences $(LysX)_nLys$ are found in different proteins of plants, animals and unicellular eukaryotes. For example, they are present in the linkers which connect N- and C-terminal parts in eukaryotic MTases [102-104]. The number of repeats ($n$) varies from 5 to 7 in this case. The sequences of the linker and the preceding protein region are highly conservative. Thus, the linker is supposed to have an important but still unknown function.

The most effective DNA transition into Z-form is observed for the sequences with alternating purine and pyrimidine nucleosides, including $5'$-$(CG)_n$-$3'$ and especially when the cytosine residues are methylated at the C5 atoms. Additionally, the transition into Z-form is stimulated by high ionic strength in solution and by DNA negative supercoiling [105]. The KG linker probably promotes Dnmt1 binding to 5′-CG-3′ islands in Z-form. However, Dnmt1 is not able to methylate Z-DNA [106]. Perhaps, the KG linker participates in Dnmt1 targeting to the regions located behind a replication fork (due to their negative supercoiling when DNA polymerase has just passed) [3].

### 5.2. Functional domains of mammalian Dnmt3 family

Dnmt3 family includes C5-DNA MTases Dnmt3a and Dnmt3b, which are considered *de novo* MTases, and Dnmt3L – a catalytically inactive protein. There are also different isoforms of the proteins in the Dnmt3 family. Dnmt3a and Dnmt3b are expressed in embryonic cells and during gametogenesis [107]. Knockout of the corresponding genes suppresses *de novo* methylation. Mouse embryos where the Dnmt3b gene is knocked out die *in utero* while mouse embryos lacking Dnmt3a gene die soon after birth [108]. Dnmt3b methylates microsatellite repeats. In humans, Dnmt3b point mutations decreasing its enzymatic activity lead to a severe disease – ICF syndrome (immunodeficiency, centromere instability, facial abnormalities syndrome) [108-110].

Like Dnmt1, the Dnmt3 family enzymes consist of the N-terminal regulatory part and the C-terminal part containing the conservative motifs typical for C5-DNA MTases (Figure 8). The catalytic domains of Dnmt1 and Dnmt3 enzymes are homologous while the N-terminal parts share no similarity. Thus, these families seem to have been evolved from different prokaryotic predecessors [111, 112]. The intramolecular interactions between the N-terminal and the C-terminal parts are absent in Dnmt3a and Dnmt3b, in contrast to Dnmt1 [12].

The N-terminal parts of Dnmt3a and Dnmt3b contain two domains:

1. cysteine-rich domain ADD (ATRX–Dnmt3–Dnmt3L), also called PHD domain (plant homeodomain);

2. PWWP domain.

There is no PWWP domain in Dnmt3L. Moreover, Dnmt3L lacks some catalytic residues and the MTase motifs IX and X in the C-terminal domain. Dnmt3L functions as a stimulator of Dnmt3a and Dnmt3b enzymatic activity. Dnmt3L knockout mice are viable but the males are sterile while the females do not produce viable offspring [113-116].

### *5.2.1. PWWP domain*

Dnmt3a and Dnmt3b contain a PWWP domain as well as some other chromatin-associated proteins. The PWWP domain is named after a conserved ProTrpTrpPro motif, though the first Pro is substituted with Ser in Dnmt3a and Dnmt3b. The second part of the motif is always the same, TrpPro [117]. PWWP domain along with chromo domain, Tudor and MBT domains belongs to the Tudor domain "Royal family" [118, 119]. The members of this family are shown to bind modified lysine residues of histones [119]. The PWWP domain consists of 100–130 amino acid residues. Its structure includes 3 motifs: a β-barrel core, an insertion between the second and the third β-strands, and a C-terminal α-helical bundle (Figure 13). Three aromatic residues form a cleft in the center of the β-barrel that is a distinctive feature of the "Royal family". The insertion motif varies in length and secondary structure among the different PWWP domains. The C-terminal α-helical bundle can contain from 1 to 5 α-helices [120].

The PWWP domain of Dnmt3b has a positively charged surface with an approximate area of 45 × 32 Å$^2$ and can bind DNA nonspecifically [117, 121]. The PWWP domain binds 30 bp duplexes with unmethylated, mono-, and dimethylated 5′-CG-3′/3′-GC-5′ sites. However, it can also bind a nonspecific duplex of the same length with the same efficiency [117]. Deletion of the PWWP domain does not influence the Dnmt3b methylation efficiency *in vitro* [117]. On the contrary, the PWWP domain of Dnmt3a is almost unable to bind DNA [121].

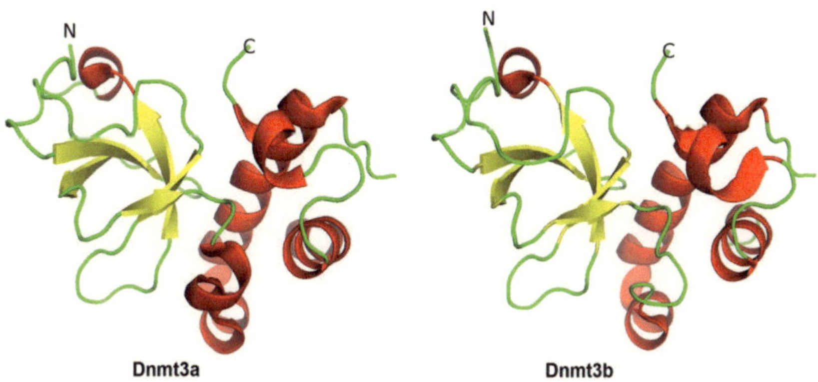


**Figure 13.** Spatial structures of the PWWP domains from human Dnmt3a (PDB code: 3llr) and Dnmt3b colored according to their secondary structure (PDB code: 3qkj). α-Helices are in red, β-strands are in yellow.

The PWWP domains of Dnmt3a and Dnmt3b are necessary for targeting these MTases to pericentromeric heterochromatin [121-123]. Deletions in the PWWP domain change the protein distribution in a nucleus and therefore result in its disability to methylate satellite repeats. However, such mutants are catalytically active since they are able to methylate DNA in other regions [121]. In humans, S282P point mutation in the PWWP domain of Dnmt3b causes the ICF syndrome [124]. In this case, the disease is likely to be caused by the enzyme improper distribution in nuclei rather than by its insufficient catalytic activity.

The PWWP domain of Dnmt3a specifically binds trimethylated Lys36 of H3 histone (H3K36m3) that increases the Dnmt3a ability to methylate nucleosomal DNA [125]. Distribution of methylated sequences in a genome correlates with the presence of H3K36m3 [126, 127]. DNA methylation and H3K36m3 serve as marks for histone deacetylation and the following gene suppression [128]. There is no crystal structure of Dnmt3a or Dnmt3b PWWP domain in complex with a histone protein or a peptide. The resolved spatial structures have a cleft that is supposed to bind methylated lysine residues. This cleft in the crystal contains a molecule of Bis-tris buffer (bis(2-hydroxyethyl)amino-tris(hydroxymethyl)methane) that is situated similar to the lysine in complexes of other PWWP domains with histone peptides containing di- or trimethylated lysine residues [120].

### 5.2.2. ADD domain

ADD domain is found only in the following proteins: ATRX (alpha thalassemia/mental retardation syndrome X-linked), Dnmt3a, Dnmt3b, and Dnmt3L. Thus, the domain is called ADD (ATRX–Dnmt3–Dnmt3L) [129]. To date, the crystal structures of ADD domain from Dnmt3a, Dnmt3L, and ATRX proteins are resolved. The structural organization of the domain remains the same in all the cases: it contains two C4-type zinc fingers [129-131]. One of them is similar to GATA binding protein 1 (GATA1) and the other one – to plant homeodomain (PHD).

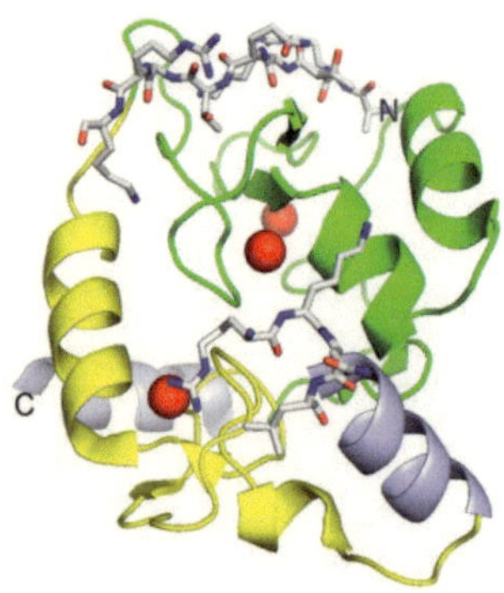


**Figure 14.** Structure of a fusion protein containing the ADD domain and a fragment of histone H3 (residues 1–9, shown in sticks representation), PDB-code: 3a1b. GATA1-like finger is in yellow, PHD finger is in green. $Zn^{2+}$ ions are shown as red spheres. The disordered linker peptide that connects the C-terminus of the histone H3 fragment and the N-terminus of ADD is not shown.

The ADD domain contains many cysteine residues which bind $Zn^{2+}$ providing thus the Dnmt3a interaction with many other proteins such as transcription factors PU.1, Myc, RP58, histone deacetylase HDAC1, heterochromatin protein HP1, histone MTases SUV39H1, SETDB1 and EZH2, methyl-CG-binding protein Mbd3, and chromatin remodeling factor Brg1 [3]. The functions of most of these interactions remain unclear. Additionally, the ADD domains of Dnmt3a, Dnmt3b, and Dnmt3L are shown to interact specifically with the N-terminal part of H3 histone when its Lys4 is not modified. This interaction stimulates Dnmt3a to methylate DNA [130-132]. Thus, the ADD domain of C5-DNA MTases can induce DNA methylation in response to specific histone modifications.

### 5.3. Domains of plant DNA methyltransferases

Plant DNA MTases are very diverse but are studied much less than the mammalian DNA MTases up to now [133]. In particular, none of the plant MTases has been crystallized.

DNA MTase Met1 from *Arabidopsis thaliana* is quite similar to mammalian Dnmt1 (Figure 15). The C-terminal domains of these enzymes which are responsible for methylation share 50% identity. Both proteins possess an extended N-terminal part that is connected with the C-terminal domain *via* KG linker. The N-terminal parts of Met1 and Dnmt1 share 24% identity [134]. There are four similar genes encoding Met1 in *A. thaliana* whereas only one gene encodes the mammalian Dnmt1. Genomes of *Daucus carota* and *Zea mays* contain two Met1 homologs. The N-terminal part of Met1 has two BAH domains. These domains seem to serve as a platform for protein–protein interactions which result in inhibition of gene expression thus providing an interconnection of DNA methylation, replication, and transcription regulation [135].

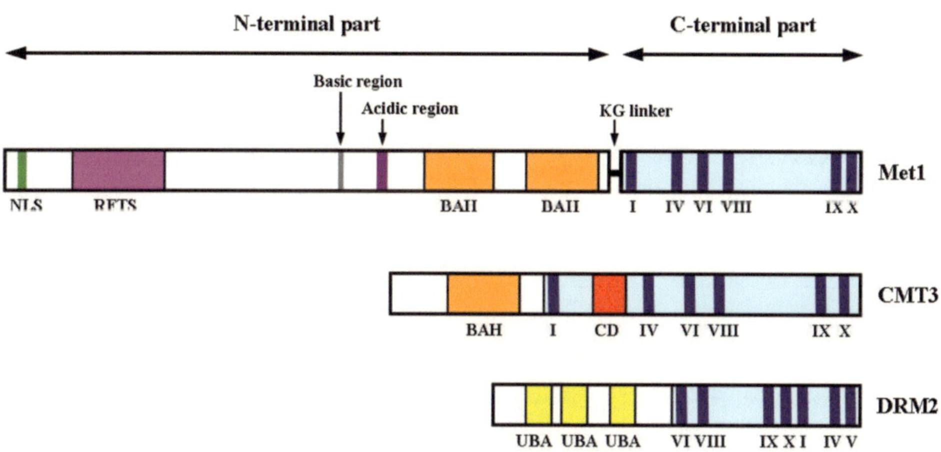


**Figure 15.** Domain architecture of different C5-DNA MTases from *A. thaliana*. Met1 – MTase similar to mammalian Dnmt1, CMT3 – chromomethyltransferase 3, DRM2 – MTase with the circular permutation of conservative motifs. The catalytic domains are marked by a light blue filling. The other domains are signed in the bottom. Roman numerals indicate the conservative motifs of C5-DNA MTases.

Dnmt3 family homologs are found in plants also. They form a DRM family (domains rearranged methyltransferase). The peculiarity of these enzymes is a circular permutation of their conservative motifs: the motifs VI–X are followed by the motifs I–V. The circular permutation of the conservative motifs is also found in some prokaryotic enzymes such as C5-DNA MTase BssHII [136]. Another characteristic of the DRM proteins is their ability to methylate 5′-CHG-3′ and 5′-CHH-3′ sites (H = A, C or T) *de novo* in an RNA-dependent manner. Such DNA methylation is supposed to take place in the presence of short RNAs that guide methylation of homologous DNA [4]. The DRM1 MTase from *Nicotiana tabacum* is shown to avoid cytosine methylation in 5′-CG-3′/3′-GC-5′ sites rather than specifically recognize any sequence. A structural basis of such an unusual functioning is not yet clarified [137].

Proteins of the DRM family are found only in flowering plants [4]. The C-terminal domains of DRM proteins share 28% identity with Dnmt3a or Dnmt3b and contain the same catalytic conservative motifs. Cysteine-rich regions of mammalian MTases (the RFTS, the CXXC, and the ADD domains) are found neither in proteins of DRM family nor in other plant homologs of C5-DNA MTases [112]. The N-terminal part of the DRM MTases contains several UBA domains (ubiquitin-associated). The presence of UBA domains seems to provide a link between DNA methylation and ubiquitin-mediated protein degradation. These domains could promote degradation of DRM molecules at specific points of the cell cycle [112]. The UBA domains are not found in any other families of DNA MTases. The UBA domains of DRM2 MTase in *A. thaliana* were experimentally shown to be required for normal RNA-directed DNA methylation. Perhaps, these domains are essential for proper localization of MTases in the cell [138].

C5-DNA MTases of chromomethylase (or chromomethyltransferase, CMT) family modify 5′-CNG-3′/3′-GNC-5′ sites (N = A, C, G or T) in plant genomes. These MTases contain chromo domains that were identified as conserved sequences between the II and the IV MTase motifs (Figure 15). The chromo domain (chromatin organization modifier) consists of 50 amino acid residues and contains three β-strands and a perpendicularly packed α-helix. This folding type belongs to OB class (oligonucleotide/oligosaccharide binding fold) and is considered to be evolutionary very old. The chromo domain is responsible for DNA binding [139]. This domain is originally found in polycomb-group proteins where it is important for the protein association with heterochromatin [140]. Therefore, CMT are thought to modify heterochromatin. The chromo domain is not found in other C5-DNA MTases. The *A. thaliana* genome contains 3 members of the CMT family: CMT1, CMT2, and CMT3. The members of this family are also found in genomes of *Oryza sativa* and *Brassica oleracea*. Function of CMT1 and CMT2 are still unknown while CMT3 seems to methylate 5′-CNG-3′/3′-GNC-5′ sites [4]. CMT3 deficiency in *A. thaliana* results in loss of DNA methylation in centromeric regions and also leads to retrotransposon activation [141, 142].

The enzymes from CMT family contain one BAH domain in its N-terminal region in contrast to the MTases from Met1 family that possess two BAH domains.

## 6. Conclusion

Precise time and space coordination of different molecular events underlies development of all living organisms, unicellular as well as multicellular. Synchronization of molecular processes can take place at a transcriptional level (when the same DNA-binding protein regulates expression of several genes) or at a post-translational level (when a multifunctional protein participates in different processes). Multifunctionality of a protein can be based on the presence of several domains in a single polypeptide chain. For example, mammalian Dnmt1, besides the catalytic domain which provides DNA methylation, contains several other domains responsible for Dnmt1 cellular localization, its interaction with other proteins, and regulation of its catalytic domain activity. Among prokaryotes, multidomain proteins are less common. Nevertheless, some bacterial DNA methyltransferases contain additional domains which are responsible for transcription regulation, topoisomerase activity *etc.*

As shown in this review, the structural and functional features of the additional domains in C5-DNA MTases are studied yet insufficiently. On the basis of the existing data, it is impossible to draw a decisive conclusion on the effect of the additional domains onto the methylating activity of C5-DNA MTases. Evidently, a complex research of multifunctional DNA MTases with multidomain organization would be most promising.

## Acknowledgements

The authors would like to thank Mrs. Anna Nazarenko for her technical assistance. The work was supported by the Russian Foundation for Basic Research (grants no. 10-04-01578 and 12-04-32103).

## Author details

A. Yu. Ryazanova[1], L. A. Abrosimova[2], T. S. Oretskaya[1,3] and E. A. Kubareva[3*]

*Address all correspondence to: kubareva@belozersky.msu.ru

1 Chemistry Department, Lomonosov Moscow State University, Moscow, Russia

2 Faculty of Bioengineering and Bioinformatics, Lomonosov Moscow State University, Moscow, Russia

3 Belozersky Institute of Physico-Chemical Biology, Lomonosov Moscow State University, Moscow, Russia

## References


[1] Jeltsch, A. (2002). Beyond Watson and Crick: DNA Methylation and Molecular Enzymology of DNA Methyltransferases. *A European Journal of Chemical Biology Chem Bio Chem*, 3(4), 274-293.

[2] Gromova, E. S., & Khoroshaev, A. V. (2003). Prokaryotic DNA Methyltransferases: the Structure and the Mechanism of Interaction with DNA. *Molekulyarnaya Biologiya*, 37(2), 300-314.

[3] Jurkowska, R. Z., Jurkowski, T. P., & Jeltsch, A. (2011). Structure and Function of Mammalian DNA Methyltransferases. *A European Journal of Chemical Biology ChemBioChem*, 12(2), 206-222.

[4] Goll, M. G., & Bestor, T. H. (2005). Eukariotic Cytosine Methyltransferases. *Annual Review of Biochemistry*, 74, 481-514.

[5] Svedruzic, Z. M. (2008). Mammalian Cytosine DNA Methyltransferase Dnmt1: Enzymatic Mechanism, Novel Mechanism-Based Inhibitors, and RNA-Directed DNA Methylation. *Current Medicinal Chemistry*, 15(1), 92-106.

[6] Jeltsch, A. (2006). Molecular Enzymology of Mammalian DNA Methyltransferases. *Current Topics in Microbiology and Immunology*, 301, 203-225.

[7] Cheng, X., & Roberts, R. J. (2001). AdoMet-Dependent Methylation, DNA Methyltransferases and Base Flipping. *Nucleic Acids Research*, 29(18), 3784-3795.

[8] Cheng, X., & Blumenthal, RM. (2008). Mammalian DNA Methyltransferases: a Structural Perspective. *Structure*, 16(3), 341-350.

[9] Song, J., Rechkoblit, O., Bestor, T. H., & Patel, D. J. (2011). Structure of DNMT1-DNA Complex Reveals a Role for Autoinhibition in Maintenance DNA Methylation. *Science*, 331(6020), 1036-1040.

[10] Zimmermann, C., Guhl, E., & Graessmann, A. (1997). Mouse DNA Methyltransferase (MTase) Deletion Mutants that Retain the Catalytic Domain Display Neither de Novo nor Maintenance Methylation Activity *in vivo*. *The Journal of Biological Chemistry*, 378(5), 393-405.

[11] Margot, J. B., Aguirre-Arteta, A. M., Di Giacco, B. V., Pradhan, S., Roberts, R. J., Cardoso, M. C., & Leonhardt, H. (2000). Structure and Function of the Mouse DNA Methyltransferase Gene: Dnmt1 Shows a Tripartite Structure. *Journal of Molecular Biology*, 297(2), 293-300.

[12] Margot, J. B., Ehrenhofer-Murray, A. E., & Leonhardt, H. (2003). Interactions within the Mammalian DNA Methyltransferase Family. *BMC Molecular Biology*, 4, 7.

[13] Fatemi, M., Hermann, A., Pradhan, S., & Jeltsch, A. (2001). The Activity of the Murine DNA Methyltransferase Dnmt1 Is Controlled by Interaction of the Catalytic Domain with the N-Terminal Part of the Enzyme Leading to an Allosteric Activation of the Enzyme after Binding to Methylated DNA. *Journal of Molecular Biology*, 309(5), 1189-1199.

[14] Wu, J. C., & Santi, D. V. (1987). Kinetic and Catalytic Mechanism of HhaI Methyltransferase. *Journal of Biological Chemistry*, 262(10), 4778-4786.

[15] Klimasauskas, S., Szyperski, T., Serva, S., & Wüthrich, K. (1998). Dynamic Modes of the Flipped-Out Cytosine During HhaI Methyltransferase-DNA Interactions in Solution. *The EMBO Journal*, 17(1), 317-324.

[16] Wang, P., Brank, A. S., Banavali, N. K., Nicklaus, M. C., Marquez, V. E., Christman, J. K., & MacKerell, A. D. (2000). Use of Oligodeoxyribonucleotides with Conformationally Constrained Abasic Sugar Targets to Probe the Mechanism of Base Flipping by HhaI DNA (Cytosine C5)-Methyltransferase. *Journal of the American Chemical Society*, 122(50), 12422-12434.

[17] Lindstrom, W. M. Jr., Flynn, J., & Reich, N. O. (2000). Reconciling Structure and Function in HhaI DNA Cytosine-C-5 Methyltransferase. *Journal of Biological Chemistry*, 275(7), 4912-4919.

[18] Vilkaitis, G., Merkiene, E., Serva, S., Weinhold, E., & Klimašauskas, S. (2001). The Mechanism of DNA Cytosine-5 Methylation. Kinetic and Mutational Dissection of HhaI Methyltransferase. *Journal of Biological Chemistry*, 276(24), 20924-20934.

[19] Svedruzic, Z. M., & Reich, N. O. (2004). The Mechanism of Target Base Attack in DNA Cytosine Carbon 5 Methylation. *Biochemistry*, 43(36), 11460-11473.

[20] Daujotyte, D., Serva, S., Vilkaitis, G., Merkiene, E., Venclovas, C., & Klimasauskas, S. (2004). HhaI DNA Methyltransferase Uses the Protruding Gln237 for Active Flipping of Its Target Cytosine. *Structure*, 12(6), 1047-1055.

[21] Horton, J. R., Ratner, G., Banavali, N. K., Huang, N., Choi, Y., Maier, M. A., Marquez, V. E., MacKerell, A. D., & Cheng, X. (2004). Caught in the Act: Visualization of an Intermediate in the DNA Base-Flipping Pathway Induced by HhaI Methyltransferase. *Nucleic Acids Research*, 32(13), 3877-3886.

[22] Merkiene, E., & Klimašauskas, S. (2005). Probing a Rate-Limiting Step by Mutational Perturbation of AdoMet Binding in the HhaI Methyltransferase. *Nucleic Acids Research*, 33(1), 307-315.

[23] Gerasimaitė, R., Merkienė, E., & Klimašauskas, S. (2011). Direct Observation of Cytosine Flipping and Covalent Catalysis in a DNA Methyltransferase. *Nucleic Acids Research*, 39(9), 3771-3780.

[24] Estabrook, R. A., Nguyen, T. T., Fera, N., & Reich, N. O. (2009). Coupling Sequence-Specific Recognition to DNA Modification. *Journal of Biological Chemistry*, 284(34), 22690-22696.

[25] Matje, D. M., Coughlin, D. F., Connolly, B. A., Dahlquist, F. W., & Reich, N. O. (2011). Determinants of Precatalytic Conformational Transitions in the DNA Cytosine Methyltransferase M.HhaI. *Biochemistry*, 50(9), 1465-1473.

[26] Renbaum, P., & Razin, A. (1992). Mode of Action of the Spiroplasma CpG Methylase M.SssI. *FEBS Letters*, 313(3), 243-247.

[27] Dryden, D. T. F. (1999). Bacterial DNA Methyltransferases. S-Adenosylmethionine-Dependent Methyltransferases: Structures and Functions. In: Cheng X., Blumenthal R.M. (ed.) Singapore: World Scientific Publishing, 283-340.

[28] O'Gara, M., Roberts, R. J., & Cheng, X. (1996). A Structural Basis for the Preferential Binding of Hemimethylated DNA by HhaI DNA Methyltransferase. *Journal of Molecular Biology*, 263(4), 597-606.

[29] Christman, J. K., Sheikhnejad, G., Marasco, C. J., & Sufrin, J. R. (1995). Methyl-2′-deoxycytidine in Single-stranded DNA Can Act in Cis to Signal de Novo DNA Methylation. *Proceedings of the National Academy of Science*, 92(16), 7347-7351.

[30] Tollefsbol, T. O., & Hutchison, C. A. 3rd. (1995). Mammalian DNA (Cytosine-5)-Methyltransferase Expressed in *Escherichia coli*, Purified and Characterized. *Journal of Biological Chemistry*, 270(31), 18543-18550.

[31] Tollefsbol, T. O., & Hutchison, C. A. 3rd. (1997). Control of Methylation Spreading in Synthetic DNA Sequences by the Murine DNA Methyltransferase. *Journal of Molecular Biology*, 269(4), 494-504.

[32] Flynn, J., Glickman, J. F., & Reich, N. O. (1996). Murine DNA Cytosine-C5 Methyltransferase: Pre-steady- and Steady-State Kinetic Analysis with Regulatory DNA Sequences. *Biochemistry*, 35(23), 7308-7315.

[33] Pradhan, S., Bacolla, A., Wells, R. D., & Roberts, R. J. (1999). Recombinant Human DNA (Cytosine-5) Methyltransferase. I. Expression, Purification, and Comparison of de Novo and Maintenance Methylation. *Journal of Biological Chemistry*, 274(46), 33002-33010.

[34] Fatemi, M., Hermann, A., Gowher, H., & Jeltsch, A. (2002). Dnmt3a and Dnmt1 Functionally Cooperate During de Novo Methylation of DNA. *European Journal of Biochemistry*, 269(20), 4981-4984.

[35] Hermann, A., Goyal, R., & Jeltsch, A. (2004). The Dnmt1 DNA-(Cytosine-C5)-Methyltransferase Methylates DNA Processively with High Preference for Hemimethylated Target Sites. *Journal of Biological Chemistry*, 279(46), 48350-48359.

[36] Goyal, R., Reinhardt, R., & Jeltsch, A. (2006). Accuracy of DNA Methylation Pattern Preservation by the Dnmt1 Methyltransferase. *Nucleic Acids Research*, 34(4), 1182-1188.

[37] Gowher, H., & Jeltsch, A. (2001). Enzymatic Properties of Recombinant Dnmt3a DNA Methyltransferase from Mouse: the Enzyme Modifies DNA in a Non-Processive Manner and Also Methylates non-CpG Sites. *Journal of Molecular Biology*, 309(5), 1201-1208.

[38] Handa, V., & Jeltsch, A. (2005). Profound Flanking Sequence Preference of Dnmt3a and Dnmt3b Mammalian DNA Methyltransferases Shape the Human Epigenome. *Journal of Molecular Biology*, 348(5), 1103-1112.

[39] Gowher, H., & Jeltsch, A. (2002). Molecular Enzymology of the Catalytic Domains of the Dnmt3a and Dnmt3b DNA Methyltransferases. *Journal of Biological Chemistry*, 277(23), 20409-20414.

[40] Reither, S., Li, F., Gowher, H., & Jeltsch, A. (2003). Catalytic Mechanism of DNA-(Cytosine-C5)-Methyltransferases Revisited: Covalent Intermediate Formation Is not Essential for Methyl Group Transfer by the Murine Dnmt3a Enzyme. *Journal of Molecular Biology*, 329(4), 675-684.

[41] Siddique, A. N., Jurkowska, R. Z., Jurkowski, T. P., & Jeltsch, A. (2011). Auto-Methylation of the Mouse DNA-(Cytosine C5)-Methyltransferase Dnmt3a at Its Active Site Cysteine Residue. *The FEBS Journal*, 278(12), 2055-2063.

[42] Jia, D., Jurkowska, R. Z., Zhang, X., Jeltsch, A., & Cheng, X. (2007). Structure of Dnmt3a Bound to Dnmt3L Suggests a Model for de Novo DNA Methylation. *Nature*, 449(7159), 248-251.

[43] Zhang, Y., Rohde, C., Tierling, S., Jurkowski, T. P., Bock, C., Santacruz, D., Ragozin, S., Reinhardt, R., Groth, M., Walter, J., & Jeltsch, A. (2009). DNA Methylation Analysis of Chromosome 21 Gene Promoters at Single Base Pair and Single Allele Resolution. *PLoS Genetics*, 5(3), e1000438.

[44] Bitinaite, J., Maneliene, Z., Menkevicius, S., Klimasauskas, S., Butkus, V., & Janulaitis, A. (1992). Alw26I, Eco31I and Esp3I- Type IIS Methyltransferases Modifying Cytosine and Adenine in Complementary Strands of the Target DNA. *Nucleic Acids Research*, 20(19), 4981-4985.

[45] Bitinaite, J., Mitkaite, G., Dauksaite, V., Jakubauskas, A., Timinskas, A., Vaisvila, R., Lubys, A., & Janulaitis, A. (2002). Evolutionary Relationship of Alw26I, Eco31I and Esp3I, Restriction Endonucleases that Recognise Overlapping Sequences. *Molecular Genetics and Genomics*, 267(5), 664-672.

[46] Kumar, R., & Rao, D. N. (2011). A Nucleotide Insertion Between Two Adjacent Methyltransferases in *Helicobacter pylori* Results in a Bifunctional DNA Methyltransferase. *Biochemical Journal*, 433(3), 487-495.

[47] Chan, S. H., Opitz, L., Higgins, L., O'Loane, D., & Xu, S. Y. (2010). Cofactor Requirement of HpyAV Restriction Endonuclease. *PLoS One*, 5(2), e9071.

[48] Shen, J. C., Rideout, W. M., & Jones, P. A. (1992). High Frequency Mutagenesis by a DNA Methyltransferase. *Cell*, 71(7), 1073-1080.

[49] Wyszynski, M., Gabbara, S., & Bhagwat, A. S. (1994). Cytosine Deamitations Catalysed by DNA Cytosine Methyltransferases Are Unlikely to Be the Major Cause of Mutational Hot-Spots at Sites of Cytosine Methylation in *E. coli*. *Proceedings of the National Academy of Science*, 91(4), 1574-1578.

[50] Bandaru, B., Wyszynski, M., & Bhagwat, A. S. (1995). HpaII Methyltransferase Is Mutagenic in *Escherichia coli*. *Journal of Bacteriology*, 177(10), 2950-2952.

[51] Yang, A. S., Shen, J. C., Zingg, J. M., Mi, S., & Jones, P. A. (1995). HhaI and HpaII DNA Methyltransferases Bind DNA Mismatches, Methylate Uracil and Block DNA Repair. *Nucleic Acids Research*, 23(8), 1380-1387.

[52] Yebra, M. J., & Bhagwat, A. S. (1995). A Cytosine Methyltransferase Converts 5-Methylcytosine in DNA to Thymine. *Biochemistry*, 34(45), 14752-14757.

[53] Zingg, J. M., Shen, J. C., Yang, A. S., Rapoport, H., & Jones, P. A. (1996). Methylation Inhibitors Can Increase the Rate of Cytosine Deamination by (Cytosine-5)-DNA Methyltransferase. *Nucleic Acids Research*, 24(16), 3267-3275.

[54] Bandaru, B., Gopal, J., & Bhagwat, A. S. (1996). Overproduction of DNA Cytosine Methyltransferase Causes Methylation and C-> T Mutations at non-Canonical Sites. *The Journal of Biological Chemistry*, 271(13), 7851-7859.

[55] Vorob'eva, O. V. (2004). (Cytosine-5)-DNA Methyltransferase SsoII as a Bifunctional Protein: Study of Its Interaction with the Methylation Site and with the Promoter Region of the Genes in the SsoII Restriction–Modification System. PhD thesis. Lomonosov Moscow State University.

[56] Shen, J. C., Zingg, J. M., Yang, A. S., Schmutte, C., & Jones, P. A. (1995). A Mutant HpaII Methyltransferase Functions as a Mutator Enzyme. *Nucleic Acids Research*, 23(21), 4275-4282.

[57] Zingg, J. M., Shen, J. C., & Jones, P. A. (1998). Enzyme-Mediated Cytosine Deamination by the Bacterial Methyltransferase M.MspI. *Biochemical Journal*, 332(1), 223-30.

[58] Selker, E. U. (1990). Premeiotic Instability of Repeated Sequences in *Neurospora crassa*. *Annual Review of Genetics*, 24, 579-613.

[59] Sharath, A. N., Weinhold, E., & Bhagwat, A. S. (2000). Reviving a Dead Enzyme: Cytosine Deaminations Promoted by an Inactive DNA Methyltransferase and an S-Adenosylmethionine Analogue. *Biochemistry*, 39(47), 14611-14616.

[60] Svedruzic, Z. M., & Reich, N. O. (2005). DNA Cytosine C5 Methyltransferase Dnmt1: Catalysis-Dependent Release of Allosteric Inhibition. *Biochemistry*, 44(27), 9472-9485.

[61] Renbaum, P., Abrahamove, D., Fainsod, A., Wilson, G. G., Rottem, S., & Razin, A. (1990). Cloning, Characterization, and Expression in *Escherichia coli* of the Gene Coding for the CpG DNA Methylase from *Spiroplasma sp.* Strain MQ1 (M.SssI). *Nucleic Acids Research*, 18(5), 1145-1152.

[62] Matsuo, K., Silke, J., Gramatikoff, K., & Schaffner, W. (1994). The CpG-Specific Methylase SssI Has Topoisomerase Activity in the Presence of $Mg^{2+}$. *Nucleic Acids Research*, 22(24), 5354-5359.

[63] Walder, R. Y., Langtimm, C. J., Catterjee, R., & Walder, J. A. (1983). Cloning of the MspI Modification Enzyme. *The Journal of Biological Chemistry*, 258(2), 1235-1241.

[64] Dubey, A. K., & Bhattacharya, S. K. (1997). Angle and Locus of the Bend Induced by the MspI DNA Methyltransferase in a Sequence-Specific Complex with DNA. *Nucleic Acids Research*, 25(10), 2025-2029.

[65] Bhattacharya, S. K., & Dubey, A. K. (2002). The N-Terminus of m5C-DNA Methyltransferase MspI Is Involved in Its Topoisomerase Activity. *European Journal of Biochemistry*, 269(10), 2491-2497.

[66] Nagornykh, M. O., Bogdanova, E. S., Protsenko, A. S., Zakharova, M. V., & Severinov, K. V. (2008). Regulation of Gene Expression in Type II Restriction-Modification Systems. *Genetika*, 44, 1-10.

[67] Protsenko, A., Zakharova, M., Nagornykh, M., Solonin, A., & Severinov, K. (2009). Transcription Regulation of Restriction-Modification System Ecl18kI. *Nucleic Acids Research*, 37(16), 5322-5330.

[68] Stankevicius, K., & Timinskas, A. (1996). Expression Autoregulation of the Eco47II Methyltransferase Gene. *Biologija*, 0, 54-56.

[69] Som, S., & Friedman, S. (1994). Regulation of EcoRII Methyltransferase: Effect of Mutations on Gene Expression and in Vitro Binding to the Promoter Region. *Nucleic Acids Research*, 22(24), 5347-5353.

[70] Som, S., & Friedman, S. (1993). Autogenous Regulation of the EcoRII Methylase Gene at the Trancriptional Level: Effect of 5-Azacytidine. *The EMBO Journal*, 12(11), 4297-4303.

[71] Som, S., & Friedman, S. (1997). Characterization of the Intergenic Region which Regulates the MspI Restriction-Modification System. *Journal of Bacteriology*, 179(3), 964-967.

[72] Butler, D., & Fitzgerald, G. F. (2001). Transcriptional Analysis and Regulation of Expression of the ScrFI Restriction-Modification System of *Lactococcus lactis subsp. cremoris* UC503. *Journal of Bacteriology*, 183(15), 4668-4673.

[73] O'Driscoll, J., Glynn, F., Cahalane, O., O'Connell-Motherway, M., Fitzgerald, G. F., & Van Sinderen, D. (2004). Lactococcal Plasmid pNP40 Encodes a Novel, Temperature-Sensitive Restriction-Modification System. *Applied and Environmental Microbiology*, 70(9), 5546-5556.

[74] O'Driscoll, J., Fitzgerald, G. F., & van Sinderen, D. (2005). A Dichotomous Epigenetic Mechanism Governs Expression of the LlaJI Restriction/Modification System. *Molecular Microbiology*, 57(6), 1532-1544.

[75] Karyagina, A., Shilov, I., Tashlitskii, V., Khodoun, M., Vasil'ev, S., Lau, P. C. K., & Nikolskaya, I. (1997). Specific Binding of SsoII DNA Methyltransferase to Its Promoter Region Provides the Regulation of SsoII Restriction-Modification Gene Expression. *Nucleic Acids Research*, 25(11), 2114-2120.

[76] Shilov, I., Tashlitsky, V., Khodoun, M., Vasil'ev, S., Alekseev, Y., Kuzubov, A., Kubareva, E., & Karyagina, A. (1998). DNA-methyltransferase SsoII Interaction with Own Promoter Region Binding Site. *Nucleic Acids Research*, 26(11), 2659-2664.

[77] Vorob'eva, O. V., Vasil'ev, S. A., Kariagina, A. S., Oretskaia, T. S., & Kubareva, E. A. (2000). Analysis of Contacts between DNA and Protein in a Complex of SsoII Methyltransferase-Promoter Region of the Gene for the SsoII Restriction-Modification System. *Molekulyarnaya Biologiya*, 34(6), 1074-1080.

[78] Karyagina, A. S., Alexeevski, A. V., Golovin, A. V., Spirin, S. A., Vorob'eva, O. V., & Kubareva, E. A. (2003). Computer Modeling of Complexes of (C5-Cytosine)-DNA Methyltransferase SsoII with Target and Regulatory DNAs. *Biophysics*, 48(1), S45-S55.

[79] Fedotova, E. A., Protsenko, A. S., Zakharova, M. V., Lavrova, N. V., Alekseevsky, A. V., Oretskaya, T. S., Karyagina, A. S., Solonin, A. S., & Kubareva, E. A. (2009). SsoII-like DNA-methyltransferase Ecl18kI: Interaction between Regulatory and Methylating Functions. *Biochemistry*, 74(1), 85-91.

[80] Fedotova, E. A. (2006). Peculiarities of Gene Expression Regulation in the SsoII Restriction–Modification System. PhD thesis. Lomonosov Moscow State University.

[81] Ryazanova, A. Yu. (2012). Structural and Functional Characterization of (Cytosine-5)-DNA Methyltransferase SsoII and Its Complexes with DNA Ligands. PhD thesis. Lomonosov Moscow State University.

[82] Cardoso, M. C., & Leonhardt, H. (1999). DNA Methyltransferase Is Actively Retained in the Cytoplasm During Early Development. *The Journal of Cell Biology*, 147(1), 25-32.

[83] Bestor, T. H. (1992). Activation of Mammalian DNA Methyltransferase by Cleavage of a Zn Binding Regulatory Domain. *The EMBO Journal*, 11(7), 2611-2617.

[84] Leonhardt, H., Page, A. W., Weier, H. U., & Bestor, T. H. (1992). A Targeting Sequence Directs DNA Methyltransferase to Sites of DNA Replication in Mammalian Nuclei. *Cell*, 71(5), 865-873.

[85] Chuang, L. S., Ian, H. I., Koh, T. W., Ng, H. H., Xu, G., & Li, B. F. (1997). Human DNA-(Cytosine-5) Methyltransferase-PCNA Complex as a Target for p21WAF1. *Science*, 277(5334), 1996-2000.

[86] Liu, Y., Oakeley, E. J., Sun, L., & Jost, J. P. (1998). Multiple Domains Are Involved in the Targeting of the Mouse DNA Methyltransferase to the DNA Replication Foci. *Nucleic Acids Research*, 26(4), 1038-1045.

[87] Takeshita, K., Suetake, I., Yamashita, E., Suga, M., Narita, H., Nakagawa, A., & Tajima, S. (2011). Structural Insight into Maintenance Methylation by Mouse DNA Methyltransferase 1 (Dnmt1). *Proceedings of the National Academy of Science*, 108(22), 9055-9059.

[88] Rountree, M. R., Bachman, K. E., & Baylin, S. B. (2000). Dnmt1 binds HDAC2 and a New Co-Repressor, DMAP1, to Form a Complex at Replication Foci. *Nature Genetics*, 25(3), 269-277.

[89] Ding, F., & Chaillet, J. R. (2002). In Vivo Stabilization of the Dnmt1 (Cytosine-5)-Methyltransferase Protein. *Proceedings of the National Academy of Science*, 99(23), 14861-14866.

[90] Margot, J. B., Cardoso, M. C., & Leonhardt, H. (2001). Mammalian DNA Methyltransferases Show Different Subnuclear Distributions. *Journal of Cellular Biochemistry*, 83(3), 373-379.

[91] Krude, T. (1995). Chromatin. Nucleosome Assembly During DNA Replication. *Current Biology*, 5(11), 1232-1234.

[92] Gasser, R., Koller, T., & Sogo, J. M. (1996). The Stability of Nucleosomes at the Replication Fork. *Journal of Molecular Biology*, 258(2), 224-239.

[93] McArthur, M., & Thomas, J. O. (1996). A Preference of Histone H1 for Methylated DNA. *The EMBO Journal*, 15(7), 1705-1714.

[94] Carotti, D., Funiciello, S., Lavia, P., Caiafa, P., & Strom, R. (1996). Different Effects of Histone H1 on de Novo DNA Methylation in Vitro Depend on Both the DNA Base Composition and the DNA Methyltransferase. *Biochemistry*, 5(36), 11660-11667.

[95] Easwaran, H. P., Schermelleh, L., Leonhardt, H., & Cardoso, M. C. (2004). Replication-Independent Chromatin Loading of Dnmt1 During G2 and M Phases. *EMBO Reports*, 5(12), 1181-1186.

[96] Syeda, F., Fagan, R. L., Wean, M., Avvakumov, G. V., Walker, J. R., Xue, S., Dhe-Paganon, S., & Brenner, C. (2011). The Replication Focus Targeting Sequence (RFTS) Domain Is a DNA-competitive Inhibitor of Dnmt1. *Journal of Biological Chemistry*, 286(17), 15344-15351.

[97] Fellinger, K., Rothbauer, U., Felle, M., Längst, G., & Leonhardt, H. (2009). Dimerization of DNA Methyltransferase 1 Is Mediated by Its Regulatory Domain. *Journal of Cellular Biochemistry*, 106(4), 521-528.

[98] Pradhan, M., Estève, P. O., Chin, H. G., Samaranayke, M., Kim, G. D., & Pradhan, S. (2008). CXXC Domain of Human Dnmt1 Is Essential for Enzymatic Activity. *Biochemistry*, 47(38), 10000-10009.

[99] Lee, J. H., Voo, K. S., & Skalnik, D. G. (2001). Identification and Characterization of the DNA Binding Domain of CpG-Binding Protein. *Journal of Biological Chemistry*, 276(48), 44669-44676.

[100] Bacolla, A., Pradhan, S., Roberts, R. J., & Wells, R. D. (1999). Recombinant Human DNA (Cytosine-5) Methyltransferase. II. Steady-State Kinetics Reveal Allosteric Activation by Methylated DNA. *Journal of Biological Chemistry*, 274(46), 33011-33019.

[101] Takeuchi, H., Hanamura, N., Hayasaka, H., & Harada, I. (1991). B-Z Transition of Poly(dG-m$^5$dC) Induced by Binding of Lys-Containing Peptides. *FEBS Letters*, 279(2), 253-255.

[102] Takeuchi, H., Hanamura, N., & Harada, I. (1994). Structural Specificity of Peptides in Z-DNA Formation and Energetics of the Peptide-Induced B-Z Transition of Poly(dG-$m^5$dC). *Journal of Molecular Biology*, 236(2), 610-617.

[103] Krzyzaniak, A., Siatecka, M., Szyk, A., Mucha, P., Rekowski, P., Kupryszewski, G., & Barciszewski, J. (2000). Specific Induction of Z-DNA Conformation by a Nuclear Localization Signal Peptide of Lupin Glutaminyl tRNA Synthetase. *Molecular Biology Reports*, 27(1), 51-54.

[104] Kim, Y. G., Park, H. J., Kim, K. K., Lowenhaupt, K., & Rich, A. (2006). A Peptide with Alternating Lysines Can Act as a Highly Specific Z-DNA Binding Domain. *Nucleic Acids Research*, 34(17), 4937-4942.

[105] Rich, A., Nordheim, A., & Wang, A. H. (1984). The Chemistry and Biology of Left-Handed Z-DNA. *Annual Review of Biochemistry*, 53-791.

[106] Bestor, T. (1987). Supercoiling-Dependent Sequence Specificity of Mammalian DNA Methyltransferase. *Nucleic Acids Research*, 15(9), 3835-3843.

[107] Okano, M., Xie, S., & Li, E. (1998). Cloning and Characterization of a Family of Novel Mammalian DNA (Cytosine-5) Methyltransferases. *Nature Genetics*, 19(3), 219-220.

[108] Okano, M., Bell, D. W., Haber, D. A., & Li, E. (1999). DNA Methyltransferases Dnmt3a and Dnmt3b Are Essential for de Novo Methylation and Mammalian Development. *Cell*, 99(3), 247-257.

[109] Hansen, R. S., Wijmenga, C., Luo, P., Stanek, A. M., Canfield, T. K., Weemaes, C. M., & Gartler, S. M. (1999). The DNMT3B DNA Methyltransferase Gene Is Mutated in the ICF Immunodeficiency Syndrome. *Proceedings of the National Academy of Science*, 96(25), 14412-14417.

[110] Xu, G. L., Bestor, T. H., Bourc'his, D., Hsieh, C. L., Tommerup, N., Bugge, M., Hulten, M., Qu, X., Russo, J. J., & Viegas-Péquignot, E. (1999). Chromosome Instability and Immunodeficiency Syndrome Caused by Mutations in a DNA Methyltransferase Gene. *Nature*, 402(6758), 187-191.

[111] Xie, S., Wang, Z., Okano, M., Nogami, M., Li, Y., He, W. W., Okumura, K., & Li, E. (1999). Cloning, Expression and Chromosome Locations of the Human DNMT3 Gene Family. *Gene*, 236(1), 87-95.

[112] Cao, X., Springer, N. M., Muszynski, M. G., Phillips, R. L., Kaeppler, S., & Jacobsen, S. E. (2000). Conserved Plant Genes with Similarity to Mammalian de Novo DNA Methyltransferases. *Proceedings of the National Academy of Science*, 97(9), 4979-4984.

[113] Hata, K., Okano, M., Lei, H., & Li, E. (2002). Dnmt3L Cooperates with the Dnmt3 Family of de Novo DNA Methyltransferases to Establish Maternal Imprints in Mice. *Development*, 129(8), 1983-1993.

[114] Bourc'his, D., Xu, G. L., Lin, C. S., Bollman, B., & Bestor, T. H. (2001). Dnmt3L and the Establishment of Maternal Genomic Imprints. *Science*, 294(5551), 2536-2539.

[115] Bourc'his, D., & Bestor, T. H. (2004). Meiotic Catastrophe and Retrotransposon Reactivation in Male Germ Cells Lacking Dnmt3L. *Nature*, 431(7004), 96-99.

[116] Webster, K. E., O'Bryan, M. K., Fletcher, S., Crewther, P. E., Aapola, U., Craig, J., Harrison, D. K., Aung, H., Phutikanit, N., Lyle, R., Meachem, S. J., Antonarakis, S. E., de Kretser, D. M., Hedger, M. P., Peterson, P., Carroll, B. J., & Scott, H. S. (2005). Meiotic and Epigenetic Defects in Dnmt3L-Knockout Mouse Spermatogenesis. *Proceedings of the National Academy of Science*, 102(11), 4068-4073.

[117] Qiu, C., Sawada, K., Zhang, X., & Cheng, X. (2002). The PWWP Domain of Mammalian DNA Methyltransferase Dnmt3b Defines a New Family of DNA-Binding Folds. *Nature Structural & Molecular Biology*, 9(3), 217-224.

[118] Maurer-Stroh, S., Dickens, N. J., Hughes-Davies, L., Kouzarides, T., Eisenhaber, F., & Ponting, C. P. (2003). The Tudor Domain 'Royal Family': Tudor, Plant Agenet, Chromo, PWWP and MBT Domains. *Trends in Biochemical Sciences*, 28(2), 69-74.

[119] Taverna, S. D., Li, H., Ruthenburg, A. J., Allis, C. D., & Patel, D. J. (2007). How Chromatin-Binding Modules Interpret Histone Modifications: Lessons from Professional Pocket Pickers. *Nature Structural & Molecular Biology*, 14(11), 1025-1040.

[120] Wu, H., Zeng, H., Lam, R., Tempel, W., Amaya, M. F., Xu, C., Dombrovski, L., Qiu, W., Wang, Y., & Min, J. (2011). Structural and Histone Binding Ability Characterizations of Human PWWP Domains. *PLoS One*, 6(6), e18919.

[121] Chen, T., Tsujimoto, N., & Li, E. (2004). The PWWP Domain of Dnmt3a and Dnmt3b Is Required for Directing DNA Methylation to the Major Satellite Repeats at Pericentric Heterochromatin. *Molecular and Cellular Biology*, 24(20), 9048-9058.

[122] Bachman, K. E., Rountree, M. R., & Baylin, S. B. (2001). Dnmt3a and Dnmt3b Are Transcriptional Repressors that Exhibit Unique Localization Properties to Heterochromatin. *The Journal of Biological Chemistry*, 276(34), 32282-32287.

[123] Ge, Y. Z., Pu, M. T., Gowher, H., Wu, H. P., Ding, J. P., Jeltsch, A., & Xu, G. L. (2004). Chromatin Targeting of de Novo DNA Methyltransferases by the PWWP Domain. *The Journal of Biological Chemistry*, 279(24), 25447-25454.

[124] Shirohzu, H., Kubota, T., Kumazawa, A., Sado, T., Chijiwa, T., Inagaki, K., Suetake, I., Tajima, S., Wakui, K., Miki, Y., Hayashi, M., Fukushima, Y., & Sasaki, H. (2002). Three Novel Dnmt3B Mutations in Japanese Patients with ICF Syndrome. *American Journal of Medical Genetics*, 112(1), 31-37.

[125] Dhayalan, A., Rajavelu, A., Rathert, P., Tamas, R., Jurkowska, R. Z., Ragozin, S., & Jeltsch, A. (2010). The Dnmt3a PWWP Domain Reads Histone 3 Lysine 36 Trimethylation and Guides DNA Methylation. *The Journal of Biological Chemistry*, 285(34), 26114-26120.

[126] Meissner, A., Mikkelsen, T. S., Gu, H., Wernig, M., Hanna, J., Sivachenko, A., Zhang, X., Bernstein, B. E., Nusbaum, C., Jaffe, D. B., Gnirke, A., Jaenisch, R., & Lander, E. S. (2008). Genome-Scale DNA Methylation Maps of Pluripotent and Differentiated Cells. *Nature*, 454(7205), 766-770.

[127] Hodges, E., Smith, A. D., Kendall, J., Xuan, Z., Ravi, K., Rooks, M., Zhang, M. Q., Ye, K., Bhattacharjee, A., Brizuela, L., McCombie, W. R., Wigler, M., Hannon, G. J., & Hicks, J. B. (2009). High Definition Profiling of Mammalian DNA Methylation by Array Capture and Single Molecule Bisulfite Sequencing. *Genome Research*, 19(9), 1593-1605.

[128] Lee, J. S., & Shilatifard, A. (2007). A Site to Remember: H3K36 Methylation a Mark for Histone Deacetylation. *Mutation Research*, 618(1-2), 130-134.

[129] Argentaro, A., Yang, J. C., Chapman, L., Kowalczyk, M. S., Gibbons, R. J., Higgs, D. R., Neuhaus, D., & Rhodes, D. (2007). Structural Consequences of Disease-Causing Mutations in the ATRX-DNMT3-DNMT3L (ADD) Domain of the Chromatin-Associated Protein ATRX. *Proceedings of the National Academy of Science*, 104(29), 11939-11944.

[130] Ooi, S. K., Qiu, C., Bernstein, E., Li, K., Jia, D., Yang, Z., Erdjument-Bromage, H., Tempst, P., Lin, S. P., Allis, C. D., Cheng, X., & Bestor, T. H. (2007). Dnmt3L Connects Unmethylated Lysine 4 of Histone H3 to de Novo Methylation of DNA. *Nature*, 448(7154), 714-717.

[131] Otani, J., Nankumo, T., Arita, K., Inamoto, S., Ariyoshi, M., & Shirakawa, M. (2009). Structural Basis for Recognition of H3K4 Methylation Status by the DNA Methyltransferase 3A ATRX-Dnmt3-Dnmt3L Domain. *EMBO Reports*, 10(11), 1235-1241.

[132] Zhang, Y., Jurkowska, R., Soeroes, S., Rajavelu, A., Dhayalan, A., Bock, I., Rathert, P., Brandt, O., Reinhardt, R., Fischle, W., & Jeltsch, A. (2010). Chromatin Methylation Activity of Dnmt3a and Dnmt3a/3L Is Guided by Interaction of the ADD Domain with the Histone H3 Tail. *Nucleic Acids Research*, 38(13), 4246-4253.

[133] Pavlopoulou, A., & Kossida, S. (2007). Plant Cytosine-5 DNA Methyltransferases: Structure, Function, and Molecular Evolution. *Genomics*, 90(4), 530-541.

[134] Finnegan, E. J., & Dennis, E. S. (1993). Isolation and Identification by Sequence Homology of a Putative Cytosine Methyltransferase from *Arabidopsis thaliana*. *Nucleic Acids Research*, 21(10), 2383-2388.

[135] Callebaut, I., Courvalin, J. C., & Mornon, J. P. (1999). The BAH (Bromo-Adjacent Homology) Domain: a Link Between DNA Methylation, Replication and Transcriptional Regulation. *FEBS Letters*, 446(1), 189-193.

[136] Xu, S., Xiao, J., Posfai, J., Maunus, R., & Benner, J. 2nd. (1997). Cloning of the BssHII Restriction-Modification System in *Escherichia coli*: BssHII Methyltransferase Contains Circularly Permuted Cytosine-5 Methyltransferase Motifs. *Nucleic Acids Research*, 25(20), 3991-3994.

[137] Wada, Y., Ohya, H., Yamaguchi, Y., Koizumi, N., & Sano, H. (2003). Preferential de Novo Methylation of Cytosine Residues in non-CpG Sequences by a Domains Rearranged DNA Methyltransferase from Tobacco Plants. *The Journal of Biological Chemistry*, 278(43), 42386-42393.

[138] Henderson, I. R., Deleris, A., Wong, W., Zhong, X., Chin, H. G., Horwitz, G. A., Kelly, K. A., Pradhan, S., & Jacobsen, S. E. (2010). The de Novo Cytosine Methyltransferase DRM2 Requires Intact UBA Domains and a Catalytically Mutated Paralog DRM3 During RNA-Directed DNA Methylation in *Arabidopsis thaliana*. *PLoS Genetics*, 6(10), e1001182.

[139] Eissenberg, J. C. (2001). Molecular Biology of the Chromo Domain: an Ancient Chromatin Module Comes of Age. *Gene*, 275(1), 19-29.

[140] Henikoff, S., & Comai, L. (1998). A DNA Methyltransferase Homolog with a Chromodomain Exists in Multiple Polymorphic Forms in *Arabidopsis*. *Genetics*, 149(1), 307-318.

[141] Lindroth, A. M., Cao, X., Jackson, J. P., Zilberman, D., McCallum, C. M., Henikoff, S., & Jacobsen, S. E. (2001). Requirement of CHROMOMETHYLASE3 for Maintenance of CpXpG Methylation. *Science*, 292(5524), 2077-2080.

[142] Bartee, L., Malagnac, F., & Bender, J. (2001). Arabidopsis CMT3 Chromomethylase Mutations Block non-CG Methylation and Silencing of an Endogenous Gene. *Genes and Development*, 15(14), 1753-1758.

Chapter 3

# Bifunctional Prokaryotic DNA-Methyltransferases

Dmitry V. Nikitin, Attila Kertesz-Farkas,
Alexander S. Solonin and Marina L. Mokrishcheva

Additional information is available at the end of the chapter

http://dx.doi.org/10.5772/51025

## 1. Introduction

Restriction-modification systems (RMS) are prokaryotic tools against invasion of foreign DNAs into cells [1]. They reduce horizontal gene transfer, thus stimulating microbial biodiversity. Usually, they consist of a restriction endonuclease (REase) and a modification DNA methyltransferase (MTase) enzyme recognising the same short 4-8 nucleotide sequence. MTase is responsible for methyl group transfer to adenine or cytosine nucleotides within the target sequence, thus preventing its hydrolysis by cognate REase. Up to now, more than 20 000 different RMS have been collected in the REBASE, the database holding all known, and many putative, RMS [2]. Many of these RMS have head-to-tail gene orientation, thus providing, by our hypothesis, the possibility of gene fusion through point mutations or genome rearrangements such as deletions, insertions, inversions or translocations. These events could be responsible for the origin of bifunctional restriction enzymes of type IIC [3] such as AloI, BcgI, BseMII, BseRI, BsgI, BspLU11III, CjeI, Eco57I, HaeIV, MmeI, PpiI, TstI and TspWGI; bifunctional MTases such as FokI and LlaI, and regulatory SsoII-related MTases [4].

In our previous work we proved the possibility of fully functional hybrid polypeptide origin through gene fusion, taking as an example Eco29kI RMS. In the given RMS, the REase gene precedes MTase gene and their Stop and Start codons overlap. By site-directed mutagenesis we joined these two ORFs into one and characterised the resulting protein, carrying both REase and MTase activities [5]. Its REase activity was decreased three times and the optima of the catalytic reaction changed, whereas MTase activity turned out to be intact [5-7]. The bifunctional enzyme could be changed as a result of evolution, leading to further divergence of its properties and functions in the cell. By our hypothesis, this example could serve as a molecular mechanism of new bifunctional RMS origin. In the current work, based on genomic data and their bioinformatics analysis, we aimed to prove that gene fusion could play an important role in evolution of metyltransferases and in origin of multidomain eukaryotic methyltransferases.

For the current work we searched protein databases as described above and found 76 new potential bifunctional MTases. Their structural organisation is presented and discussed in the report. Beside this, we analysed structural organisation of 627 non-putative prokaryotic DNA-methyltransferases available out of 980 methyltransferases collected up to now in REBASE. The most frequently observed structural type, other than "canonical" MTases, represents SsoII-related methyltransferases, capable to serve as transcriptional autoregulatory proteins. These data provide additional evidences that gene fusion might play an important role in evolution of methyltransferases, restriction-modification systems and other DNA-modifying proteins. We discuss the general consequences of a hypothetical protein fusion event with methyltransferases and RMS enzymes.

### 1.1. Method used

For this study 10619 methyltransferases and 3250 restriction enzyme sequences were downloaded from the REBASE database [2] and searched against the non-redundant protein database which was downloaded from the NCBI's ftp site. The similarity search was carried out by BLAST version 2.2.23+ [8] on a Linux server using the BLAST default parameters. The local pairwise alignments hits were then filtered using the following criteria: a match to a methyltransferase enzyme was kept if its E-value was less than 1e-140, the sequence identity of the aligned region was greater than 80% and the subject sequence was at least twice longer than the query. By this algorithm we found 272 candidate hits. A match to a restriction enzyme was kept if its E-value was less than 1e-140, the sequence identity within the aligned region was greater than 80% and the length of the subject sequence was at least 1.5 times longer than the query. By this algorithm we found 28 candidate matches. The candidate matches then were manually analysed.

## 2. Research course

*Methyltransferase fusions with a restriction endonuclease*

Newly found potential bifunctional restriction and modification enzymes are presented in Table 1. With our BLAST search we succeeded to filter from NCBI database 22 fusions of a DNA methyltransferase with a restriction endonuclease, carrying both endonuclease and methyltransferase domains in one polypeptide. As can be seen from Table 1, the enzymes were grouped according to their domain organisation as it was presented in Conserved Domain Database [9]. As could be judged from their domain organisation, 20 new bifunctional REases are thought to represent the fusion of a REase with MTase and target recognition subunits of the type I restriction-modification systems (R-M-S structure), having similar organisation with the known type IIC bifunctional enzymes such as AloI [10], CjeI [11], MmeI [12], PpiI [13], TstI [13] and TspGWI [14]. Type I RMS enzymes are multisubunit proteins that function as a single protein complex, consisting of R, M and S subunits [3]. The S subunit is the specificity subunit that determines which DNA sequence is recognised. The R subunit is essential for cleavage (restriction) and the M subunit catalyses the methylation reaction. Their protein products are marked as HsdS, HsdR and HsdM, respectively. Covalent linking of these subunits in one polypeptide is not thought to interfere with their catalytic activities, giving an opportunity for successful fusion. Currently, the REBASE contains more than 8000 entries corresponding to Type I RMS. Hypothetically, any of these RMS could be joint, naturally or artificially, giving a new bifunctional RMS.

One RMS from *Bacteroides sp.* D22, probably originated from the fusion of type III enzymes. It has conserved motifs similar to Eco57I protein, which consists of Mod and Res subunits of type III enzymes [15]. Type III systems are composed of two genes (mod and res) encoding protein subunits that function in one protein complex either in DNA recognition and modification, Mod, or restriction, Res [3]. As in the case of the type I enzymes, in-frame fusion might not affect their normal functioning, thus, being also favourable for new bifunctional protein origin.

One of the found RMS from *Arthrospira maxima* CS-328 has a different domain organisation, belonging to R-M type of structure (type II REase and MTase fusion). It could be suggested that it originated from fusion of head-to-tail oriented Type II REase and MTase genes. The principal possibility of a new bifunctional RMS origin by this mechanism was proven by in-frame joining of type IIEco29kI REase and MTase genes [5]. The resulting RMS was capable of defending host cells from phage invasion, although 100 times less effectively than the wild type. In a similar way, a new bifunctional RMS could appear from other head-to-tail oriented RMS of type II such as AccI, BanI, Bsp6I, BsuBI, Cfr9I, DdeI, EagI, EcoPI, EcoP15, EcoRI, FnuDI, HaeIII, HgiBI, HgiCI, HgiCII, HgiDI, HgiEI, HgiGI, HhaII, HincII, HindIII, HinfI, HpaI, MboII, MwoI, NcoI, NdeI, NgoMI, NgoPII, NlaIII, PaeR7I, RsrI, SalI, Sau3A, Sau96I, TaqI, TthHB8I, XbaI, and XmaI [16]. Type II restriction enzymes and modification enzymes work separately and their fusion could create steric difficulties for their functionality. In fact, in the case of the RM.Eco29kI enzyme, its REase activity decreased three times in comparison with initial R.Eco29kI nuclease. This is perhaps why it is the only found example of natural bifunctional RMS originating from type II RMS.

| **RMS** |
|---|
| ZP_01728785.1, 1307 aa, type II restriction-modification enzyme, *Cyanothece sp.* CCY0110] |
| YP_892534, 1285 aa, restriction and modification enzyme, *Campylobacter fetus subsp. fetus* 82-40. |
| YP_001482568, 1190 aa, hypothetical protein C8J_0992, *Campylobacter jejuni subsp. Jejuni* 81116. |
| ZP_00368052, 1343 aa, type I restriction modification enzyme, *Campylobacter coli* RM2228. |
| ADC28633, 1364 aa, restriction modification enzyme, *Campylobacter jejuni subsp. Jejuni* IA3902. |
| ZP_01967949,1255 aa, hypothetical protein RUMTOR_01515, *Ruminococcus torques* ATCC |
| 27756. |

ZP_06253288, 1297 aa, putative type I restriction modification DNA specificity domain protein, *Prevotella copri* DSM 18205.

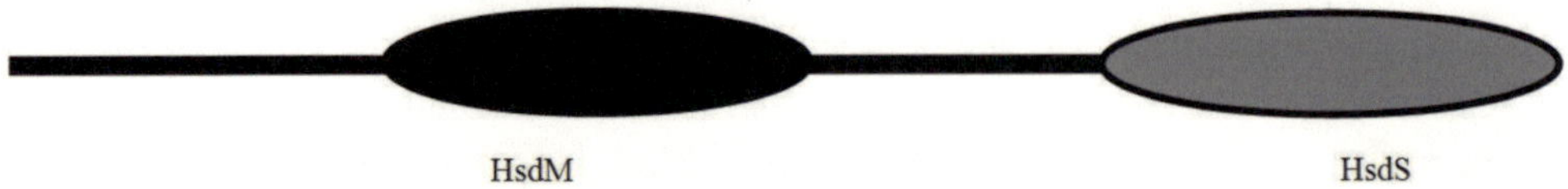


ZP_06373928, 1080 aa, hypothetical protein, *Campylobacter jejuni subsp. jejuni* 1336.

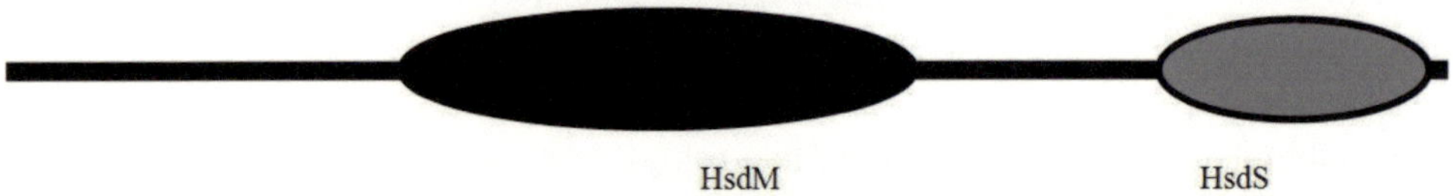


YP_002344446, 1339 aa, restriction modification enzyme, *Campylobacter jejuni subsp. Jejuni* NCTC 11168.

YP_003633850, 1134 aa, restriction modification system DNA specificity domain protein, *Brachyspira murdochii* DSM 12563.

ZP_06409683, 889 aa, putative type II restriction-modification enzyme, *Clostridium hathewayi* DSM 13479.

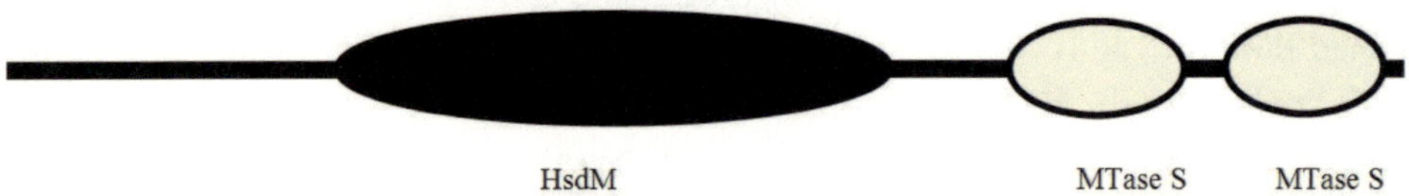


ZP_06998902.1, 1053 aa, type IIS restriction endonuclease, *Bacteroides sp.* D22.

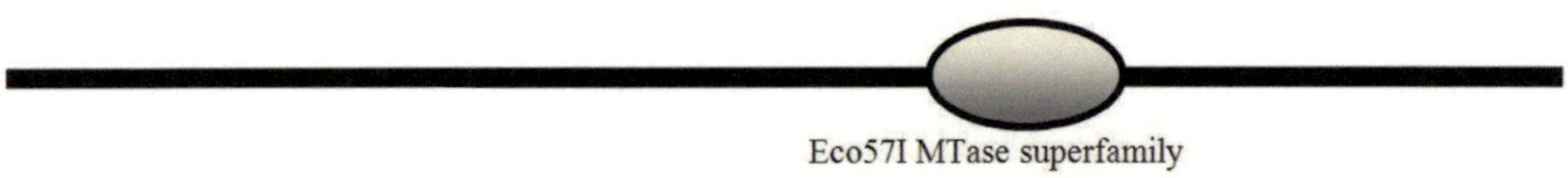


ZP_03658113, 1171 aa, type II restriction-modification enzyme, *Helicobacter cinaedi* CCUG 18818.

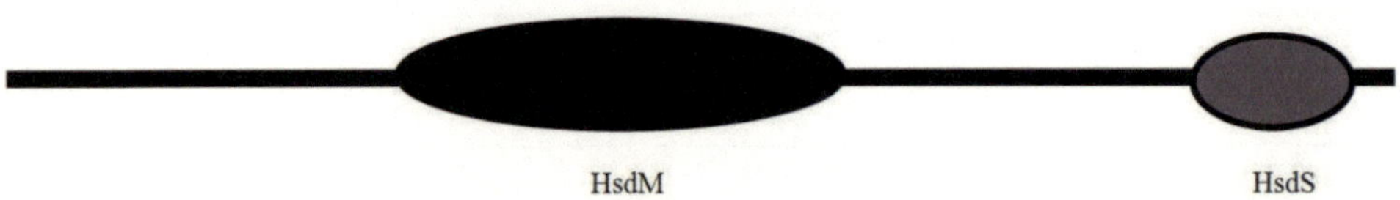


ZP_03656081, 1322 aa, restriction modification enzyme, *Helicobacter canadensis* MIT 98-5491.

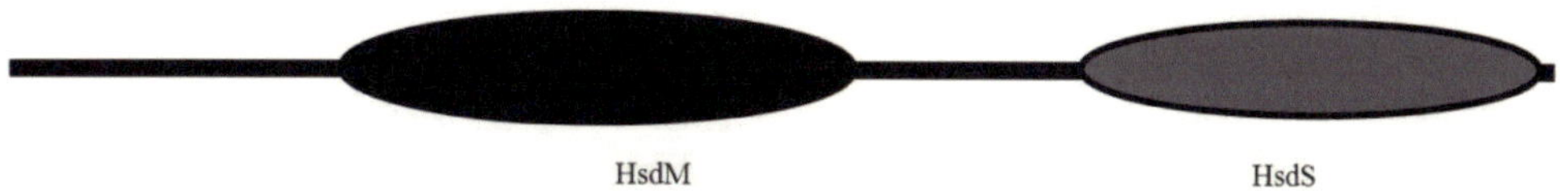


NP_860965, 1164 aa, type I restriction/modification enzyme, *Helicobacter hepaticus* ATCC 51449.

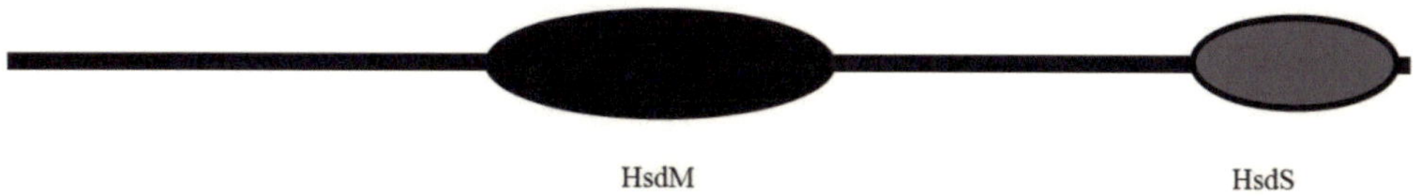


YP_003127864, 1068 aa, N-6 DNA Methylase, *Methanocaldococcus fervens* AG86.

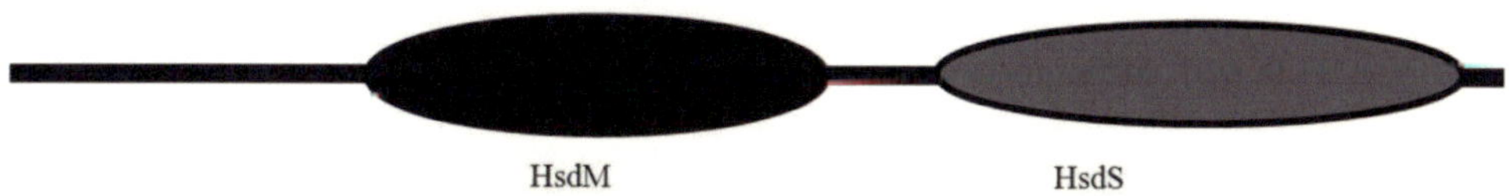


YP_001783948, 1110 aa, N-6 DNA Methylase, *Haemophilus somnus* 2336.

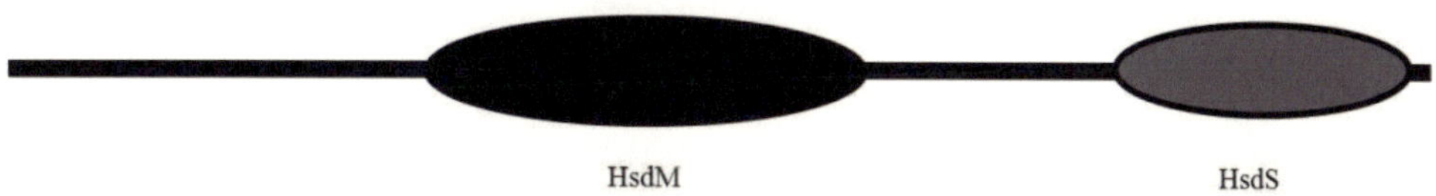


ZP_04582604, 894 aa, type II restriction-modification enzyme, *Helicobacter winghamensis* ATCC BAA-430.

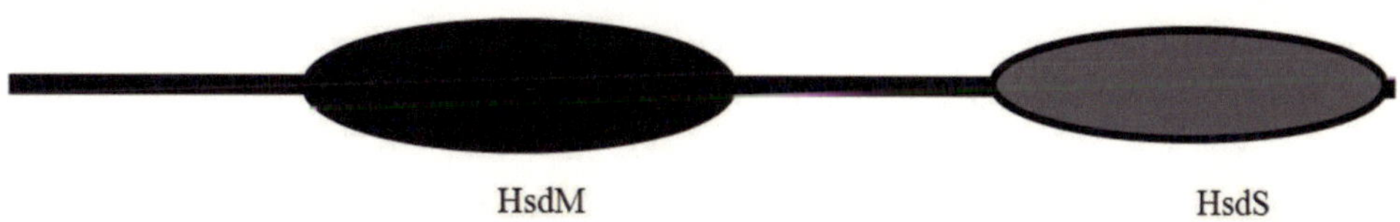


ZP_01253792, 1020 aa, type II restriction-modification enzyme, *Psychroflexus torquis* ATCC 700755.

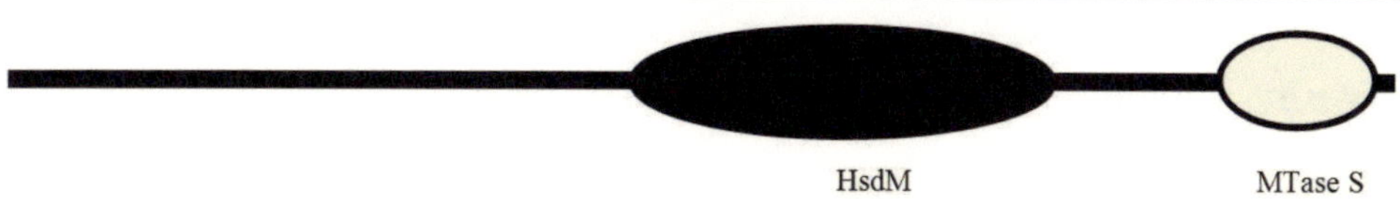


ZP_07401090, 737 aa, type II restriction-modification enzyme, *Campylobacter coli* JV20.

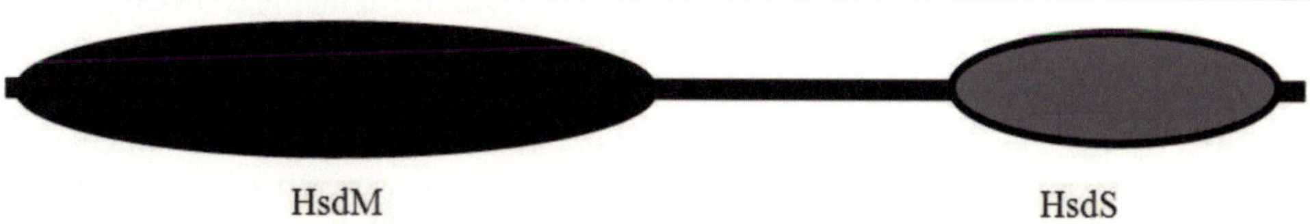

ZP_06009534, 727 aa, restriction and modification enzyme, *Campylobacter fetus subsp. venerealis* str. Azul-94.

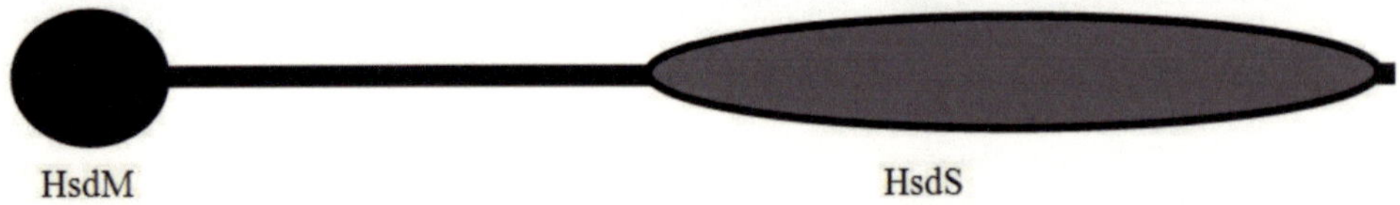


**RM**

ZP_03272741.1, 1473 aa, protein of unknown function DUF559, *Arthrospira maxima* CS-328.

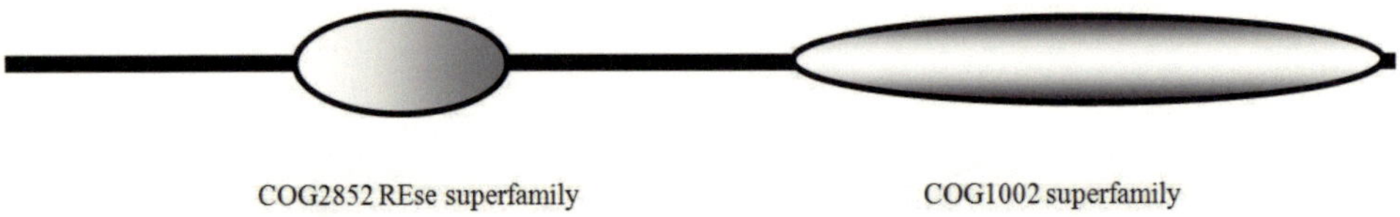


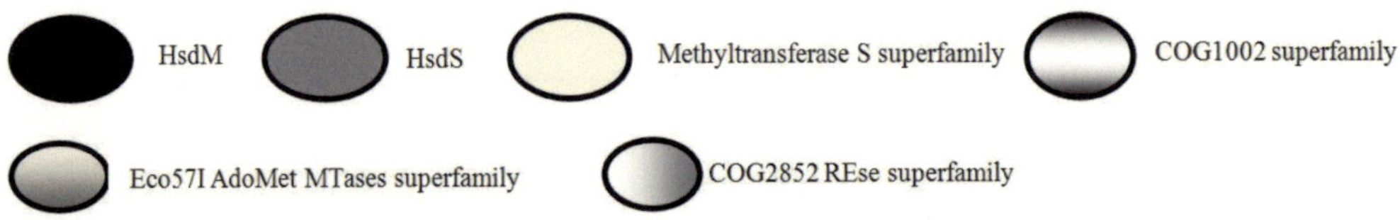


**Table 1.** Methyltransferase fusions with a restriction endonuclease. Domains are predicted and presented as in Conserved Domain Database [9]. Different domains are shown by different fillings and their classification is shown under the table. Short description for each found protein includes Gene Bank accession number, length in amino acids, current name in the database and host strain information.

The newly found potential type IIC proteins are good candidates to expand on the current list of 12 bifunctional enzymes: AloI[10], BcgI [17], BseMII [18], BseRI [19], BspLU11III [20], CjeI[11], Eco57I [15], HaeIV [21], MmeI [12], PpiI [13], TstI [13] and TspGWI [14]. Taking into consideration intensiveness with what new microbial genomes have been sequencing during the last decade, new bifunctional RMS could be discovered very soon.

## 3. Fusions between two DNA methyltransferases

As shown in Table 2, in contrast to the situation with bifunctional MTase - REase fusions, among 54 newly found fusions between two methyltransferases 49, apparently, are joining of two different methyltransferase ORFs (M-M structure) and 5 of methyltransferase (HsdM) and target recognition subunit (HsdS, M-S structure). 11 M-M type proteins represent interesting examples of dcm and dam methyltransferase fusion. In this case dam corresponds not only to one particular MTase, but to a conserved domain common for DNA adenine methyltransferases, as adopted from the Conserved Domain Database web site [9]. In a similar way, dcm corresponds to a conserved domain common for DNA cytosine methyltransferases. These MTases catalyse methyl group transfers to different nucleotide bases, adenine in the case of dam, and cytosine in the case of dcm. It could be suggested that originally they belonged to two different genes, and were joint in-frame occasionally. The post-segregation killing effect of restriction-modification enzymes prevents RMS from being lost [22], thus promoting maintenance of a fused ORF and its spreading in bacterial populations. The next chapter will be devoted to a more detailed analysis of this effect. The other 23 bifunctional MTases of M-M type probably originated from a similar joining of two dam methyltransferase genes (Table 2). Further evolution of bifunctional MTases depends on their involvement in RMS functioning. If both activities are critical for the RMS work, for example, modifying two different bases of an asymmetric recognition sequence [23], they will be maintained as elements of this RMS. If the activity of at least one MTase domain of the bifunctional enzyme is redundant, it could accumulate mutations and, after many generations, reduce or gain new substrate specificity and function in the cell history.

| **MS** |
|---|
| CBL28228.1, 825 aa, Type I restriction-modification system methyltransferase subunit, *Synergistetes bacterium* SGP1. |
| ZP_04875770, 760 aa, N-6 DNA Methylase family, *Aciduliprofundum boonei* T469. |
| YP_002961053, 777 aa, hypothetical protein MCJ_005510, *Mycoplasma conjunctivae* HRC/581. |

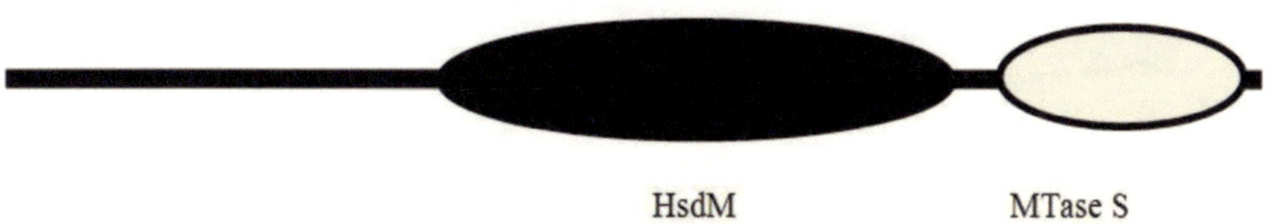


| |
|---|
| YP_002004068, 785 aa, N-6 DNA methylase, *Candidatus phytoplasma mali*. |

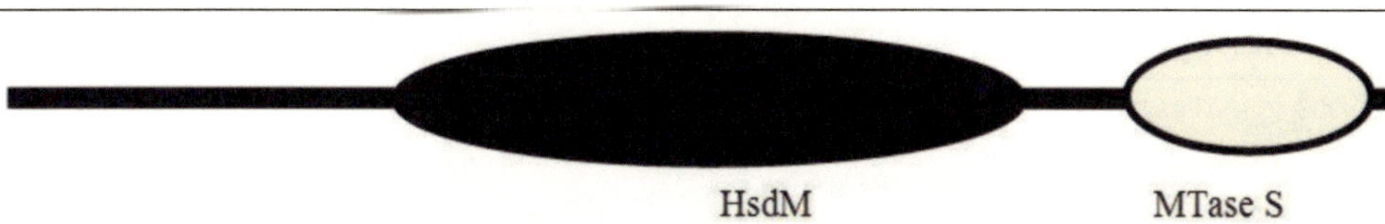


| |
|---|
| ZP_04643292, 907 aa, putative restriction-modification enzyme, *Lactobacillus gasseri* 202-4. |

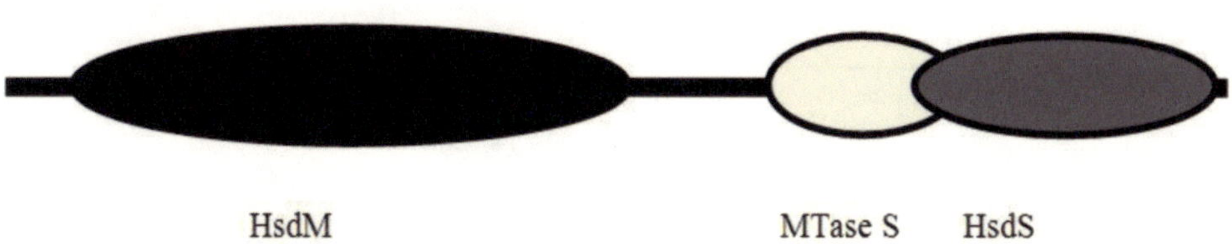


| **MM** |
|---|
| YP_006537.1, 754 aa, DNA methyltransferase Dmt, *Enterobacteria* phage P1. |
| ZP_07502038, 862 aa, putative DNA methyltransferase, *Escherichia coli* M605. |

ZP_07381018, 808 aa, DNA adenine methylase, *Pantoea sp*. AB.

ZP_06715601, 722 aa, DNA C5 cytosine methyltransferase, *Edwardsiella tarda* ATCC 23685.

ZP_02701644, 819 aa, DNA methyltransferase Dmt, *Salmonella enterica subsp. enterica* serovar Newport str. SL317.

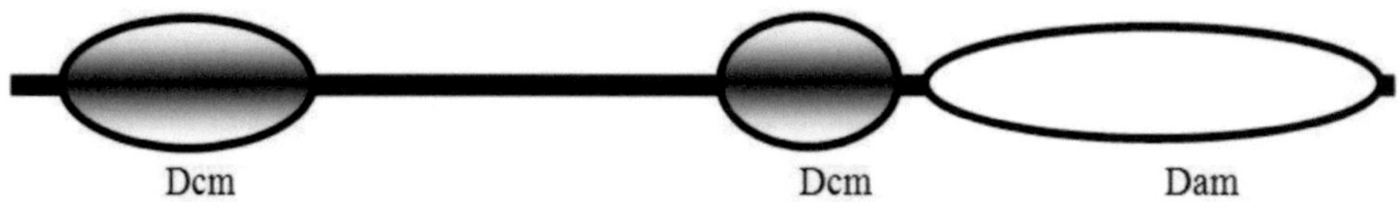


YP_003237972, 1013 aa putative DNA methyltransferase, *Escherichia coli* O111:H- str. 11128.

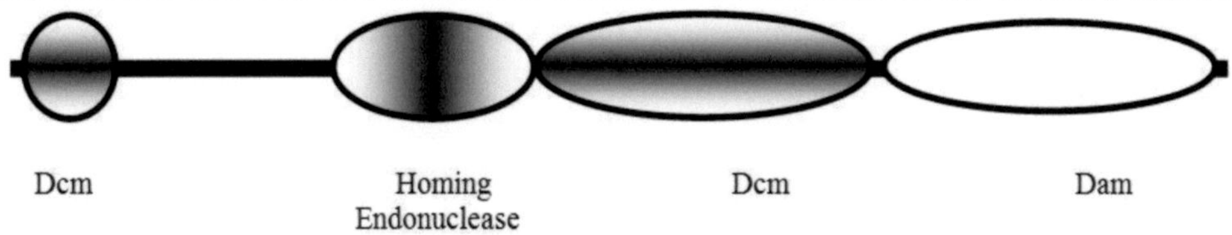


AF503408_62, 672 aa, adenine DNA methyltransferase Dam, *Enterobacteria* phage P7.

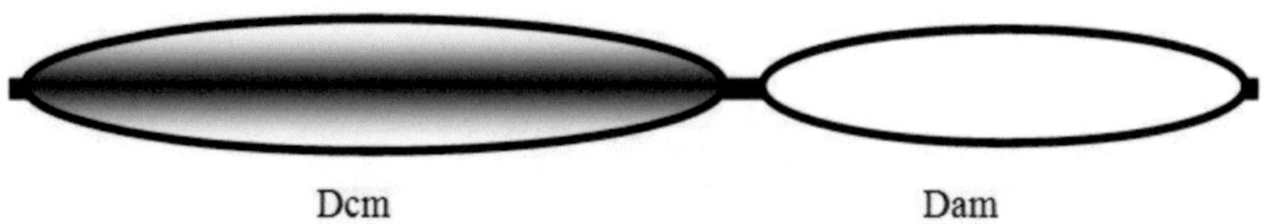


AF458984_2, 952 aa, N6 adenine and C5 cytosine DNA methyltransferase, *Acinetobacter lwoffii*.

AAQ72364, 1007 aa, methylase fusion protein, *Geobacillus stearothermophilus*.

AAS09913, 1068 aa, BsmBI M1-M2 methyltransferase fusion protein, *Geobacillus stearothermophilus.*

AF458983_2, 1061 aa, N6 adenine and C5 cytosine DNA methyltransferase, *Hafnia alvei*.

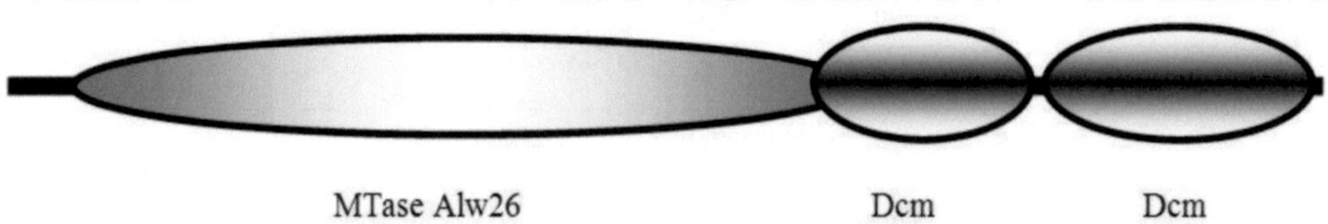


ACZ62643, 687 aa, BtsCIM Methylase, *Ureibacillus thermosphaericus*.

ZP_05132801, 653 aa, DNA methyltransferase, *Clostridium sp*. 7_2_43FAA.

ZP_02080986, 664 aa, hypothetical protein CLOLEP_02452, *Clostridium leptum* DSM 753.

P29347, 653 aa, Adenine-specific methyltransferase StsI, *Streptococcus sanguinis*.

YP_002744130, 627 aa, DNA adenine Methylase, *Streptococcus equi subsp. zooepidemicus*.

YP_002746827, 620 aa, DNA adenine Methylase, *Streptococcus equi subsp. equi* 4047.

ZP_04008314, 618 aa, adenine DNA methyltransferase, *Lactobacillus salivarius* ATCC 11741.

| |
|---|
| ZP_00231287, 608 aa, DNA methyltransferase, *Listeria monocytogenes* str. 4b H7858. |
| ZP_03958097, 625 aa, possible site-specific DNA methyltransferase, *Lactobacillus ruminis* ATCC 25644. |
| YP_003532979, 617 aa, adenine methyltransferase, *Erwinia amylovora* CFBP1430. |
| YP_002650601, 617 aa, adenine specific DNA methyltransferase, *Erwinia pyrifoliae* Ep1/96. |
| ZP_06871587, 670 aa, adenine methyltransferase, *Fusobacterium nucleatum subsp. nucleatum* ATCC 23726. |
| ZP_04573763, 670 aa, adenine methyltransferase, *Fusobacterium* sp. 7_1. |
| ZP_06560574, 722 aa, DNA adenine methylase, *Megasphaera genomosp*. type_1 str. 28L. |
| ZP_06290558, 729 aa, modification methylase, *Peptoniphilus lacrimalis* 315-B. |
| ZP_04452030, 711 aa, hypothetical protein GCWU000182_01325, *Abiotrophia defectiva* ATCC 49176. |
| ZP_05861343, 722 aa, putative adenine methylase, *Jonquetella anthropi* E3_33 E1. |
| ZP_04977178, 722 aa, adenine methyltransferase, *Mannheimia haemolytica* PHL213. |
| ACZ68466, 710 aa, modification Methylase, *Staphylococcus aureus*. |
| ADD81212, 700 aa, DNA methyltransferase, *Enterococcus faecalis*. |
| ZP_07642163, 716 aa, modification Methylase, *Streptococcus mitis* SK597. |
| ZP_01834649, 716 aa, adenine methyltransferase, *Streptococcus pneumonia* SP23-BS72. |
| NP_602723, 496 aa, adenine-specific methyltransferase, *Fusobacterium nucleatum subsp. nucleatum* ATCC 25586. |

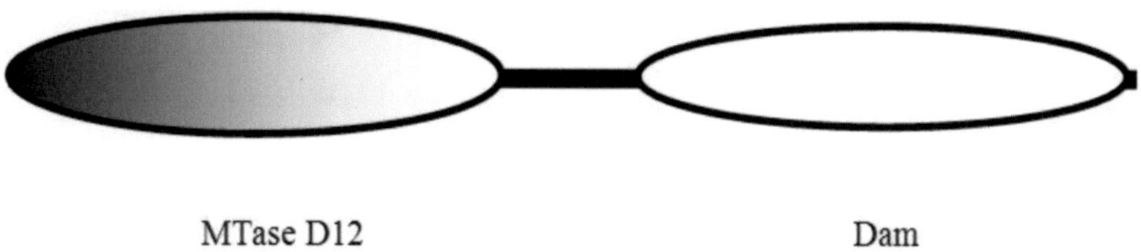


| |
|---|
| ZP_05849684.1, 752 aa, twin-argninine leader-binding protein DmsD, *Haemophilus influenzae* NT127. |
| AAT40808, 518 aa, type III restriction-modification system methyltransferase-like protein, *Haemophilus influenzae*. |
| ZP_04736658.1, 724 aa, putative type III restriction/modification system modification Methylase, *Neisseria gonorrhoeae* PID332. |
| ZP_01788156.1, 687 aa, twin-argninine leader-binding protein DmsD, *Haemophilus influenzae* 3655. |
| YP_001292975.1, 724 aa, twin-argninine leader-binding protein DmsD, *Haemophilus influenzae* PittGG. |
| YP_001291080.1, 713 aa, putative type III restriction/modification system modification methylase, *Haemophilus influenzae* PittEE. |
| ZP_01789924.1, 681 aa, twin-argninine leader-binding protein DmsD, *Haemophilus influenzae* PittAA. |
| ZP_04736658.1, 724 aa, putative type III restriction/modification system modification methylase, *Neisseria gonorrhoeae* PID332. |

| |
|---|
| ZP_04719045.1, 736 aa, putative type III restriction/modification system modification methylase, *Neisseria gonorrhoeae* 35/02. |
| YP_975326.1, 744 aa, putative type III restriction/modification system modification methylase, *Neisseria meningitidis* FAM18. |
| ZP_05849684.1, 752 aa, twin-argninine leader-binding protein DmsD, *Haemophilus influenzae* NT127. |
| ZP_05986443.1, 701 aa, type III restriction/modification enzyme, methylase subunit, *Neisseria lactamica* ATCC 23970. |
| ABI85522.1, 717 aa, DNA methylase M.Hin1056ModP-2, *Haemophilus influenzae*. |
| YP_207780.1, 756 aa, putative type III restriction/modification system modification methylase, *Neisseria gonorrhoeae* FA 1090. |
| ZP_05986443.1, 701 aa, type III restriction/modification enzyme, *Neisseria lactamica* ATCC 23970. |

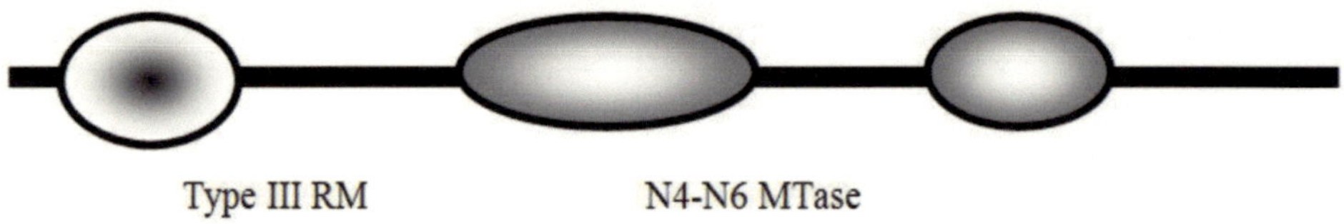


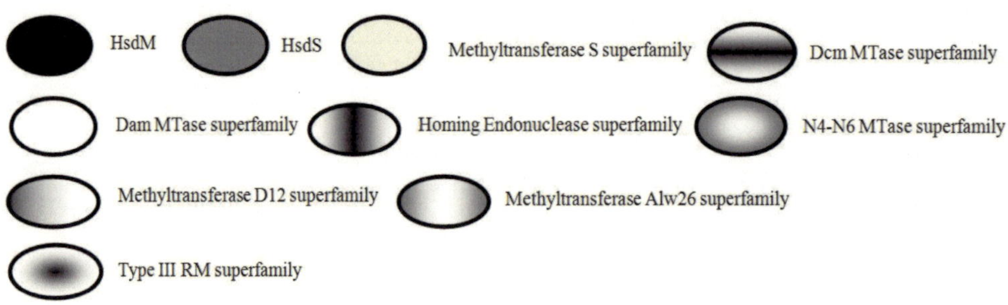


**Table 2.** Fusions between two DNA methyltransferases. Domains are predicted and presented as in Conserved Domain Database [9]. Different domains are shown by different fillings and their classification is shown under the table. Short description for each found protein includes Gene Bank accession number, length in amino acids, current name in the database and host strain information.

For example, DNMT1, a DNA methyltransferase 1 from *H. sapiens* [24], contains a conserved domain of m5C MTases at its C-terminal domain. The N-terminal and central parts of the enzyme include several different domains such as DMAP binding domain, replication foci domain, zinc finger domain and two bromo adjacent homology domains (Figure 1 a). It could be suggested that several gene fusion events were involved in its evolutionary. This hypothesis is supported by existence of simpler homologs of DNMT1 such as, for example, M.AimAII (Figure 1 b) and M.AimAI (Figure 1 d) from *Ascobolus immersus,* and M.NcrNI from *Neurospora crassa* (Figure 1 c), looking like not completely assembled DNMT1 with one or several domains missing. 15 other M-M type bifunctional MTases from Table 2 represent the fusion of a conserved pfam12564 type III RMS 60 aa domain with pfam01555 N4-N6 MTase domain, characteristic both for N4 cytosine-specific and N6 adenine-specific DNA methylases. The pfam01555 conserved domain could be found both in type II MTases, such as M.KpnI, and type III Mod proteins, such as EcoP1I and EcoP15I. In contrast, a 60 aa conserved pfam12564 domain could be found only in several type III enzymes. Its addition could influence the biochemical properties of the corresponding proteins. To establish the character of its influence experimentally in the future, it would be necessary to compare the biochemical properties of MTases containing the pfam12564 60 aa sequence, with MTases not containing it.

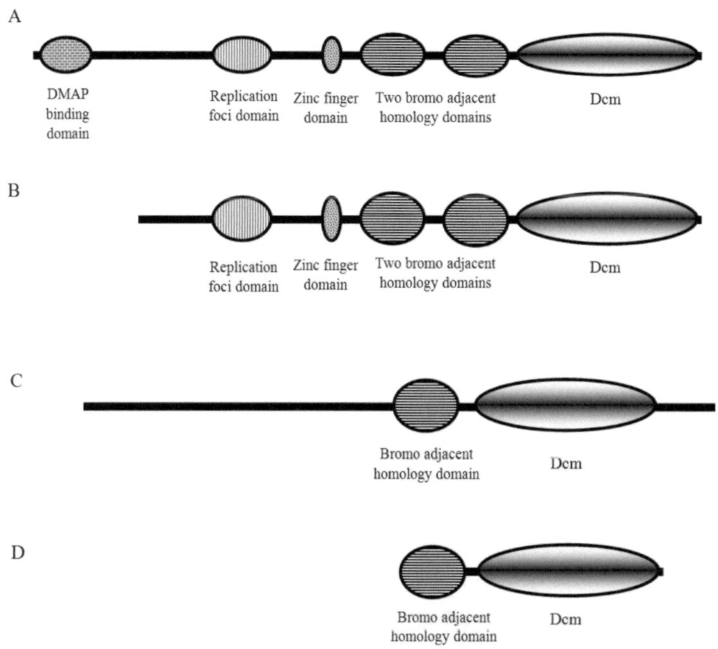


**Figure 1.** Domain organisation of DNMT1, a DNA methyltransferase 1 from *H. sapiens* (a); M.AimAII, a methyltransferase from *Ascobolus immersus* (b), M.NcrNI from *Neurospora crassa* (c) and M.AimAI from *Ascobolus immersus* (d). Domains are predicted and presented as in Conserved Domain Database [9]. Different domains are shown by different fillings.

## 4. Fusion of RMS enzymes with a hypothetical protein

Figure 2 shows the consequences of a RMS protein fusion with a hypothetical protein, X. The upper part of the figure represents normal RMS functioning, when host DNA is protected by an MTase and foreign DNA is degraded by a cognate REase. In the case of RMS loss, MTase and REase enzymes will be diluted following cell divisions, host DNA will become unprotected and, finally, degraded by the residual REase activity.

This effect is known as post-segregation killing [22] and is possibly due to REase activity lasting longer than MTase activity after the RMS loss. The lower part of the figure illustrates the situation of the fusion of some protein X with one of the RMS enzymes. If this joining will not affect seriously the enzyme activities, the RMS will continue to protect cells from foreign DNA invasion. In the case of RMS loss, the same mechanism will lead to host DNA degradation. In this way, a fused protein with RMS enzymes will be supported and spread among bacterial populations. In fact, during a BLAST search we could see close homologues (>98%) of bifunctional enzymes such as, for example, CjeI, spread among numerous strains of the *Campylobacter* group of microorganisms. These observations could illustrate our hypothesis. Another example of the propagation of a RMS-fused protein is provided by M.SsoII-related enzymes. These MTases represent fusion of a regulatory protein with a C5-cytosine methyltransferase [4] and can be found in 63 different microbial taxa.

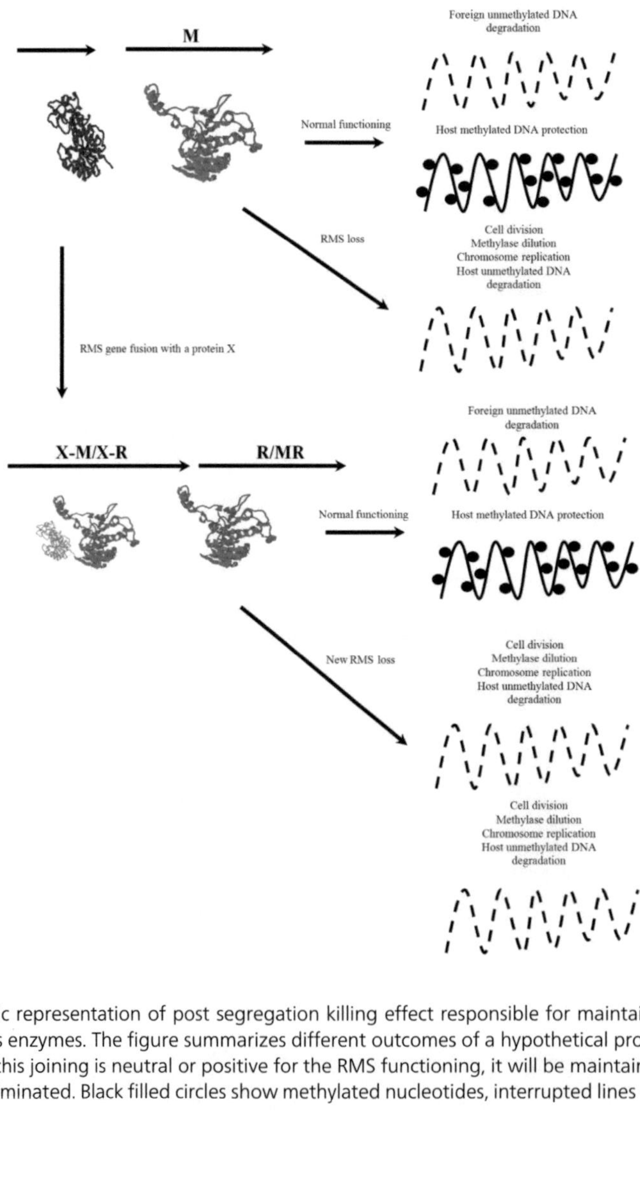


**Figure 2.** Schematic representation of post segregation killing effect responsible for maintaining RMS and proteins joint with one of its enzymes. The figure summarizes different outcomes of a hypothetical protein X joining to one of a RMS enzymes. If this joining is neutral or positive for the RMS functioning, it will be maintained and spread; if detrimental, it will be eliminated. Black filled circles show methylated nucleotides, interrupted lines - degraded DNA.

In another case, if fusion with a hypothetical protein is detrimental for the activity of one of the RMS enzymes, an outcome will depend on which of the enzymes is affected. If an MTase activity will be reduced, the corresponding RMS will be eliminated due to host DNA degradation by cognate REase. If a REase activity is disturbed, the corresponding RMS will become non-functional, will not be supported by post-segregation killing mechanism and, after many generations, could disappear or take on different functions in the cell. Another, less probable, scenario is possible if a joining with a hypothetical protein would improve the properties of RMS enzymes. In this situation, the corresponding RMS would protect host cells more effectively and that would increase their selective advantage over competitive microbial populations, which, in turn, could lead to a wider distribution of the RMS carrying the fused protein.

## 5. Domain organisation of non-putative DNA methyltransferases from REBASE

We analyse structural organisation of 627 non-putative prokaryotic DNA-methyltransferases collected up to now in REBASE, a major database of restriction-modification enzymes [2]. We succeeded to download sequences of 627 prokaryotic methyltransferases out of 980 non-putative MTases enlisted in REBASE on 01.12.2011 (for their detailed description see Supplementary materials). Out of 627, 190 sequences belong to dcm type of DNA-methyltransferases; 172 - to N6-N4 type; 99 - to HsdM type and 78 - to dam-related enzymes according to Conserved Domain Database [9]. We found that the most frequently observed structure, other than "canonical" methyltransferases with conserved motives responsible for binding with AdoMet and a methyl group transfer, represents C5-methyltransferase core domain fusion with a regulatory DNA-binding protein and up to now includes 18 potential enzymes (Table 3). These SsoII-related methyltransferases carry additional DNA-binding HTH-domains and they are capable to serve as transcriptional autorepressors [4]. Among these 18 SsoII-like MTases HTH-motif can be located in majority of cases on N-terminal part, and in three proteins - in the middle of their polypeptide chains (M.Esp1396I, M.PflMI and M.SfiI; Table 3). Ability for autoregulation was not confirmed for majority of these SsoII-like MTases and will require some experimental proofs, which could be considered as perspective future directions of research. The fact of SsoII-like enzymes propagation among different bacterial taxa could illustrate well our analysis of a RMS protein fusion with a hypothetical protein, described in the previous chapter.

M.AseI, Type II methyltransferase, recognition sequence ATTAAT, GenBank ADO24185, 552 aa

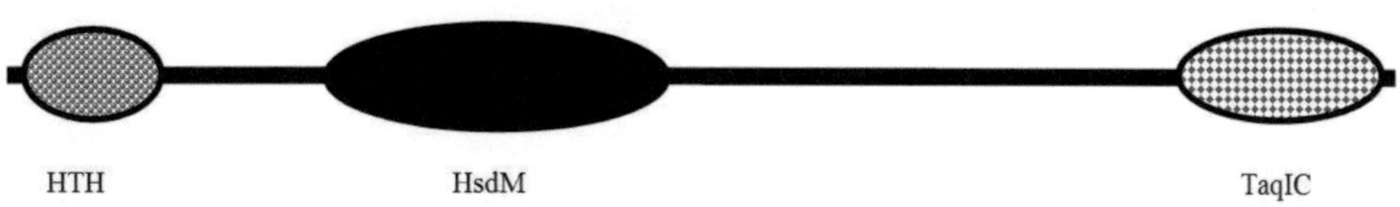

M.AvaII, Type II methyltransferase, recognition sequence GGWCC, GenBank BA000019, 477 aa

M.BadAII, Type II methyltransferase, recognition sequence CCNGG, GenBank AP009256, 383 aa

M.Csp68KI, Type II methyltransferase, recognition sequence GGWCC, GenBank CP000806, 461 aa

M.Ecl18kI, Type II methyltransferase, recognition sequence CCNGG, GenBank Y16897, 379 aa

M.Eco47II, Type II methyltransferase, recognition sequence GGNCC, GenBank X82105, 417 aa

M.Kpn2kI, Type II methyltransferase, recognition sequence CCNGG, GenBank AF300473, 379 aa

M.MspI, Type II methyltransferase, recognition sequence CCGG, GenBank X14191, 418 aa

M.Sau96I, Type II methyltransferase, recognition sequence GGNCC, GenBank X53096, 430 aa

M1.ScrFI, Type II methyltransferase, recognition sequence CCNGG, GenBank U89998, 389 aa

M.SenPI, Type II methyltransferase, recognition sequence CCNGG, GenBank U65460, 379 aa

M.SinI, Type II methyltransferase, recognition sequence GGWCC, GenBank J03391, 461 aa

M.SsoII, Type II methyltransferase, recognition sequence CCNGG, GenBank M86545, 379 aa

M.StyD4I, Type II methyltransferase, recognition CCNGG, GenBank D73442, 379 aa

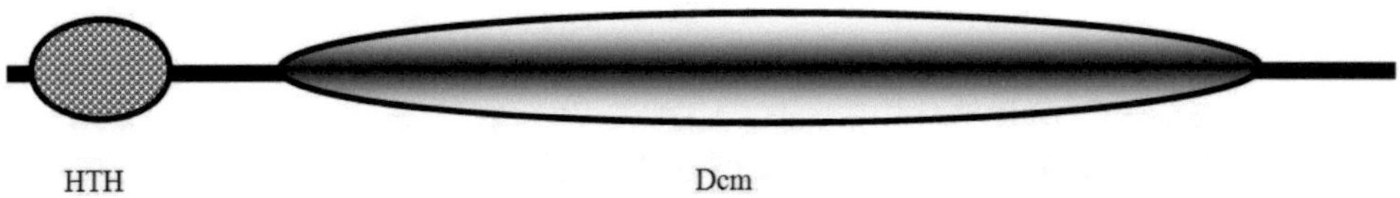


M.Esp1396I, Type II methyltransferase, recognition sequence CCANNNNNTGG, GenBank AF527822, 332 aa

M.PflMI, orphan methyltransferase, recognition sequence CCANNNNNTGG, GenBank ADZ31427, 363 aa

M.SfiI, Type II methyltransferase, recognition sequence GGCCNNNNNGGCC, GenBank AF039750, 421 aa

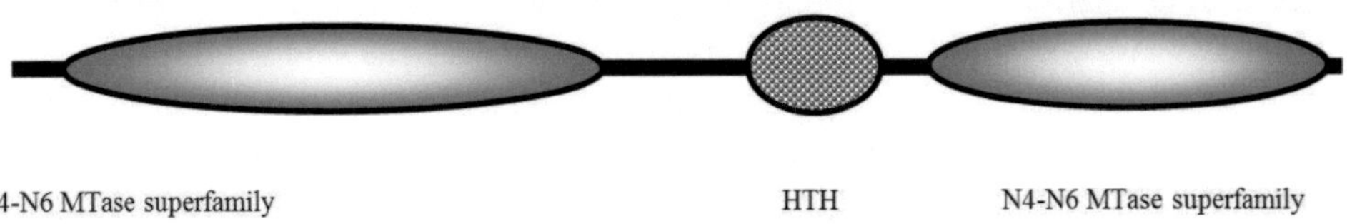


M1.SfaNI, Type II methyltransferase, recognition sequence GCATC, GenBank GU565605, 700 aa

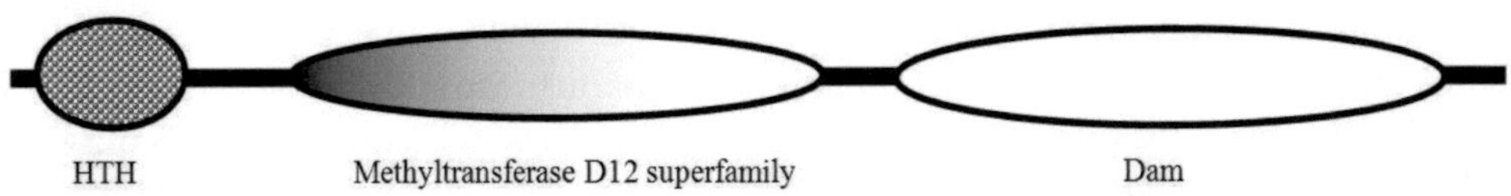


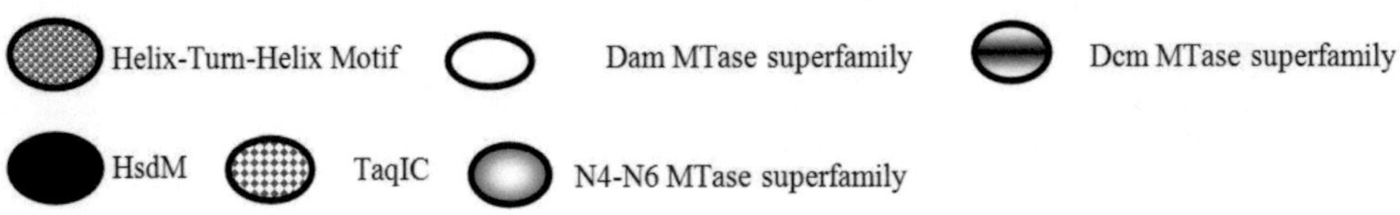


**Table 3.** Domain organisation of SsoII-like prokaryotic DNA methyltransferases, collected in REBASE. Domains are predicted and presented as in Conserved Domain Database [9]. Different domains are shown by different fillings.

## 6. Conclusion

Here we report finding 76 new bifunctional methyltransferases. The majority of the found joint proteins with a nuclease are thought to be fusions of a restriction nuclease with methylase and target recognition subunits of type I restriction-modification systems (R-M-S structure). The majority of the found joint proteins between two methylases appears to be dam-dcm and dam-dam enzyme fusions (M-M structure). Similar proteins could serve as structural intermediates for multidomain eukaryotic methyltransferase evolution. We suggest that a hypothetical protein fusion with a restriction-modification enzyme can promote its propagation in bacterial populations. Altogether, our data illustrate a role of gene fusion in restriction-modification enzyme evolution.

*Abbreviations*

ORF - open reading frame; REase - restriction endonuclease; MTase - methyltransferase; RMS - restriction-modification system; TRD - target recognition domain; aa - amino acids.

## Author details

Dmitry V. Nikitin[1,2*], Attila Kertesz-Farkas[2], Alexander S. Solonin[1] and Marina L. Mokrishcheva[1]

*Address all correspondence to: dvnikitin@rambler.ru

1 Institute of Biochemistry and Physiology of Microorganisms, Russian Academy of Sciences, Russia

2 ICGEB, Area Science Park, Italy

## References

[1] Williams, R. (2003). Restriction endonucleases: classification, properties, and applications. *Molecular Biotechnology*, 23, 225-243.

[2] Vincze, T., Posfai, J., & Macelis, D. (2010). REBASE-a database for DNA restriction and modification: enzymes, genes and genomes. *Nucleic Acids Research*, 38, 234-236.

[3] Roberts, R. J., Belfort, M., Bestor, T., et al. (2003). A nomenclature for restriction enzymes, DNA methyltransferases, homing endonucleases and their genes. *Nucleic Acids Research*, 31, 1805-1812.

[4] Karyagina, A., Shilov, I., Tashlitskii, V., Khodoun, M., Vasil'ev, S., Lau, P., & Nikolskaya, I. (1997). Specific binding of SsoII DNA methyltransferase to its promoter region provides the regulation of SsoII restriction-modification gene expression. *Nucleic Acids Research*, 25, 2114-2120.

[5] Mokrishcheva, M., Solonin, A. S., & Nikitin, D. (2011). Fused eco29kIR- and M genes coding for a fully functional hybrid polypeptide as a model of molecular evolution of restriction-modification systems. *BMC Evolutionary Biology*, 11, 35.

[6] Nikitin, D., Mokrishcheva, M., Denjmukhametov, M., Pertzev, A., Zakharova, M., & Solonin, A. (2003). The construction of an overproducing strain, purification and biochemical characterization of the 6His-Eco29kI restriction endonuclease. *Protein Expression and Purification*, 30, 26-31.

[7] Nikitin, D., Mokrishcheva, M., & Solonin, A. (2007). 6His-Eco29kI methyltransferase methylation site and kinetic mechanism characterization. *Biochimica Biophysica Acta*, 1774, 1014-1019.

[8] Altschul, S. F., Gish, W., Miller, W., Myers, E. W., & Lipman, D. J. (1990). Basic local alignment search tool. *Journal of Molecular Biology*, 215, 403-410.

[9] Marchler-Bauer, A., Lu, S., Anderson, J., et al. (2011). CDD: a Conserved Domain Database for the functional annotation of proteins. *Nucleic Acids Research*, 39, 225-229.

[10] Cesnaviciene, E., Petrusiyte, M., Kazlauskiene, R., Maneliene, Z., Timinskas, A., Lubys, A., & Janulaitis, A. (2001). Characterization of AloI, a Restriction-modification System of a New Type. *Journal of Molecular Biology*, 314, 205-216.

[11] Vitor, J., & Morgan, R. (1995). Two novel restriction endonucleases from Campylobacter jejuni. *Gene*, 157, 109-110.

[12] Morgan, R., Bhatia, T., Lovasco, L., & Davis, T. (2008). MmeI: a minimal Type II restriction-modification system that only modifies one DNA strand for host protection. *Nucleic Acids Research*, 36, 6558-6570.

[13] Jurenaite-Urbanaviciene, S., Serksnaite, J., Kriukiene, E., Giedriene, J., Venclovas, C., & Lubys, A. (2007). Generation of DNA cleavage specificities of type II restriction endonucleases by reassortment of target recognition domains. *Proceedings of National Academy of Sciences USA*, 104, 10358-10463.

[14] Zylicz-Stachula, A., Bujnicki, J., & Skowron, P. M. (2009). Cloning and analysis of a bifunctional methyltransferase/restriction endonuclease TspGWI, the prototype of a Thermus sp. enzyme family. *BMC Molecular Biology*, 10, 52.

[15] Rimseliene, R., Maneliene, Z., Lubys, A., & Janulaitis, A. (2003). Engineering of restriction endonucleases: using methylation activity of the bifunctional endonuclease Eco57I to select the mutant with a novel sequence specificity. *Journal of Molecular Biology*, 327, 383-391.

[16] Wilson, G. G. (1991). Organization of restriction-modification systems. *Nucleic Acids Research*, 19, 2539-2566.

[17] Kong, H., Roemer, S., Waite-Rees, P., Benner, J., Wilson, G., & Nwankwo, D. (1994). Characterization of BcgI, a New Kind of Restriction-Modification System. *Journal of Biological Chemistry*, 269, 683-690.

[18] Jurenaite-Urbanaviciene, S., Kazlauskiene, R., Urbelyte, V., Maneliene, Z., Petrusyte, M., Lubys, A., & Janulaitis, A. (2001). Characterization of BseMII, a new type IV restriction-modification system, which recognizes the pentanucleotide sequence 5'-CTCAG(N)(10/8)/. *Nucleic Acids Research*, 29, 895-903.

[19] Mushtaq, R., Naeem, S., Sohail, A., & Riazuddin, S. (1993). BseRI a novel restriction endonuclease from a Bacillus species which recognizes the sequence 5'...GAGGAG... 3'. *Nucleic Acids Research*, 21, 3585.

[20] Lepikhov, K., Tchernov, A., Zheleznaja, L., Matvienko, N., Walter, J., & Trautner, T. A. (2001). Characterization of the type IV restriction modification system BspLU11III from Bacillus sp. LU11. *Nucleic Acids Research*, 29, 4691-4698.

[21] Piekarowicz, A., Golaszewska, M., Sunday, A., Siwińska, M., & Stein, D. (1999). The HaeIV restriction modification system of Haemophilus aegyptius is encoded by a single polypeptide. *Journal of Molecular Biology*, 293, 1055-1065.

[22] Kobayashi, I., Nobusato, A., Kobayashi-Takahashi, N., & Uchiyama, I. (1999). Shaping the genome- restriction-modification systems as mobile genetic elements. *Current Opinion in Genetics and Development*, 9, 649-656.

[23] Madhusoodanan, U. K., & Rao, D. N. (2010). Diversity of DNA methyltransferases that recognize asymmetric target sequences. *Critical Reviews in Biochemistry and Molecular Biology*, 45, 125-145.

[24] Yen, R., Vertino, P., Nelkin, B., et al. (1992). Isolation and characterization of the cDNA encoding human DNA methyltransferase. *Nucleic Acids Research*, 20, 2287-2291.

Section 3

# Protein Arginine Methylation in Mammals

Chapter 4

# Deciphering Protein Arginine Methylation in Mammals

Ruben Esse, Paula Leandro, Isabel Rivera, Isabel Tavares de Almeida, Henk J Blom and Rita Castro

Additional information is available at the end of the chapter

http://dx.doi.org/10.5772/51984

## 1. Introduction

The myriad of different post-translation modifications (PTMs) of proteins augments the information encoded by the human genome, from about 25,000 genes to over 1 million proteins that compose the human proteome [1, 2]. PTMs involve the chemical modification of target amino acid residues and, among others, include the addition of a methyl group to arginine residues, or arginine methylation, which is one of the most extensive protein modifications occurring in mammalian cells. During the last years, arginine methylation has attracted growing attention due to its impact on cellular function. Attesting to its biological importance, protein arginine methylation appears to be an evolutionarily ancient modification. Arginine methylation is now recognized as a widespread PTM that occurs on multiple classes of proteins with distinct cellular localizations. The arginine residue is unique among amino acids, since its guanidine group contains five potential hydrogen bond donors (Figure 1) positioned for interactions with hydrogen bond acceptors as DNA, RNA and proteins. Each addition of a methyl group removes a hydrogen donor, so the methylation of arginine residues in proteins will readily modulate their binding interactions and thus their physiological functions. Here, we provide an introduction to protein arginine methylation and discuss the current state of knowledge regarding this modification in mammals. In addition, we provide insight into how protein arginine methylation relates with the homocysteine metabolism. Lastly, we briefly discuss how protein arginine methylation may be disturbed in the context of hyperhomocysteinemia, sharing some of our recent results.

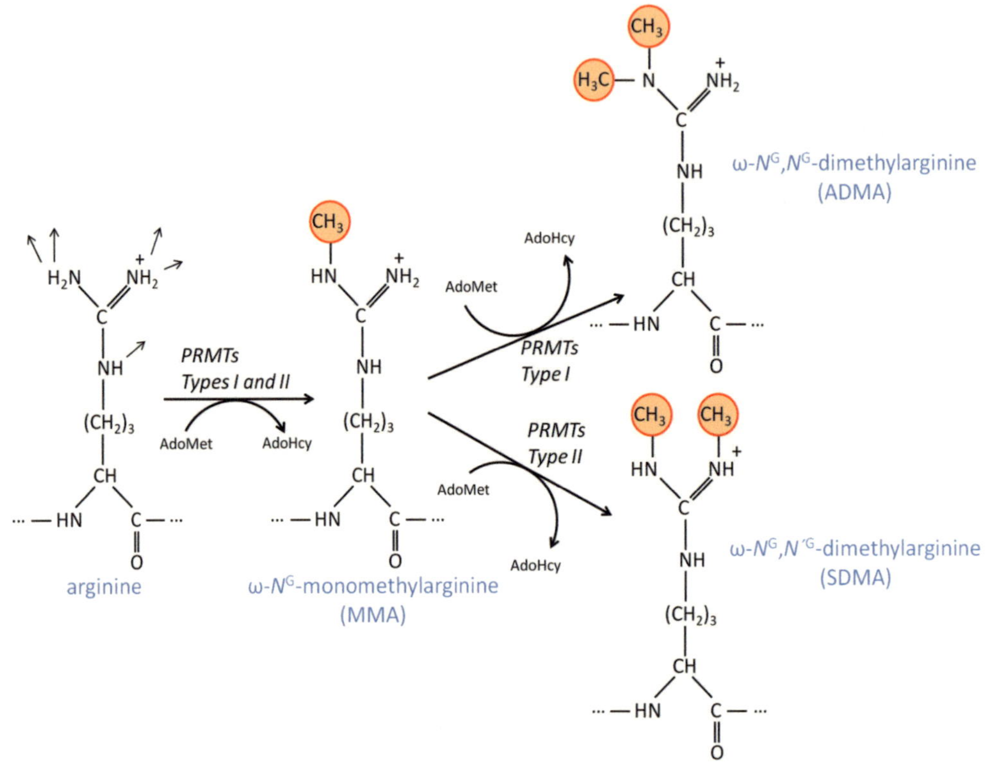


**Figure 1.** Methylation of the arginine side chain in proteins by protein arginine methyltransferases (PRMTs). The arginine residue holds 5 potential hydrogen bond donors. Mammalian PRMTs use the methyl group from a molecule of S-adenosyl-L-methionine (AdoMet) to form ω-NG-monomethylarginine (MMA). Subsequently, type I PRMTs add a methyl group to the same nitrogen atom forming ω-$N^G$,$N^G$-dimethylarginine (ADMA), whereas type II PRMTs generate ω-$N^G$,$N'^G$-dimethylarginine (SDMA).

## 2. The mammalian PRMTs: A brief overview

Methylation of arginine is catalyzed by protein arginine methyltransferases (PRMTs). PRMTs catalyze the transfer of methyl groups from the universal methyl donor, S-adenosyl-L-methionine (AdoMet), to the guanidine nitrogen atom of the target arginine residues within proteins [3].

The first documented protein with arginine methylation activity, then termed protein methylase I, was purified from calf thymus [4, 5]. Additional family members were subsequently identified and purified from different tissues and cell lines [6-16]. In mammals, PRMTs are grouped in two major classes: type I and type II. Both PRMT types catalyze the transfer of a single methyl group from AdoMet to an arginine residue in the target protein, producing ω-$N^G$-monomethylarginine (MMA) (Figure 1). However, differences exist when adding the second methyl group: type I members add it on the same previously methylated nitrogen, forming ω-$N^G$,$N^G$-dimethylarginine (ADMA), whereas type II members add it to the other N-terminal nitrogen of the arginine residue, yielding ω-$N^G$,$N'^G$-dimethylarginine (SDMA). Therefore, three distinct types of methylated arginine residues (MMA, ADMA and SDMA) are present on a horde of different proteins in the cytosol, nucleus and organelles of mammalian cells, ADMA being the most prevalent [3].

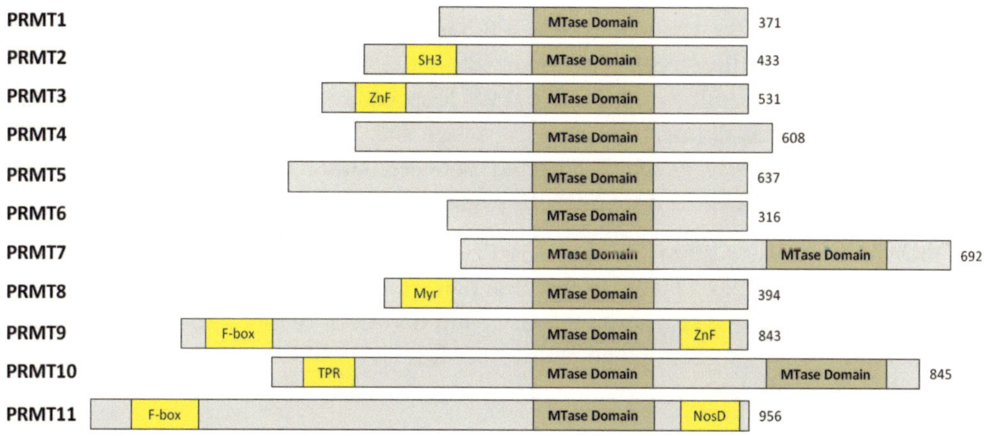


**Figure 2.** Schematic representation of the human protein arginine methyltransferase (PRMTs) family. For each member, the length of the longest isoform is indicated on the right. All members of the family possess at least one conserved MTase domain with signature motifs I, post-I, II, and III and a THW loop. Additional domains are marked in yellow boxes: SH3, ZnF (zinc finger), Myr (myristoylation), F-box, TPR (tetratricopeptide) and NosD (nitrous oxidase accessory protein). Adapted from [17].

To date, the human PRMT family includes eleven enzymes, termed from PRMT1 to PRMT11. Six are classified as type I (PRMT1, PRMT2, PRMT3, PRMT4, PRMT6 and PRMT8), and two as type II (PRMT5 and PRMT9). The classification of PRMT7 is controversial, as described below. The remaining two proteins, PRMT10 and PRMT11, were identified by their homology with PRMT7 and PRMT9, respectively, but their PRMT activity has not been sustained by experimental evidence [18, 19]. The genes encoding the different PRMTs are all located on different chromosomes, except the ones coding for PRMTs 1 and 4, which are both located in chromosome 19. Different splice variants coding for the corresponding isoforms are recognized for all PRMTs. Moreover, different cellular localizations are observed among them.

Although the human PRMT members vary in length from 316 to 956 amino acid residues, they all contain a highly conserved catalytic core region of around 300 residues (Figure 2). However, each PRMT presents a unique N-terminal region of variable length and distinct domain motifs, as for example PRMT3 and PRMT8 that bear a zinc finger (ZnF) and a myristoylation domain, respectively. Interestingly PRMT7 and PRMT10 exhibit a second catalytic domain. Until present, only the 3D structures of PRMT1, PRMT3 and PRMT5 were solved by X-ray crystallography [20-22]. These structures revealed that, also at the structural level, the catalytic core is highly conserved. Three structural regions were identified, namely, a methyltransferase (MTase) domain, a β-barrel domain unique to the PRMT family and a dimerization arm. The MTase domain is located in the N-terminal region of the catalytic core. It consists of a α/β Rossmann fold, typical of AdoMet-dependent methyltransferases, containing the conserved motifs I, post-I, II and III [23]. Motif I includes in its C-terminal part the signature sequences for most classes of MTases (GxGxG) involved in AdoMet binding. A relevant structural element localized in the MTase domain is the double-E loop (containing two invariant glutamate (E) residues). The C-terminal part of the catalytic core is a β-barrel domain containing 10 β-strands and a THW (threonine-histidine-tryptophan) loop (the most highly conserved sequence of this domain). Within the overall structure, the THW loop is located next to the double-E loop in the AdoMet binding domain, forming the active site. The dimerization arm is formed by a three-helix segment, which is inserted between strands 6 and 7 of the β-barrel domain and is responsible for dimerization, essential for enzyme activity [21].

Most PRMTs methylate arginine residues localized within glycine- and arginine-rich (GAR) sequences, but there are exceptions to this rule [24]. For instance, PRMT4 cannot methylate GAR motifs, and PRMT5 methylates both GAR and non-GAR motifs. Other factors, such as the accessibility of the target arginine and the conformation of the involved sequence, also govern substrate methylation.

PRMT1 was the first mammalian PRMT to be cloned [25] and is the predominant type I enzyme [26] found in all embryonic and adult tissues examined so far [27]. Due to alternative splicing, there are seven isoforms of the protein, all varying in their N-terminal domain, which are expressed in a tissue-specific manner and have distinct subcellular localization patterns [28]. PRMT1 has broad substrate specificity with over 40 targets, most being RNA processing proteins, and multiple interacting partners [29]. Targeted PRMT1 knockout in mice results in embryonic lethality, thus showing that loss of PRMT1 activity is incompatible with life [30].

PRMT2 transcripts have been found in most human tissues, with highest levels in heart, prostate, ovary and neuronal system [10, 31]. PRMT2 was found predominantly in the nucleus and to a lower degree in the cytoplasm of mammalian cells [17]. Only recently, based on the observation that it catalyzes the formation of MMA and ADMA residues on histone H4, PRMT2 was recognized as a type I enzyme [32]. PRMT2 may act in cooperation with PRMT8, since its SH3 domain binds the N-terminal domain of the latter enzyme [33]. Some of the known targets of PRMT2, besides the aforementioned histone H4 [32], are the STAT3 (signal transducer and activator of transcription 3) protein [34], the estrogen receptor alpha [35], the androgen receptor [31], the retinoblastoma gene product [36], and the heterogeneous nuclear ribonucleoprotein (hnRNP) E1B-AP5 [37]. In contrast with PRMT1 knockouts, *PRMT2 null* mice are viable and grow normally [34].

PRMT3 was first identified as a PRMT1-binding partner. It is widely expressed in human tissues and has a predominantly cytosolic subcellular localization [9]. PRMT3 possesses a zinc finger domain that assists in its binding to ribosomal proteins, including the S2 protein of the small ribosomal subunit. Mouse embryos with a targeted disruption of PRMT3 are small in size but survive after birth and attain a normal size in adulthood [38].

PRMT4, or CARM1, was first identified as a steroid receptor coactivator [11], providing the first evidence that protein arginine methylation participates in the regulation of gene expression (please, see sections *3.2.1 and 3.2.2.1.*). PRMT4 is ubiquitously expressed, exhibits a nuclear localization, and presents restricted substrate specificity. Specifically, in addition to nuclear hormone receptors and histones, it targets splicing factors [39, 40] and ATP-remodeling factors [41]. As opposed to most PRMTs, and as already referred, PRMT4 does not methylate GAR sequences. PRMT4 participates in many biological processes, including early T cell development [42], adipocyte differentiation [43], endochondral ossification [44], and proliferation and differentiation of pulmonary epithelial cells [45]. Embryos of *PRMT4 null* mice are small in size and die perinatally, thus showing the importance of PRMT4 activity to life [46].

PRMT5 was the first PRMT type II to be identified. PRMT5 is widely expressed in mammals, and more extensively in heart, muscle and testis [12]. PRMT5 is located both in the nucleus and in the cytoplasm [47]. Interestingly, PRMT5 is localized in the Golgi apparatus (GA) and its loss disrupts the GA structure, thereby suggesting that this enzyme plays a role in the maintenance of GA architecture [47]. In addition, PRMT5 is involved in the maintenance of the spliceosome integrity [48, 49]. PRMT5 targets histones, transcriptional elongation factors, chromatin remodelers and co-repressors [50]. In mice, loss of PRMT5 results in early embryonic lethality [51].

PRMT6 is the smallest family member (316 amino acids) and is localized predominantly in the nucleus [13]. Little is known about its properties, besides the fact that it produces asymmetrically dimethylated arginine residues. Similarly, PRMT6 functions are not completely understood. However, a role for PRMT6 in the regulation of cell proliferation and senescence, through transcriptional repression of tumor suppressor genes, has just been reported [52].

PRMT7 is present mainly in thymus, dendritic cells and testis [15, 53]. It has both nuclear and cytosolic localizations [15]. PRMT7 is involved in the modulation of sensitivity to DNA damaging agents [54, 55], methylation of male germline imprinted genes [56], and embryonic stem cell pluripotency [57]. Although Lee and colleagues characterized PRMT7 as a type II enzyme capable of forming SDMA [15], this finding was recently contested. In fact, Zurita-Lopez and coworkers have just reported that PRMT7 produces exclusively MMA residues, constituting the sole mammalian PRMT member with this type of methyltransferase activity [58].

PRMT8 is the type I PRMT with the highest degree of homology with PRMT1, but, unlike the latter, is mostly found in brain [14, 33]. PRMT8 possesses a myristoylation motif at its N-terminal end, which facilitates electrostatic interactions with membrane lipids and renders its distinct plasma membrane localization [14, 33]. Interestingly, its activity is regulated by the conformation of its N-terminal end, and removal of this domain results in enhancement of its enzymatic activity [33]. PRMT8 targets the pro-oncoprotein encoded by the Ewing sarcoma (EWS) gene, which contains a GAR motif in its C-terminal terminus [59].

PRMT9 was identified as a putative arginine methyltransferase and was classified as a type II PRMT due to its ability to catalyze the formation of MMA and ADMA [16]. However, there is limited sequence homology between PRMT9 and other human PRMTs [17]. Like most of the PRMTs, PRMT9 is widely expressed in mammalian tissues. PRMT9 has both nuclear and cytoplasmatic localization [17]. Several PRMT9 isoforms are recognized and alternate splicing may be an important mechanism to regulate methylation by PRMT9 [16]. So far, the only known substrates for PRMT9 are histones, the maltose binding protein and several peptides [16]. Disruption of the PRMT9 activity has been associated with inflammation of the middle ear, indicating the importance of methylation in disease [60, 61].

PRMT10 and PRMT11 were identified by their homology with PRMT7 and PRMT9, respectively, but, as referred to above, their PRMT activity has not been sustained by experimental evidence.

## 3. Physiological roles of protein arginine methylation

Following the advent of improved sensitivity conquered with mass spectrometry, current proteomic technologies have been uncovering an increasingly large fraction of the human proteome as substrates for PRMTs. Additionally, advances in molecular biology techniques and the generation of mice with targeted deletion of the various members of the PRMTs family have been disclosing the functional relevance of this PTM. As new substrates are being characterized, a broadening spectrum of PRMT-regulated cellular processes is being realized. So far, targeted cellular processes can be loosely categorized in RNA processing, transcriptional regulation, DNA repair and signal transduction.

### 3.1. RNA processing

Most proteins targeted by PRMTs are RNA-binding proteins (RBPs) harboring GAR motifs, which are involved in all aspects of RNA metabolism [29]. During eukaryotic transcription, RBPs associate with the nascent pre-mRNA allowing a series of RNA processing events to take place, including 5′-end capping, splicing, 3′-end cleavage and polyadenylation [62].

The importance of protein arginine methylation for RNA processing was first revealed by the observation that in HeLa cells splicing reactions were completely inhibited by a pan SDMA-specific antibody [63]. Subsequent studies have shown that a number of spliceosomal proteins are subject to both asymmetrical and symmetrical dimethylation, uncovering the crucial role of protein arginine methylation in the assembly of the spliceosome [64-66]. Other RBPs (hnRNP1, fibrillarin, nucleolin, HuD and HuR) have also been shown to contain methylated arginine residues [67-70]. Importantly, several of these RBPs lack proper subcellular localization if hypomethylated [71, 72]. For instance, asymmetrical dimethylation of specific arginine residues comprising the nuclear poly(A) binding protein prevents its transport to the cytoplasm [73].

### 3.2. Transcriptional regulation

Protein arginine methylation was initially detected in histones and studied mainly in relation to transcriptional regulation. More recently, the presence of methylated arginines in a large number of non-histonic proteins that also impact on transcriptional regulation was recognized.

#### *3.2.1. Histone arginine methylation*

Methylation of histones at arginine residues has been very well documented and subject to periodic review [74-76]. Therefore, a comprehensive review of histone arginine methylation would go beyond the scope of this paper and will be depicted in general terms only.

A few arginine residues within the N-terminal tail of histones H3, H4 and H2A are subject to methylation. The N-terminal tail of histone H3 contains several arginine residues that are targeted by different PRMTs,[1] while only one residue in histone H4 (H4R3) is subject to arginine methylation.[2] Since the first residues of the N-terminal tails of histones H4 and H2A are identical, residue 3 of histone H2A may be methylated in the same manner as H4R3 [76]. Interestingly, histone asymmetrical dimethylation generally activates gene transcription, while generation of SDMA is normally a repressive mark, although exceptions to this rule exist [75]. Arginine methylation occurring in histone tails may either affect other PTMs or influence the docking of key transcriptional effector molecules [76].

#### *3.2.2. Arginine methylation of non-histonic proteins*

In addition to histones, PRMTs also target other proteins that are involved in the transcriptional control of gene expression in mammals. These proteins include several types of transcription factors, transcription elongation factors, methyl DNA-binding proteins, and RNA polymerase II, as presented in the following sub-sections. In each, we choose to use some illustrative examples, rather than present an exhaustive list of all non-histonic targets for PRMTs that impact transcriptional regulation.

##### *3.2.2.1. Transcription factors*

Transcriptional coregulators are well recognized targets of PRMTs. Methylation of nuclear hormone receptors (NRs) illustrate well how arginine methylation of transcriptional coregulators may affect gene transcription. NRs are a large group of structurally related transcription factors that are responsible for mediating the biological effects of hormones. Transcription activation by NRs is a multistep process involving transcriptional coactivator proteins, as CREB-binding protein (CBP) and p300. These two co-activators have similar structures, sharing one N-terminal KIX domain that displays several arginine residues that are subject of methylation by PRMT4 [83]. CBP/p300 exhibits HAT (histone acetyl transfer-

---

1 In histone H3, residues 17 (H3R17) and 26 (H3R26) are methylated by PRMT4 [77], H3R2 is methylated by PRMT6 [78], and H3R8 is methylated by PRMT5 [79].

2 In histone H4, one arginine residue (H4R3) is subject to methylation. Asymmetric dimethylation of this residue is catalyzed by PRMT1, PRMT6 and PRMT8 [80-82], while symmetric dimethylation is catalyzed by PRMT5 and PRMT7 [56, 79].

ase) and HMT (histone methyl transferase) activities. Both CBP/p300 and PRMT4 are recruited to DNA by the NR bound to its ligand, where they stimulate transcription by remodeling chromatin through subsequent histone acetylation and methylation in the vicinity of hormone response element (HRE). Notably, it was shown that CBP/p300 activates NR-dependent gene transcription only if methylated in their KIX domain [83].

Peroxisome proliferator-activated receptor-gamma coactivator (PGC) 1 alpha (PGC-1$\alpha$) is other example of a coactivator of NRs whose activity was clearly shown to be dependent on PRMT activity. PGC-1$\alpha$ signaling is extremely important in the heart, where PGC-1$\alpha$ is highly expressed and controls cardiac energy pathways during development and in response to stressors. Interestingly, it was shown that PRMT1 activates PGC-1$\alpha$ through its methylation at several arginine residues [84]. Remarkably, experimentally based evidence has recently linked decreased levels of methyl-PGC-1$\alpha$ due to decreased PRMT1 activity to cardiomyopathy in mice [85].

Arginine methylation may also impact transcriptional activity by targeting transcription factors that bind directly to DNA, like the STAT1 protein. STAT1 (signal transducer and activator of transcription) is a member of the STAT family and mediates the cellular response to cytokines and growth factors thus regulating many aspects of growth, survival and differentiation of cells. After activation by cytoplasmic phosphorylation, STAT1 migrates to the nucleus, where it binds to the enhancer elements of response genes. The N-terminal region of STAT1 comprises a conserved arginine residue that was shown to be a PRMT1 target [86]. Inhibition of PRMT1 activity hinders the DNA binding activity of STAT1 and STAT1-mediated transcription.

#### *3.2.2.2. Transcription elongation factors*

Activity of PRMTs may also affect transcription by marking transcription elongation factors, like Spt5. The Spt5 protein displays several KOW domains, which contain consensus sites for arginine methylation and overlap the RNA polymerase II binding domain. Notably, Spt5 can be methylated in its RNA polymerase II binding domain by PRMT1 or PRMT5 and this methylation may cause transcriptional pausing [87].

#### *3.2.2.3. Methyl DNA-binding proteins*

PRMTs may also participate in the DNA methylation system of chromatin control. DNA methylation, an important regulator of gene transcription, occurs within a CpG context in differentiated mammalian cells. MBD2 is a methyl DNA-associated protein that docks methylated CpGs in DNA and negatively affects gene transcription by recruiting proteins that repress chromatin. Interestingly, both PRMT1 and PRMT5 methylate MBD2, thereby impairing the transcription repression function of MBD2 [88].

#### *3.2.2.4. RNA polymerase II*

In eukaryotic cells, the C-terminal domain (CTD) of RNA polymerase II provides a platform to recruit different regulators of the transcription apparatus. Recently, arginine methylation of a single residue in the CTD (R1810) was documented and implied in the regulation of transcription driven by RNA polymerase II [89].

### 3.3. DNA repair

Genome integrity is constantly subject to monitoring by a complicated and entangled network of mechanisms collectively termed as DNA damage response (DDR). Some proteins integrating this system are known targets of PRMTs. Mre11 is part of a complex that is critically implicated in homologous recombination repair of DNA double strand breaks. This protein harbors a GAR motif that is methylated by PRMT1, allowing its association with nuclear structures and recruitment to sites of DNA damage [90], as well as its exonuclease activity [91]. PRMT5-induced methylation of Rad9, a cell cycle checkpoint protein, enables activation of Chk1, an important downstream checkpoint effector, and loss of Rad9 methylation leads to S/M and G2/M checkpoint defects [92]. DNA polymerase beta, which participates in DNA base excision repair, is methylated by PRMT6, which enhances its binding to DNA and its processivity [93].

### 3.4. Signal transduction

In addition to regulating numerous nuclear processes, arginine methylation is involved in conveying information from the cell surface, through the cytoplasm, to the nucleus. For instance, the implication of protein arginine methylation in interferon (IFN) signaling has been substantiated by the fact that PRMT1 interacts with the cytoplasmic domain of the type I IFN receptor [94], and that its depletion impairs the biological activity of type I IFN [95]. The involvement of arginine methylation within T cell receptor signaling cascades is also gaining prominence. In fact, stimulation of T helper cells induces arginine methylation of several cytoplasmic proteins, which when inhibited causes signaling defects in CD4 T cells and severe immunosuppression [96]. PRMT1-mediated methylation also impacts insulin signaling and glucose uptake in skeletal muscle cells [97]. Estrogen rapid signaling is similarly mediated by PRMT1, which targets estrogen receptor alpha (ER-$\alpha$) [98]. PRMT1 also methylates FoxO1, a member of the mammalian forkhead transcription factors of class O (FoxO) subfamily [99]. These transcription factors are involved in many vital processes (e.g. apoptosis, cell-cycle control, glucose metabolism, oxidative stress resistance and longevity) and, in response to insulin or several growth factors, are negatively regulated through phosphorylation by serine-threonine kinase Akt/protein kinase B (Akt/PKB) (that results in their export from the nucleus to the cytoplasm) [100]. PRMT1 methylates FoxO1 at arginine residues within the Akt consensus motif, blocking the Akt-mediated phosphorylation and augmenting FoxO1 target gene expression [99]. Another Akt-target protein is BCL-2, antagonist of cell death, which is also methylated by PRMT1 on its consensus phosphorylation motif [101]. Methylation-phosphorylation switches are presently regarded as paradigms operating in signal transduction pathways and other physiological processes, since numerous other examples of this crosstalk have been described. The implication of PRMTs other than PRMT1 in signaling routes has not been well studied. The association of PRMT8 with the plasma membrane provides a clue that this enzyme may facilitate the triggering of a signaling pathway [14]. A recent study has uncovered that PRMT5 regulates the amplitude of the RAS to extracellular signal-regulated kinase (ERK) signal transduction cascade, impacting on cell fate decision [102].

# 4. Modulation of PRMTs activity

PRMTs associate with proteins that may change their activity or substrate specificity. Examples of proteins that enhance the activity of a specific PRMT are: BTG1 (B-cell translocation gene 1 protein), BTG2 (B-cell translocation gene 2 protein) and hCAF1 (chemokine receptor 4-associated factor 1), which associate with PRMT1 [25, 103]; the chromatin remodelers BRG and BRM, which enhance PRMT5 activity [79]; and BORIS (brother of the regulator of imprinted sites), which has been reported to elevate PRMT7 activity [56]. In contrast, tumor suppressor DAL-1 inhibits the activity of PRMT3 *in vitro* and *in vivo* [104]. PRMT4 association with other proteins within the nucleosomal methylation activator complex (NUMAC) enhances its ability to methylate nucleosomal histone H3, while the free enzyme preferentially methylates free core histone H3 [41]. Similarly, PRMT5 association with COPR5 shifts its preferential target from H3R8 to H4R3 [105].

PRMT activity may also be modulated by PTMs. For instance, several PRMTs are automethylated, but the relevancy of this phenomenon is not acquainted [33]. PRMT4 phosphorylation during mitosis prevents its homodimerization, thereby decreasing its activity [106]. Additionally, PRMT4 phosphorylation abolishes the binding of AdoMet and thus its activity, and promotes its cytoplasm localization [107].

# 5. The reversibility of protein arginine methylation: A fast-growing field of knowledge

An important question under recent investigation was whether demethylation reactions occurred to reverse the effects of protein arginine methylation. Initial studies indicated that this PTM was a permanent mark on proteins. As such, the only way to reverse the effects of the presence of this methyl mark would be to degrade the protein to its amino acid components and then make a new unmethylated version by protein synthesis [108]. However, the long-standing notion that arginine methylation is a stable covalent mark has been challenged in recent years due to the discovery of two types of enzymes that can remove methyl groups from arginine residues in histones by demethylation and citrullination (Figure 3).

The first evidence of demethylation of arginine residues came from a study by Chang and coworkers [110] that reported that JMJD6, a Jumonji domain-containing protein, demethylates H3R2 and H4R3 residues that are either asymmetrically or symmetrically dimethylated (Figure 3A). Mass spectrometry of a peptide containing dimethylated arginine residues, which was incubated with JMJD6 and then immunoprecipitated with a monomethylarginine specific antibody, revealed that the enzyme catalyzed the loss of one methyl group

http://dx.doi.org/10.5772/51984

from the methylated substrate. Current view holds that JMJD6 may be a bifunctional enzyme, catalyzing either demethylation or lysyl-hydroxylation reactions [111].

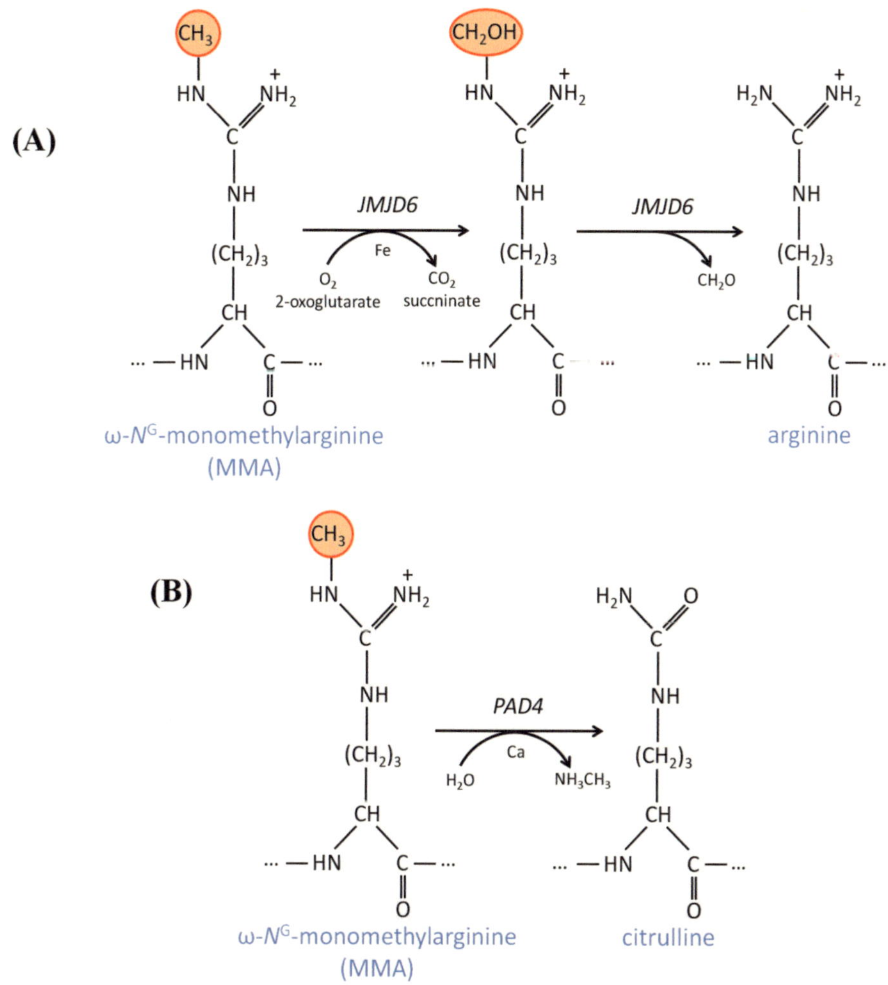


**Figure 3.** Reversing or annulling protein arginine methylation: demethylation and citrullination reactions. (A) Demethylation of a monomethylarginine (MMA) residue by JMJD6. (B) Citrullination of a MMA residue by PAD4. This reaction antagonizes arginine methylation, since it is not reversible. Adapted from [109].

Monomethylated arginine residues may be converted to citrulline by deimination, a modification catalyzed by peptidylarginine deiminases (PADs). In this process, the guanidinium side chain of an arginine residue is hydrolyzed and methylamine released [112] (Figure 3B). To date, five human PAD homologs have been identified and designated as PAD1-4 and PAD6. Most mechanistic studies on PADs have been performed with PAD4. PADs may be activated by calcium, which seems to be essential for the catalysis to occur [113, 114]. Citrulline residues are found with great extent in histones H2A, H3, and H4 [115]. Importantly, the sites of deimination by PAD4 overlap those of arginine methylation on these histones [112], and an increase in histone citrulline levels correlates with a decrease in methylated arginine levels [116, 117]. However, PADs only catalyze the deimination of MMA residues, and no enzyme has been identified that can convert citrulline back to arginine. Thus, citrullination blocks remethylation, adding a new layer to the regulation of protein arginine methylation [118, 119].

## 6. The disposal of methylated arginine residues / ADMA and vascular disease

Proteolysis of arginine-methylated proteins results in free MMA, ADMA and SDMA, which are secreted to the extracellular space [120]. These metabolites can then be taken up by other cells via carriers of the cationic amino acid family [121] or eliminated by renal excretion [122]. In addition, ADMA can be hydrolyzed to citrulline and dimethylamine, by dimethylarginine dimethylaminohydrolase (DDAH), which is present in kidney, liver and vasculature [123]. Interestingly, MMA and ADMA are endogenous inhibitors of nitric oxide (NO) production in endothelial cells. Due to the paramount role of NO on the homeostasis of the vascular endothelium, ADMA, which is present in plasma in much larger quantities than MMA, has emerged as a novel risk factor in the setting of endothelial dysfunction and vascular disease [124]. As stated before, PRMTs are ubiquitously expressed and participate in crucial cellular processes. Thus, deregulation of these enzymes is likely implicated in the pathogenesis of a number of different diseases, including cardiovascular disease. In addition to the intricate set of potential interactions between protein arginine methylation and cardiovascular disease, we must add ADMA, an additional player that may impact the cardiovascular system.

## 7. Protein arginine hypomethylation in the context of hyperhomocysteinemia: "Another brick in the wall"?

As illustrated in Figure 1, the methyl group responsible for the establishment of protein arginine methylation patterns by PRMTs originates from AdoMet, an intermediate in the homocysteine metabolism. Therefore, protein arginine methylation and homocysteine metabolism are biochemically linked (Figure 4). In addition to protein arginine methylation, AdoMet serves as the methyl donor for more than one hundred cellular methyl transfer reactions, including the methylation of other residues in proteins (namely, histidine and lysine), DNA and RNA. Following the transfer of the methyl group, AdoMet is converted into S-adenosyl homocysteine (AdoHcy). AdoHcy is further converted into homocysteine and adenosine by AdoHcy hydrolase, which is widely distributed in mammalian tissues [125]. This reaction is reversible and strongly favors AdoHcy synthesis rather than its hydrolysis; however, both homocysteine and adenosine are rapidly removed under physiological condi-

http://dx.doi.org/10.5772/51984

tions, favoring the hydrolysis reaction [126]. Nevertheless, if homocysteine accumulates, AdoHcy will accumulate as well [125].

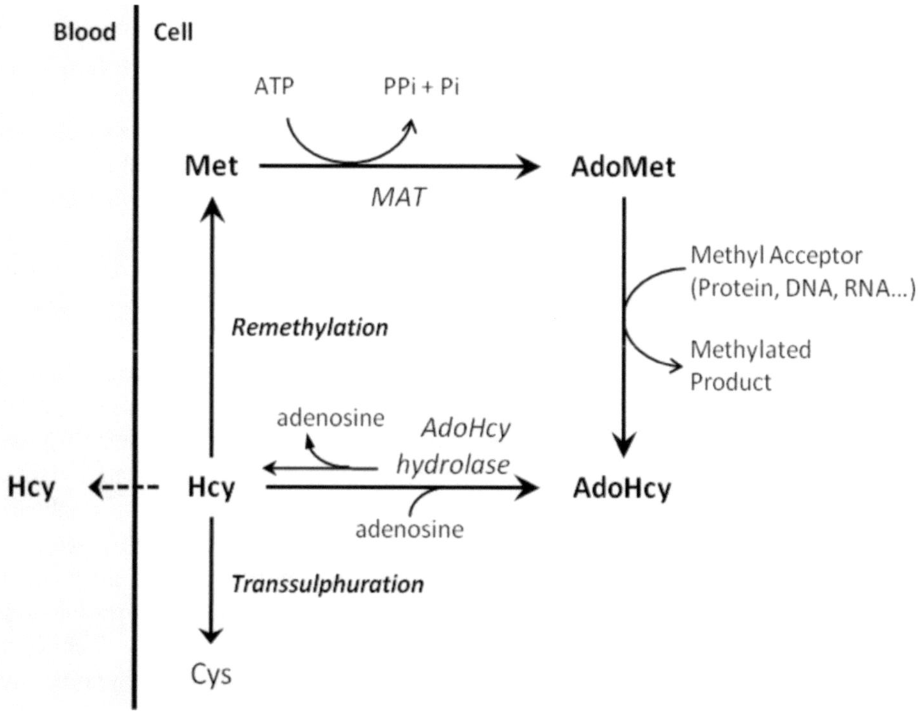


**Figure 4.** Simplified homocysteine metabolism. Homocysteine (Hcy) results from methionine metabolism as a by-product of cellular transmethylation reactions. Methionine (Met) is the "entry" point of this pathway and is provided by diet and protein breakdown. S-Adenosylmethionine (AdoMet) is first synthesized from Met by methionine adenosyltransferase (MAT). AdoMet is the methyl group donor in a wide variety of transmethylation reactions, being converted to S-Adenosylhomocysteine (AdoHcy). AdoHcy is subsequently hydrolyzed to Hcy and adenosine by AdoHcy hydrolase. Hcy can then be converted to cysteine (Cys) through the transsulphuration pathway, remethylated back to methionine or exported.

Despite recent controversy, elevated levels of homocysteine in plasma (or hyperhomocysteinemia) are accepted as a risk factor for cardiovascular disease [127, 128]. Notably, despite several potential mechanisms underlying this association having been the focus of intense research, the subject remains to be fully understood [125]. Our group has been actively studying whether a hypomethylating environment associated with hyperhomocysteinemia contributes to the vascular toxicity of homocysteine [129-133]. AdoHcy is a competitive inhibitor of most AdoMet-dependent methyltransferases, since it binds to their active sites with higher affinity than AdoMet [134]. As such, the ratio AdoMet/AdoHcy is taken as an index of cellular methylation capacity. As mentioned above, if homocysteine accumulates, AdoHcy will accumulate as well. Thus, increased homocysteine may be regarded as a cellular hypomethylation effector, via AdoHcy accumulation.

We have demonstrated that patients with vascular disease present increased levels of both plasma homocysteine and intracellular AdoHcy, together with decreased DNA methylation [129]. Other studies also supported a role for hyperhomocysteinemia in modulating epigenetic mechanisms [135-138]. Additionally, we confirmed, *in vitro*, the AdoHcy ability to decrease global DNA methylation status [131]. Currently, we are studying whether, in addition to DNA, protein arginine methylation extend is are also decreased by AdoHcy accumulation. Supporting this possibility, results from kinetic studies regarding competitive inhibition of several methyltransferases by AdoHcy sustain that this metabolite is a stronger inhibitor of PRMT1 than of DNA methyltransferase 1, the enzyme responsible for the maintenance of DNA methylation patterns [6, 139]. Interestingly, we observed that intracellular AdoHcy accumulation lowered ADMA production by human vascular endothelial cells accumulation [133]. This observation led us to postulate that this effect was due to AdoHcy-induced protein arginine hypomethylation. Supporting this possibility, we subsequently found decreased levels of protein-incorporated ADMA in human vascular endothelial cells under AdoHcy intracellular accumulation ([140] and Esse R et *al.*, manuscript 1 under submission). Moreover, we observed that this effect was more pronounced than the parallel reduction in global DNA methylation patterns. Therefore, we have concluded that AdoHcy build-up affects protein arginine methylation to a higher extent than DNA methylation. Importantly, this observation suggests that protein arginine methylation is more easily affected than DNA methylation in the context of hyperhomocysteinemia. Very recently, we have also assessed protein arginine methylation status in an animal model of diet-induced hyperhomocysteinemia and found that increased homocysteine is associated with protein arginine hypomethylation, although in a tissue-dependent manner ([141] and Esse R *et al.*, manuscript 2 under submission). Specifically, we found global protein arginine hypomethylation in heart and in brain from hyperhomocysteinemic rats, while methylation of hepatic proteins was not affected. Currently, we are undertaking both *in vitro* and *in vivo* studies to identify proteins sensitive to AdoHcy-induced hypomethylation, and to assess the impact of its different methylation states on vascular homeostasis. Actually, differential methylation of proteins may well play a role in pathologies related to elevated homocysteine, including vascular disease.

## 8. Conclusions

The field of protein arginine methylation has been enjoying widespread interest in the scientific community, owing to the recent development of molecular biology techniques and mass spectrometry instrumentation. It is now clear that this common PTM impacts crucial biological functions, including RNA processing, transcriptional regulation, DNA repair and signal transduction. Yet, information is still scant regarding some important issues of protein arginine methylation, namely its regulation by other PTMs, how it affects interaction with the protein ligands, and what are the factors governing the specificity of the different PRMTs towards the target protein. Importantly, protein arginine methylation, which was considered a static modification during a long time, is now recognized as a reversible and dynamic modification, increasing the complexity of the interplay between DNA, proteins and vital cellular process. Nevertheless, the characterization of enzymes that reverse and block protein arginine methylation has just commenced. Moreover, the pathological implications of protein arginine methylation disturbance have not been exhaustively explored. The methyl group marking of arginine residues originates from AdoMet, an intermediate in homocysteine metabolism. Thus, the metabolism of this amino acid and protein arginine methylation are biochemically linked. Homocysteine elevation relates with an increased risk of vascular disease and others pathologies. Notably, the potential detrimental effect of increased circulating homocysteine on protein arginine methylation status may constitute an additional molecular mechanism contributing to disease, and, as such, warrants further investigation.

## Acknowledgments

This work was supported by Fundação para a Ciência e a Tecnologia (FCT, Portugal) grants (SFRH/BD/48585/2008 to RE, and PTDC/SAU-ORG/112683/2009 to RC).

## Author details

Ruben Esse[1], Paula Leandro[1,2], Isabel Rivera[1,2], Isabel Tavares de Almeida[1,2], Henk J Blom[3,4] and Rita Castro[1,2*]

*Address all correspondence to: rcastro@ff.ul.pt

1 Institute for Medicines and Pharmaceutical Sciences (iMed.UL), Faculty of Pharmacy, University of Lisbon, Lisbon, Portugal

2 Department of Biochemistry and Human Biology, Faculty of Pharmacy, University of Lisbon, Lisbon, Portugal

3 Metabolic Unit, Department of Clinical Chemistry, VU University Medical Center, Amsterdam,, The Netherlands

4 Institute for Cardiovascular Research ICaR-VU, VU University Medical Center, Amsterdam, The Netherlands

## References

[1] Human Genome Sequencing Consortium. Finishing the euchromatic sequence of the human genome. Nature. 2004;431:931-945.

[2] Jensen ON. Modification-specific proteomics: characterization of post-translational modifications by mass spectrometry. Curr Opin Chem Biol. 2004;8:33-41.

[3] Bedford MT, Richard S. Arginine methylation an emerging regulator of protein function. Mol Cell. 2005;18:263-272.

[4] Paik WK, Kim S. Enzymatic methylation of protein fractions from calf thymus nuclei. Biochem Biophys Res Commun. 1967;29:14-20.

[5] Paik WK, Kim S. Protein methylase I. Purification and properties of the enzyme. J Biol Chem. 1968;243:2108-2114.

[6] Ghosh SK, Paik WK, Kim S. Purification and molecular identification of two protein methylases I from calf brain. Myelin basic protein- and histone-specific enzyme. J Biol Chem. 1988;263:19024-19033.

[7] Rawal N, Rajpurohit R, Paik WK, Kim S. Purification and characterization of S-adenosylmethionine-protein-arginine N-methyltransferase from rat liver. Biochem J. 1994;300:483-489.

[8] Liu Q, Dreyfuss G. In vivo and in vitro arginine methylation of RNA-binding proteins. Mol Cell Biol. 1995;15:2800-2808.

[9] Tang J, Gary JD, Clarke S, Herschman HR. PRMT 3, a type I protein arginine N-methyltransferase that differs from PRMT1 in its oligomerization, subcellular localization, substrate specificity, and regulation. J Biol Chem. 1998;273:16935-16945.

[10] Katsanis N, Yaspo ML, Fisher EM. Identification and mapping of a novel human gene, HRMT1L1, homologous to the rat protein arginine N-methyltransferase 1 (PRMT1) gene. Mamm Genome. 1997;8:526-529.

[11] Chen D, Ma H, Hong H, Koh SS, Huang SM, Schurter BT, Aswad DW, Stallcup MR. Regulation of transcription by a protein methyltransferase. Science. 1999;284:2174-2177.

[12] Pollack BP, Kotenko SV, He W, Izotova LS, Barnoski BL, Pestka S. The human homologue of the yeast proteins Skb1 and Hsl7p interacts with Jak kinases and contains protein methyltransferase activity. J Biol Chem. 1999;274:31531-31542.

[13] Frankel A, Yadav N, Lee J, Branscombe TL, Clarke S, Bedford MT. The novel human protein arginine N-methyltransferase PRMT6 is a nuclear enzyme displaying unique substrate specificity. J Biol Chem. 2002;277:3537-3543.

[14] Lee J, Sayegh J, Daniel J, Clarke S, Bedford MT. PRMT8, a new membrane-bound tissue-specific member of the protein arginine methyltransferase family. J Biol Chem. 2005;280:32890-32896.

[15] Lee JH, Cook JR, Yang ZH, Mirochnitchenko O, Gunderson SI, Felix AM, Herth N, Hoffmann R, Pestka S. PRMT7, a new protein arginine methyltransferase that synthesizes symmetric dimethylarginine. J Biol Chem. 2005;280:3656-3664.

[16] Cook JR, Lee JH, Yang ZH, Krause CD, Herth N, Hoffmann R, Pestka S. FBXO11/PRMT9, a new protein arginine methyltransferase, symmetrically dimethylates arginine residues. Biochem Biophys Res Commun. 2006;342:472-481.

[17] Wolf SS. The protein arginine methyltransferase family: an update about function, new perspectives and the physiological role in humans. Cell Mol Life Sci. 2009;66:2109-2121.

[18] Krause CD, Yang ZH, Kim YS, Lee JH, Cook JR, Pestka S. Protein arginine methyltransferases: evolution and assessment of their pharmacological and therapeutic potential. Pharmacol Ther. 2007;113:50-87.

[19] Pal S, Sif S. Interplay between chromatin remodelers and protein arginine methyltransferases. J Cell Physiol. 2007;213:306-315.

[20] Zhang X, Zhou L, Cheng X. Crystal structure of the conserved core of protein arginine methyltransferase PRMT3. EMBO J. 2000;19:3509-3519.

[21] Zhang X, Cheng X. Structure of the predominant protein arginine methyltransferase PRMT1 and analysis of its binding to substrate peptides. Structure. 2003;11:509-520.

[22] Sun L, Wang M, Lv Z, Yang N, Liu Y, Bao S, Gong W, Xu R. M. Structural insights into protein arginine symmetric dimethylation by PRMT5. Proc Natl Acad Sci U S A. 2011;108:20538-20543.

[23] Kozbial PZ, Mushegian AR. Natural history of S-adenosylmethionine-binding proteins. BMC Struct Biol. 2005;5:19.

[24] Najbauer J, Johnson BA, Young AL, Aswad DW. Peptides with sequences similar to glycine, arginine-rich motifs in proteins interacting with RNA are efficiently recognized by methyltransferase(s) modifying arginine in numerous proteins. J Biol Chem. 1993;268:10501-10509.

[25] Lin WJ, Gary JD, Yang MC, Clarke S, Herschman HR. The mammalian immediate-early TIS21 protein and the leukemia-associated BTG1 protein interact with a protein-arginine N-methyltransferase. J Biol Chem. 1996;271:15034-15044.

[26] Tang J, Frankel A, Cook RJ, Kim S, Paik WK, Williams KR, Clarke S, Herschman HR. PRMT1 is the predominant type I protein arginine methyltransferase in mammalian cells. J Biol Chem. 2000;275:7723-7730.

[27] Pawlak MR, Scherer CA, Chen J, Roshon MJ, Ruley HE. Arginine N-methyltransferase 1 is required for early post implantation mouse development, but cells deficient in the enzyme are viable. Mol Cell Biol. 2000;20:4859-4869.

[28] Goulet I, Gauvin G, Boisvenue S, Cote J. Alternative splicing yields protein arginine methyltransferase 1 isoforms with distinct activity, substrate specificity, and subcellular localization. J Biol Chem. 2007;282:33009-33021.

[29] Pahlich S, Zakaryan RP, Gehring H. Protein arginine methylation: Cellular functions and methods of analysis. Biochim Biophys Acta. 2006;1764:1890-1903.

[30] Yu Z, Chen T, Hebert J, Li E, Richard S. A mouse PRMT1 null allele defines an essential role for arginine methylation in genome maintenance and cell proliferation. Mol Cell Biol. 2009;29:2982-2996.

[31] Meyer R, Wolf SS, Obendorf M. PRMT2, a member of the protein arginine methyltransferase family, is a coactivator of the androgen receptor. J. Steroid Biochem. Mol Biol. 2007;107:1-14.

[32] Lakowski TM, Frankel A. Kinetic analysis of human protein arginine N-methyltransferase 2: formation of monomethyl- and asymmetric dimethyl-arginine residues on histone H4. Biochem J. 2009;421:253-261.

[33] Sayegh J, Webb K, Cheng D, Bedford MT, Clarke SG. Regulation of protein arginine methyltransferase 8 (PRMT8) activity by its N-terminal domain. J Biol Chem. 2007;282:36444-36453.

[34] Iwasaki H, Kovacic JC, Olive M, Beers JK, Yoshimoto T, Crook MF, Tonelli LH, Nabel EG. Disruption of protein arginine N-methyltransferase 2 regulates leptin signaling and produces leanness in vivo through loss of STAT3 methylation. Circ Res. 2010;107:992-1001.

[35] Qi C, Chang J, Zhu Y, Yeldandi AV, Rao SM, Zhu YJ. Identification of protein arginine methyltransferase 2 as a coactivator for estrogen receptor alpha. J Biol Chem. 2002;277:28624-28630.

[36] Yoshimoto T, Boehm M, Olive M, Crook MF, San H, Langenickel T, Nabel EG. The arginine methyltransferase PRMT2 binds RB and regulates E2F function. Exp Cell Res. 2006;312:2040-2053.

[37] Kzhyshkowska J, Schutt H, Liss M, Kremmer E, Stauber R, Wolf H, Dobner T. Heterogeneous nuclear ribonucleoprotein E1B-AP5 is methylated in its Arg-Gly-Gly (RGG) box and interacts with human arginine methyltransferase HRMT1L1. Biochem J. 2001;358:305-314.

[38] Swiercz R, Cheng D, Kim D, Bedford MT. Ribosomal protein rpS2 is hypomethylated in PRMT3-deficient mice. J Biol Chem. 2007;282:16917-16923.

[39] Cheng D, Cote J, Shaaban S, Bedford MT. The arginine methyltransferase CARM1 regulates the coupling of transcription and mRNA processing. Mol Cell 2007;25:71-83.

[40] Feng Q, Yi P, Wong J, O'Malley BW. Signaling within a coactivator complex: methylation of SRC-3/AIB1 is a molecular switch for complex disassembly. Mol Cell Biol. 2006;26:7846-7857.

[41] Xu W, Cho H, Kadam S, Banayo EM, Anderson S, Yates JR 3rd, Emerson BM, Evans RM. A methylation-mediator complex in hormone signaling. Genes Dev. 2004;18:144-156.

[42] Kim J, Lee J, Yadav N, Wu Q, Carter C, Richard S, Richie E, Bedford MT. Loss of CARM1 results in hypomethylation of thymocyte cyclic AMP-regulated phosphoprotein and deregulated early T cell development. J Biol Chem. 2004;279:25339-25344.

[43] Yadav N, Cheng D, Richard S, Morel M, Iyer VR, Aldaz CM, Bedford MT. CARM1 promotes adipocyte differentiation by coactivating PPAR gamma. EMBO Rep. 2008;9:193-198.

[44] Ito T, Yadav N, Lee J, Furumatsu T, Yamashita S, Yoshida K, Taniguchi N, Hashimoto M, Tsuchiya M, Ozaki T, Lotz M, Bedford MT, Asahara H. Arginine methyltransferase CARM1/PRMT4 regulates endochondral ossification. BMC Dev Biol. 2009;9:47. (doi:10.1186/1471-213X-9-47)

[45] O'Brien KB, berich-Jorda M, Yadav N, Kocher O, Diruscio A, Ebralidze A, Levantini E, Sng NJ, Bhasin M, Caron T, Kim D, Steidl U, Huang G, Halmos B, Rodig SJ, Bedford MT, Tenen DG, Kobayashi S. CARM1 is required for proper control of proliferation and differentiation of pulmonary epithelial cells. Development. 2010;137:2147-2156.

[46] Yadav N, Lee J, Kim J, Shen J, Hu MC, Aldaz CM, Bedford MT. Specific protein methylation defects and gene expression perturbations in coactivator-associated arginine methyltransferase 1-deficient mice. Proc Natl Acad Sci U S A. 2003;100:6464-6468.

[47] Zhou Z, Sun X, Zou Z, Sun L, Zhang T, Guo S, Wen Y, Liu L, Wang Y, Qin J, Li L, Gong W, Bao S. PRMT5 regulates Golgi apparatus structure through methylation of the golg in GM130. Cell Res. 2010;20:1023-1033.

[48] Friesen WJ, Paushkin S, Wyce A, Massenet S, Pesiridis GS, Van DG, Rappsilber J, Mann M, Dreyfuss G. The methylosome, a 20S complex containing JBP1 and pICln, produces dimethylarginine-modified Sm proteins. Mol Cell Biol. 2001;21:8289-8300.

[49] Meister G, Fischer U. Assisted RNP assembly: SMN and PRMT5 complexes cooperate in the formation of spliceosomal UsnRNPs. EMBO J. 2002;21:5853-5863.

[50] Karkhanis V, Hu YJ, Baiocchi RA, Imbalzano AN, Sif S. Versatility of PRMT5-induced methylation in growth control and development. Trends Biochem Sci. 2011;36:633-641.

[51] Tee WW, Pardo M, Theunissen TW, Yu L, Choudhary JS, Hajkova P, Surani MA. Prmt5 is essential for early mouse development and acts in the cytoplasm to maintain ES cell pluripotency. Genes Dev. 2010;24:2772-2777.

[52] Stein C, Riedl S, Rüthnick D, Nötzold RR, Bauer UM. The arginine methyltransferase PRMT6 regulates cell proliferation and senescence through transcriptional repression of tumor suppressor genes. Nucleic Acids Res. 2012; Aug 16. [Epub ahead of print]

[53] Miranda TB, Miranda M, Frankel A, Clarke S. PRMT7 is a member of the protein arginine methyltransferase family with a distinct substrate specificity. J Biol Chem. 2004;279:22902-22907.

[54] Bleibel WK, Duan S, Huang RS, Kistner EO, Shukla SJ, Wu X, Badner JA, Dolan ME. Identification of genomic regions contributing to etoposide-induced cytotoxicity. Hum Genet. 2009;125:173-180.

[55] Verbiest V, Montaudon D, Tautu MT, Moukarzel J, Portail JP, Markovits J, Robert J, Ichas F, Pourquier P. Protein arginine (N)-methyl transferase 7 (PRMT7) as a potential target for the sensitization of tumor cells to camptothecins. FEBS Lett. 2008;582:1483-1489.

[56] Jelinic P, Stehle JC, Shaw P. The testis-specific factor CTCFL cooperates with the protein methyltransferase PRMT7 in H19 imprinting control region methylation. PLoS Biol. 2006;4:e355.

[57] Buhr N, Carapito C, Schaeffer C, Kieffer E, Van DA, Viville S. Nuclear proteome analysis of undifferentiated mouse embryonic stem and germ cells. Electrophoresis. 2008;29:2381-2390.

[58] Zurita-Lopez CI, Sandberg T, Kelly R, Clarke SG. Human protein arginine methyltransferase 7 (PRMT7) is a type III enzyme forming omega-NG-monomethylated arginine residues. J Biol Chem. 2012;287:7859-7870.

[59] Kim JD, Kako K, Kakiuchi M, Park GG, Fukamizu A. EWS is a substrate of type I protein arginine methyltransferase, PRMT8. Int J Mol Med. 2008;22:309-315.

[60] Hardisty-Hughes RE, Tateossian H, Morse SA, Romero MR, Middleton A, Tymowska-Lalanne Z, Hunter AJ, Cheeseman M, Brown SD. A mutation in the F-box gene, Fbxo11, causes otitis media in the Jeff mouse. Hum Mol Genet. 2006;15:3273-3279.

[61] Segade F, Daly KA, Allred D, Hicks PJ, Cox M, Brown M, Hardisty-Hughes RE, Brown SD, Rich SS, Bowden DW. Association of the FBXO11 gene with chronic otitis media with effusion and recurrent otitis media: the Minnesota COME/ROM Family Study. Arch Otolaryngol Head Neck Surg. 2006;132:729-733.

[62] Licatalosi DD, Darnell RB. RNA processing and its regulation: global insights into biological networks. Nat Rev Genet. 2010;11:75-87.

[63] Boisvert FM, Cote J, Boulanger MC, Cleroux P, Bachand F, Autexier C, Richard S. Symmetrical dimethylarginine methylation is required for the localization of SMN in Cajal bodies and pre-mRNA splicing. J Cell Biol. 2002;159:957-969.

[64] Brahms H, Raymackers J, Union A, de Keyser F, Meheus L, Lührmann R. The C-terminal RG dipeptide repeats of the spliceosomal Sm proteins D1 and D3 contain symmetrical dimethylarginines, which form a major B-cell epitope for anti-Sm autoantibodies. J Biol Chem. 2000;275:17122-17129.

[65] Brahms H, Meheus L, de Brabandere V, Fischer U, Lührmann R. Symmetrical dimethylation of arginine residues in spliceosomal Sm protein B/B' and the Sm-like protein LSm4, and their interaction with the SMN protein. RNA. 2001;7:1531-1542.

[66] Miranda TB, Khusial P, Cook JR, Lee JH, Gunderson SI, Pestka S, Zieve GW, Clarke S. Spliceosome Sm proteins D1, D3, and B/B' are asymmetrically dimethylated at arginine residues in the nucleus. Biochem Biophys Res Commun. 2004;323:382-387.

[67] McBride AE, Weiss VH, Kim HK, Hogle JM, Silver PA. Analysis of the yeast arginine methyltransferase Hmt1p/Rmt1p and its in vivo function. Cofactor binding and substrate interactions. J Biol Chem. 2000;275:3128-3136.

[68] Côté J, Boisvert FM, Boulanger MC, Bedford MT, Richard S. Sam68 RNA binding protein is an in vivo substrate for protein arginine N-methyltransferase 1. Mol Biol Cell. 2003;14:274-287.

[69] Yu MC, Bachand F, McBride AE, Komili S, Casolari JM, Silver PA. Arginine methyltransferase affects interactions and recruitment of mRNA processing and export factors. Genes Dev. 2004;18:2024-2035.

[70] Fujiwara T, Mori Y, Chu DL, Koyama Y, Miyata S, Tanaka H, Yachi K, Kubo T, Yoshikawa H, Tohyama M. CARM1 regulates proliferation of PC12 cells by methylating HuD. Mol Cell Biol. 2006;26:2273-2285.

[71] Lukong KE, Richard S. Arginine methylation signals mRNA export. Nat Struct Mol Biol. 2004;11:914-915.

[72] Smith WA, Schurter BT, Wong-Staal F, David M. Arginine methylation of RNA helicase a determines its subcellular localization. J Biol Chem. 2004;279:22795-22798.

[73] Fronz K, Güttinger S, Burkert K, Kühn U, Stöhr N, Schierhorn A, Wahle E. Arginine methylation of the nuclear poly(a) binding protein weakens the interaction with its nuclear import receptor, transportin. J Biol Chem. 2011;286:32986-32994.

[74] Bannister AJ, Schneider R, Kouzarides T. Histone methylation: dynamic or static? Cell. 2002;109:801-806.

[75] Wysocka J, Allis CD, Coonrod S. Histone arginine methylation and its dynamic regulation. Front Biosci. 2006;11:344-355.

[76] Di Lorenzo A, Bedford MT. Histone arginine methylation. FEBS Lett. 2011;585:2024-2031.

[77] Schurter BT, Koh SS, Chen D, Bunick GJ, Harp JM, Hanson BL, Henschen-Edman A, Mackay DR, Stallcup MR, Aswad DW. Methylation of histone H3 by coactivator-associated arginine methyltransferase 1. Biochemistry. 2001;40:5747-5756.

[78] Guccione E, Bassi C, Casadio F, Martinato F, Cesaroni M, Schuchlautz H, Lüscher B, Amati B. Methylation of histone H3R2 by PRMT6 and H3K4 by an MLL complex are mutually exclusive. Nature. 2007;449:933-937.

[79] Pal S, Vishwanath SN, Erdjument-Bromage H, Tempst P, Sif S. Human SWI/SNF-associated PRMT5 methylates histone H3 arginine 8 and negatively regulates expression of ST7 and NM23 tumor suppressor genes. Mol Cell Biol. 2004;24:9630-9645.

[80] Wang H, Huang ZQ, Xia L, Feng Q, Erdjument-Bromage H, Strahl BD, Briggs SD, Allis CD, Wong J, Tempst P, Zhang Y. Methylation of histone H4 at arginine 3 facilitating transcriptional activation by nuclear hormone receptor. Science. 2001;293:853-857.

[81] Hyllus D, Stein C, Schnabel K, Schiltz E, Imhof A, Dou Y, Hsieh J, Bauer UM. PRMT6-mediated methylation of R2 in histone H3 antagonizes H3 K4 trimethylation. Genes Dev. 2007;21:3369-3380.

[82] Iberg AN, Espejo A, Cheng D, Kim D, Michaud-Levesque J, Richard S, Bedford MT. Arginine methylation of the histone H3 tail impedes effector binding. J Biol Chem. 2008;283:3006-3010.

[83] Xu W, Chen H, Du K, Asahara H, Tini M, Emerson BM, Montminy M, Evans RM. A transcriptional switch mediated by cofactor methylation. Science. 2001;294:2507-2511.

[84] Teyssier C, Ma H, Emter R, Kralli A, Stallcup MR. Activation of nuclear receptor coactivator PGC-1 alpha by arginine methylation. Genes Dev. 2005;19:1466-73.

[85] Garcia MM, Guéant-Rodriguez RM, Pooya S, Brachet P, Alberto JM, Jeannesson E, Maskali F, Gueguen N, Marie PY, Lacolley P, Herrmann M, Juillière Y, Malthiery Y, Guéant JL. Methyl donor deficiency induces cardiomyopathy through altered methylation/acetylation of PGC-1alpha by PRMT1 and SIRT1. J Pathol. 2011;225:324-335.

[86] Mowen KA, Tang J, Zhu W, Schurter BT, Shuai K, Herschman HR, David M. Arginine methylation of STAT1 modulates IFNalpha/beta-induced transcription. Cell. 2001;104:731-741.

[87] Kwak YT, Guo J, Prajapati S, Park KJ, Surabhi RM, Miller B, Gehrig P, Gaynor RB. Methylation of SPT5 regulates its interaction with RNA polymerase II and transcriptional elongation properties. Mol Cell. 2003;11:1055-1066.

[88] Tan CP, Nakielny S. Control of the DNA methylation system component MBD2 by protein arginine methylation. Mol Cell Biol. 2006;26:7224-7235.

[89] Sims RJ 3rd, Rojas LA, Beck D, Bonasio R, Schüller R, Drury WJ 3rd, Eick D, Reinberg D. The C-terminal domain of RNA polymerase II is modified by site-specific methylation. Science. 2011;332:99-103.

[90] Boisvert FM, Hendzel MJ, Masson JY, Richard S. Methylation of MRE11 regulates its nuclear compartmentalization. Cell Cycle. 2005;4:981-989.

[91] Boisvert FM, Dery U, Masson JY, Richard S. Arginine methylation of MRE11 by PRMT1 is required for DNA damage checkpoint control. Genes Dev. 2005;19:671-676.

[92] He W, Ma X, Yang X, Zhao Y, Qiu J, Hang H. A role for the arginine methylation of Rad9 in checkpoint control and cellular sensitivity to DNA damage. Nucleic Acids Res. 2011;39:4719-4727.

[93] El-Andaloussi N, Valovka T, Toueille M, Steinacher R, Focke F, Gehrig P, Covic M, Hassa PO, Schär P, Hübscher U, Hottiger MO. Arginine methylation regulates DNA polymerase beta. Mol Cell. 2006;22:51-62.

[94] Abramovich C, Yakobson B, Chebath J, Revel M. A protein-arginine methyltransferase binds to the intracytoplasmic domain of the IFNAR1 chain in the type I interferon receptor. EMBO J. 1997;16:260-266.

[95] Altschuler L, Wook JO, Gurari D, Chebath J, Revel M. Involvement of receptor-bound protein methyltransferase PRMT1 in antiviral and antiproliferative effects of type I interferons. J Interferon Cytokine Res. 1999;19:189-195.

[96] Parry RV, Ward SG. Protein arginine methylation: a new handle on T lymphocytes? Trends Immunol. 2010;31:164-169.

[97] Iwasaki H, Yada T. Protein arginine methylation regulates insulin signaling in L6 skeletal muscle cells. Biochem Biophys Res Commun. 2007;364:1015-1021.

[98] Le Romancer M, Treilleux I, Leconte N, Robin-Lespinasse Y, Sentis S, Bouchekioua-Bouzaghou K, Goddard S, Gobert-Gosse S, Corbo L. Regulation of estrogen rapid signaling through arginine methylation by PRMT1. Mol Cell. 2008;31:212-221.

[99] Yamagata K, Daitoku H, Takahashi Y, Namiki K, Hisatake K, Kako K, Mukai H, Kasuya Y, Fukamizu A. Arginine methylation of FOXO transcription factors inhibits their phosphorylation by Akt. Mol Cell. 2008;32:221-231.

[100] Kops GJ, de Ruiter ND, De Vries-Smits AM, Powell DR, Bos JL, Burgering BM. Direct control of the Forkhead transcription factor AFX by protein kinase B. Nature. 1999;398:630-634.

[101] Sakamaki J, Daitoku H, Ueno K, Hagiwara A, Yamagata K, Fukamizu A. Arginine methylation of BCL-2 antagonist of cell death (BAD) counteracts its phosphorylation and inactivation by Akt. Proc Natl Acad Sci U S A. 2011;108:6085-6090.

[102] Andreu-Pérez P, Esteve-Puig R, de Torre-Minguela C, López-Fauqued M, Bech-Serra JJ, Tenbaum S, García-Trevijano ER, Canals F, Merlino G, Avila MA, Recio JA. Protein arginine methyltransferase 5 regulates ERK1/2 signal transduction amplitude and cell fate through CRAF. Sci Signal. 2011;4:ra58.

[103] Robin-Lespinasse Y, Sentis S, Kolytcheff C, Rostan MC, Corbo L, Le Romancer M. hCAF1, a new regulator of PRMT1-dependent arginine methylation. J Cell Sci. 2007;120:638-647.

[104] Singh V, Miranda TB, Jiang W, Frankel A, Roemer ME, Robb VA, Gutmann DH, Herschman HR, Clarke S, Newsham IF. DAL-1/4.1B tumor suppressor interacts with protein arginine N-methyltransferase 3 (PRMT3) and inhibits its ability to methylate substrates in vitro and in vivo. Oncogene. 2004;23:7761-7771.

[105] Lacroix M, El Messaoudi S, Rodier G, Le Cam A, Sardet C, Fabbrizio E. The histone-binding protein COPR5 is required for nuclear functions of the protein arginine methyltransferase PRMT5. EMBO Rep. 2008;9:452-458.

[106] Higashimoto K, Kuhn P, Desai D, Cheng X, Xu W. Phosphorylation-mediated inactivation of coactivator-associated arginine methyltransferase 1. Proc Natl Acad Sci U S A. 2007;104:12318-12323.

[107] Feng Q, He B, Jung SY, Song Y, Qin J, Tsai SY, Tsai MJ, O'Malley BW. Biochemical control of CARM1 enzymatic activity by phosphorylation. J Biol Chem. 2009;284:36167-36174.

[108] Bedford MT, Clarke SG. Protein arginine methylation in mammals: who, what, and why. Mol Cell. 2009;33:1-13.

[109] Ng SS, Yue WW, Oppermann U, Klose RJ. Dynamic protein methylation in chromatin biology. Cell Mol Life Sci. 2009;66:407-22.

[110] Chang B, Chen Y, Zhao Y, Bruick RK. JMJD6 is a histone arginine demethylase. Science. 2007;318:444-7.

[111] Webby CJ, Wolf A, Gromak N, Dreger M, Kramer H, Kessler B, Nielsen ML, Schmitz C, Butler DS, Yates JR 3rd, Delahunty CM, Hahn P, Lengeling A, Mann M, Proudfoot NJ, Schofield CJ, Böttger A. Jmjd6 catalyses lysyl-hydroxylation of U2AF65, a protein associated with RNA splicing. Science. 2009;325:90-93.

[112] Thompson PR, Fast W. Histone citrullination by protein arginine deiminase: is arginine methylation a green light or a roadblock? ACS Chem Biol. 2006;1:433-441.

[113] Arita K, Hashimoto H, Shimizu T, Nakashima K, Yamada M, Sato M. Structural basis for Ca(2+)-induced activation of human PAD4. Nat Struct Mol Biol. 2004;11:777-783.

[114] Kearney PL, Bhatia M, Jones NG, Yuan L, Glascock MC, Catchings KL, Yamada M, Thompson PR. Kinetic characterization of protein arginine deiminase 4: a transcriptional corepressor implicated in the onset and progression of rheumatoid arthritis. Biochemistry. 2005;44:10570-10582.

[115] Nakashima K, Hagiwara T, Yamada M. Nuclear localization of peptidylarginine deiminase V and histone deimination in granulocytes. J Biol Chem. 2002;277:49562-49568.

[116] Cuthbert GL, Daujat S, Snowden AW, Erdjument-Bromage H, Hagiwara T, Yamada M, Schneider R, Gregory PD, Tempst P, Bannister AJ, Kouzarides T. Histone deimination antagonizes arginine methylation. Cell. 2004;118:545-553.

[117] Wang Y, Wysocka J, Sayegh J, Lee YH, Perlin JR, Leonelli L, Sonbuchner LS, McDonald CH, Cook RG, Dou Y, Roeder RG, Clarke S, Stallcup MR, Allis CD, Coonrod SA. Human PAD4 regulates histone arginine methylation levels via demethylimination. Science. 2004;306:279-283.

[118] Hidaka Y, Hagiwara T,Yamada M. Methylation of the guanidino group of arginine residues prevents citrullination by peptidylarginine deiminase IV. FEBS Lett. 2005;579:4088-4092.

[119] Raijmakers R, Zendman AJ, Egberts WV, Vossenaar ER, Raats J, Soede-Huijbregts C, Rutjes FP, van Veelen PA, Drijfhout JW, Pruijn GJ. Methylation of arginine residues interferes with citrullination by peptidylarginine deiminases in vitro. J Mol Biol. 2007;367:1118-1129.

[120] Boger RH. The emerging role of asymmetric dimethylarginine as a novel cardiovascular risk factor. Cardiovasc Res. 2003;59:824-833.

[121] Closs EI, Basha FZ, Habermeier A, Forstermann U. Interference of L-arginine analogues with L-arginine transport mediated by the y+ carrier hCAT-2B. Nitric Oxide. 1997;1:65-73.

[122] Carello KA, Whitesall SE, Lloyd MC, Billecke SS, D'Alecy LG. Asymmetrical dimethylarginine plasma clearance persists after acute total nephrectomy in rats. Am J Physiol Heart Circ Physiol. 2006;290:H209-216.

[123] Palm F, Onozato ML, Luo Z, Wilcox CS. Dimethylarginine dimethylaminohydrolase (DDAH): expression, regulation, and function in the cardiovascular and renal systems. Am J Physiol Heart Circ Physiol. 2007;293:H3227-H3245.

[124] Antoniades C, Shirodaria C, Leeson P, Antonopoulos A, Warrick N, Van-Assche T, Cunnington C, Tousoulis D, Pillai R, Ratnatunga C, Stefanadis C, Channon KM. Association of plasma asymmetrical dimethylarginine (ADMA) with elevated vascular superoxide production and endothelial nitric oxide synthase uncoupling: implications for endothelial function in human atherosclerosis. Eur Heart J. 2009;30:1142-1150.

[125] Handy DE, Castro R, Loscalzo J. Epigenetic modifications: basic mechanisms and role in cardiovascular disease. Circulation. 2011;123:2145-2156.

[126] Finkelstein JD. Methionine metabolism in mammals. J Nutr Biochem. 1990;1:228-237.

[127] Joseph J, Handy DE, Loscalzo J. Quo vadis: whither homocysteine research? Cardiovasc Toxicol. 2009;9:53-63.

[128] Blom HJ, Smulders Y. Overview of homocysteine and folate metabolism. With special references to cardiovascular disease and neural tube defects. J Inherit Metab Dis. 2011;34:75-81.

[129] Castro R, Rivera I, Struys EA, Jansen EE, Ravasco P, Camilo ME, Blom HJ, Jakobs C, Tavares de Almeida I. Increased homocysteine and S-adenosylhomocysteine concentrations and DNA hypomethylation in vascular disease. Clin Chem. 2003;49:1292-1296.

[130] Castro R, Rivera I, Ravasco P, Camilo ME, Jakobs C, Blom HJ, de Almeida IT. 5,10-methylenetetrahydrofolate reductase (MTHFR) 677C-->T and 1298A-->C mutations are associated with DNA hypomethylation. J Med Genet. 2004; 41:454-458.

[131] Castro R, Rivera I, Martins C, Struys EA, Jansen EE, Clode N, Graça LM, Blom HJ, Jakobs C, de Almeida IT. Intracellular S-adenosylhomocysteine increased levels are associated with DNA hypomethylation in HUVEC. J Mol Med 2005;83:831-836.

[132] Castro R, Rivera I, Blom HJ, Jakobs C, Tavares de Almeida I. Homocysteine metabolism, hyperhomocysteinaemia and vascular disease: an overview. J Inherit Metab Dis. 2006;29:3-20.

[133] Barroso M, Rocha MS, Esse R, Gonçalves I Jr, Gomes AQ, Teerlink T, Jakobs C, Blom HJ, Loscalzo J, Rivera I, de Almeida IT, Castro R. Cellular hypomethylation is associated with impaired nitric oxide production by cultured human endothelial cells. Amino Acids. 2012;42:1903-1911.

[134] Ueland PM. Pharmacological and biochemical aspects of S-adenosylhomocysteine and S-adenosylhomocysteine hydrolase. Pharmacol Rev. 1982;34:223-253.

[135] Yi P, Melnyk S, Pogribna M, Pogribny IP, Hine RJ, James SJ. Increase in plasma homocysteine associated with parallel increases in plasma S-adenosylhomocysteine and lymphocyte DNA hypomethylation. J Biol Chem. 2000;275:29318-29323.

[136] Friso S, Choi SW, Girelli D, Mason JB, Dolnikowski GG, Bagley PJ, Olivieri O, Jacques PF, Rosenberg IH, Corrocher R, Selhub J. A common mutation in the 5,10-methylenetetrahydrofolate reductase gene affects genomic DNA methylation through an interaction with folate status. Proc Natl Acad Sci U S A. 2002;99:5606-5611.

[137] James SJ, Melnyk S, Pogribna M, Pogribny IP, Caudill MA. Elevation in S-adenosylhomocysteine and DNA hypomethylation: potential epigenetic mechanism for homocysteine-related pathology. J Nutr. 2002;132:2361S-2366S.

[138] Ingrosso D, Cimmino A, Perna AF, Masella L, De Santo NG, De Bonis ML, Vacca M, D'Esposito M, D'Urso M, Galletti P, Zappia V. Folate treatment and unbalanced methylation and changes of allelic expression induced by hyperhomocysteinaemia in patients with uraemia. Lancet. 2003;361:1693-1699.

[139] Flynn J, Reich N. Murine DNA (cytosine-5-)-methyltransferase: steady-state and substrate trapping analyses of the kinetic mechanism. Biochemistry. 1998;37:15162-15169.

[140] Esse R, Rocha MS, Barroso M, Goncalves Jr I, Leandro P, Teerlink T, Jakobs C, Blom HJ, Castro R, Tavares de Almeida I. S-Adenosyl homocysteine accumulation decreases global protein arginine methylation status in cultured human endothelial cells. J Inherit Metab Dis. 2010;33:S35.

[141] Esse R, Imbard A, Rocha MS, Teerlink T, Castro R, Tavares de Almeida I, Blom HJ. Diet-induced hyperhomocysteinemia in rats affects protein arginine methylation in a tissue-specific manner. J Inherit Metab Dis. 2012;35:S51.

Section 4

# Cancer Research Through Study of Methylation Cell Processes

Chapter 5

# Methylation in Tumorigenesis

Melissa A. Edwards, Pashayar P. Lookian,
Drew R. Neavin and Mark A. Brown

Additional information is available at the end of the chapter

http://dx.doi.org/10.5772/52867

## 1. Introduction

The development, maturation, and maintenance of tissues and organisms are anchored in distinct programs for protein expression which define the identities and roles of individual cell lines [1, 2]. These programs are maintained in a heritable state by epigenetic mechanisms that convey cellular memory [3, 4]. In this way, the global synchronization of patterns in gene expression broadly dictates developmental consequences [5, 6]. At the foundation of such gene regulation are coordinated cascades that affect the packaging of DNA into chromatin, thereby establishing the degree of DNA accessibility to transcriptional complexes [7-10]. These pathways include histone methylation, methylation of transcriptional regulators, DNA methylation, histone replacement, chromatin remodeling, and other alterations to histone tails [11-16]. Abnormalities in these epigenetic events are commonly associated with tumorigenesis and subsequent clinical outcomes [17-23].

From tightly regulated transcription to mitosis, chromatin is an elastic repository of the genome [24]. In this state, a chromosome is sequentially condensed through a succession of organized compaction while limited regions of DNA are selectively made available to transcriptional complexes [25, 26]. Hence, chromatin exists in a dynamic state into which approximately 2 m of DNA is packaged in the nucleus while maintaining an extraordinary level of utility [25, 26]. At its core, chromatin is established in a series of nucleosomes, their basic structural unit [25, 27], comprised of 146 base pairs of DNA, wrapped 1.7 times around an octamer of histones and interspersed by regions of roughly 50 base pairs [28]. The key histones participating in the assembly of a nucleosome include histones H2A, H2B, H3 and H4. These histones form hetero-dimers resulting in each being twice represented in the nucleosomal unit [29-31]. Structurally, histones are are highly conserved, including a folded core followed by an unstructured tail [30, 31]. A globular domain forms the histone core as a helix-turn-helix motif, which allows dimerization [31]. In contrast, the tails of histones do not exist in defined conformations except when attached to their cognate proteins [31]. Within the sequence of histone tail domains is a large representation of conserved amino acid residues including lysine, arginine, and serine [31, 32]. Under normal conditions, histone tails have a net basic charge facilitating their interaction with the poly-anionic backbone of DNA, thereby contributing to the stability of nucleosomes [31]. Consequently, chromatin structure and transcriptional regulation are commonly mediated through post-translational modifications that impact specific residues within the sequence of these tails [33, 34]. Modifications to tail residues can regulate the accessibility of nuclear factors to regions of DNA or induce the recruitment of such factors involved in chromatin structural and transcriptional regulatory pathways [33, 34].

The Histone-DNA interface is formed principally by inelastic hydrogen bonds between the phosphate oxygen of DNA and the main chain amide of the histone. Electrostatic interactions between basic side chains and negatively charged phosphate groups and other nonpolar interactions further strengthen the association between histones and DNA [35]. While this, in theory, should facilitate the establishment of nucleosomes upon any DNA sequence, there are likely specific sequence parameters for nucleosomal placement [36]. The composition of the DNA sequences, by which the histone core is enveloped, is likely a major factor contributing to the positioning of core histones and the dynamic comportment of the nucleosome under the influence of the SWI/SNF ATPase and sequence-specific transcription factors [37]. The most broadly characterized nucleosomal assembly is the 30 nm fiber [38], which is anchored by linker histones [39-41] and the relative juxtaposition of each nucleosome [42], establishing close physical proximity while generating only marginal internucleosomal attraction energy [38, 43-45]. Hence, this architecture allows a great degree of variation in condensation without producing serious topological changes. Chromatin exists in a series of more densely compacted structures [46], which are commonly driven by interaction with non-histone, structural proteins [47].

In recent decades, a number of process which impact the structure and/or function of chromatin including post-translational modifications of histones, DNA methylation, incorporation of histone variants, and ATP-dependent chromatin remodelling have been the subjects of intense study. The findings of these studies clearly show that chromatin modifications and the complexes involved with their facilitation are linked to the control of many biological processes which depend upon the level of chromatin accessibility [48-51]. Such processes include chromosome segregation during mitosis, X chromosome inactivation, gene expression, DNA repair, and chromatin condensation during apoptosis [23, 52-56].

Chromatin modifications convey epigenetic regulation of protein expression without alterations in DNA sequence. Disturbing the equilibrium of epigenetic networks has been shown to be associated with numerous pathological events, including syndromes involving chromosomal instability, neurological disorders, and tumorigenesis [57-59]. Advances in knowledge related to epigenetic inheritance and chromatin structure/regulation have paved the way for promising novel therapeutics directed against the specific factors that are responsible [60]. Of particular importance in the role of chromatin modifications in human disease are methylation of DNA, histone targets, and other regulatory targets.

## 2. DNA methylation in tumorigenesis

Methylation of DNA is a covalent modification that occurs at cytosines within CpG-rich regions of DNA and is catalyzed by DNA methyltransferases [61, 62]. The methylation of DNA affects the binding of proteins to their cognate DNA sequences [61, 63]. Such addition of methyl groups can prevent the binding of basal transcriptional machinery and ubiquitous transcription factors [61]. Thus, DNA methylation contributes to epigenetic inheritance, allele-specific expression, inactivation of the X chromosome, genomic stability and embryonic development. It is through these pathways that progressive DNA methylation is thought to be an agent for both normal aging as well as neoplasias [64, 65]. The majority of methylated CpG islands are located within repetitive elements including centromeric repeats, satellite sequences and gene repeats. These CpG regions are often found at the 5' end of genes where DNA methylation affects transcription by recruiting methyl-CpG binding domain (MBD) proteins that function as adaptors between methylated DNA and chromatin-modifying enzymes [66]. There is a clear relationship between DNA methylation and other silencing mechanisms including histone modifications and chromatin remodeling [65, 66]. In fact, several studies suggest that DNA methylation affects genes that are already suppressed by other mechanisms [65].

Changes in the pattern of DNA methylation have been correlated with altered histone post-translational modifications and genetic lesions [67]. Either hypermethylation or hypomethylation have been identified in almost all types of cancer cells examined, to date [18, 21, 68]. Hypomethylation at centromeric repeat sequences has been linked to genomic instability [18] whereas local hypermethylation of individual genes has been associated with aberrant gene silencing [21]. In oncogenic cells, hypermethylation is often correlated with the repression of tumor suppressor genes while hypomethylation is associated with the activation of genes required for invasion and metastasis [68, 69]. In neoplastic tissues, the incidence of hypermethylation in genes with promoter associated CpG islands in markedly increased which, in turn, is associated with repression of tumor suppressors [70]. Although the complete mechanistic pathway for DNA methylation in cancers is still being determined, aberrant methylation in tumors is already being examined as an instrument for diagnosis [21, 70]. For example, techniques, such as the polymerase chain reaction amplification of bisulfite-modified DNA, have enabled the study of patterns of DNA methylation [71-73]. These methods are currently being improved and adapted for cancer cell identification, profiling of tumor-suppressor-gene expression, and prognostic factors that are linked to CpG island hypermethylation [74]. Likewise, reversal of hypermethylation by several indiscriminant demethylating compounds has been approved for therapeutic intervention associated with blood-borne cancers [21].

Detection of DNA methylation has recently been added to the armory of preventative/diagnostic medicine for the prevention and treatment of colorectal cancer [75]. This represents the most common form of gastrointestinal cancer and is a leading killer among all malignancies. The colonoscopy is broadly employed for detection of lesions which often give rise to colorectal tumors. The invasiveness of this procedure and consequent lack of patient cooperation with recommended colonoscopies is a limiting factor in the efficacy of this procedure as a preventative. Fortunately, epigenetic screening has arisen as a new tier in preventative medicine targeting colorectal cancer. Specifically, DNA methylation is associated with gene-silencing related to onset of colorectal cancer. Given that these changes are detectable prior to tumorigenesis, target-specific screening of DNA methylation represents a promising front in the war against colorectal cancer [75].

Similar to colorectal cancer, the role of DNA methylation in prostate cancers has been the subject of numerous studies [76-78]. Indeed, aberrant hyper/hypo methylation has been linked in numerous prostate-specific malignant processes ranging from early tumorigenesis to late stage, androgen independent tumors [79]. The identification of specific targets which are down-regulated as a result of hypermethylation at their promoters has lead to the development of methylation biomarkers for early detection [80]. These targets of inactivation by promoter hypermethylation include Ras-association domain family 1A (RASSF1A), GSTP1, and retinoic acid receptor beta2 (RARbeta2). Though the role of hypomethylation in prostate cancer is less understood, there are several recent studies which link it to alterations in the expression of genes associated with early and late stage prostate tumors [81-83].

Additional studies indicate that hyper/hypomethylation of specific promoter regions is associated with tumorigenesis in a broad range of tissues including lung, breast, thyroid, head and neck squamous cell carcinomas, and hepatocellular carcinomas [84-86]. There are ongoing studies in dozens of other tissue types indicating a role for hyper/hypomethylation in a broadening range of cancers. Thus, aberrant alterations in methylation promise to provide a broad-spectrum mechanism for early detection and prognostication of tumors.

## 3. Histone methylation in tumorigenesis

Modifications to histone tails comprise the broadest range of variation in epigenetic controls, encompassing more than four dozen known sites of alteration [87]. Histone proteins are the targets of many forms of post-translational modification such as citrullination, acetylation, phosphorylation, SUMOylation, ADP-ribosylation and methylation (Figure 1) [87, 88]. These alterations are translated into biological consequences by impacting the structure of the nucleosome as well as facilitating the recruitment of specific regulatory complexes. The combination of different histone modifications in concert communicates a "histone code" that is interpreted in the form of distinct nuclear events [89].

Histone methylation is has been observed to be a mark that imparts long-term epigenetic memory [90]. Histone lysine methylation is a central factor in such processes as X chromosome inactivation, DNA methylation, transcriptional regulation, and the formation of heterochromatin [91, 92]. This modification, catalyzed by histone methyltransferases, often facilitates the regulation of protein expression in a residue-dependent manner [90]. The de-

http://dx.doi.org/10.5772/52867

gree of achievable specificity is increased by the breadth of biological outcomes which are dependent upon whether a residue is mono-, di-, or tri-methylated [93-95]. Likewise, is has also been widely observed that histone lysine methylation works concomitantly with many transient histone modifications, thereby further enhancing the degree of information which can be communicated by this epigenetic modification [15].

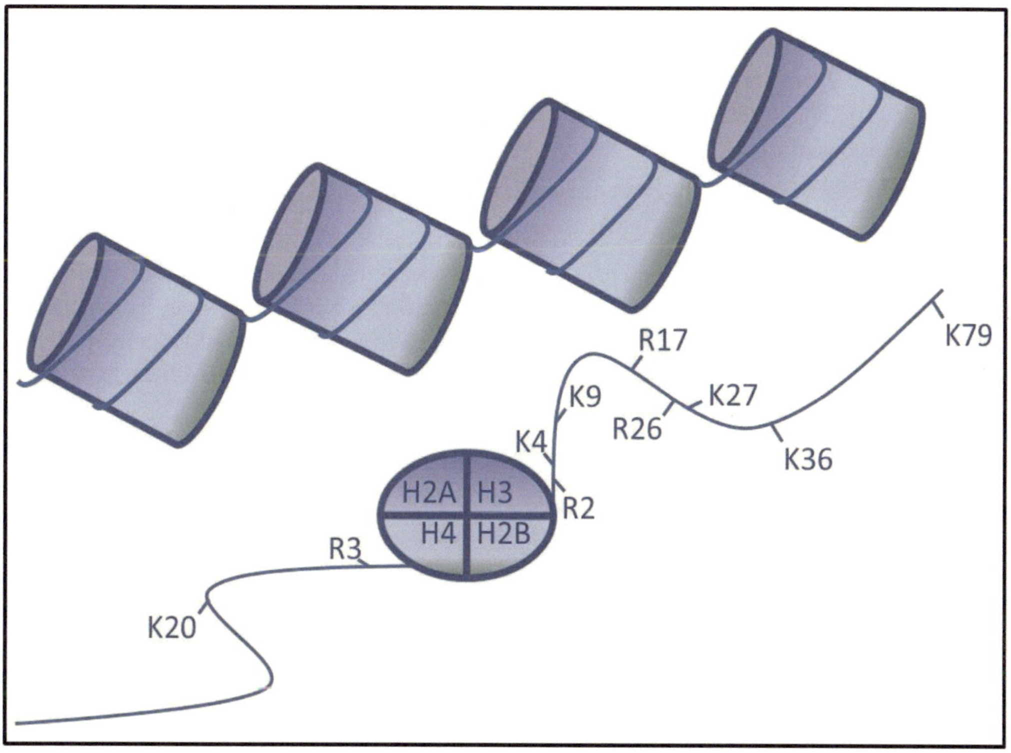


**Figure 1.** Common sites of Histone Methylation

Almost all histone lysine methyltransferases are dependent upon a SET domain for catalyzing the transfer of methyl groups. The SET domain is present in many proteins that control a range of biological processes, including several involved in development and proper cell cycle progression [7, 96]. Promoter associated, residue-specific histone methylation often correlates with distinct patterns of protein expression [96]. The bulk of known modifications occur on histone H3 which thereby serves as a central conduit of epigenetic regulation. Lysine methylation at histone H3, lysine 9 (H3K9), H3K27, and H4K20 is most often associated with gene silencing, whereas methylation of H3K4, H3K36, or H3K79 is commonly linked to the activation of transcription [7, 96]. Accumulating evidence points to histone methylation in the recruitment of chromatin remodeling complexes, such as CHD1, an ATP-dependent chromatin remodeling factor that binds specifically to methylated the forms of H3K4 [97]. While histone lysine methylation was previously believed to be a permanent mark, a number of enzymes have now been identified that are capable of reversing histone methylation in a site-specific manner [98-100].

The presence of histone variants creates yet another tier to the potential of epigenetic mechanisms to communicate cellular information [53]. Variants affect the nucleosomal architecture as well as the proclivity of local chromatin to be remodeled. Thus, the inclusion of histone variants may modify nucleosome mobility, stability, and/or potential patterns of histone modifications. These, in turn, impact higher order structure and downstream events [101-104]. For example, a specialized H3-like variant CENP-A, replaces H3 in centromeric nucleosomes to establish a distinct architecture that is essential for proper segregation of the chromosomes [105]. In recent years, there have been an increasing number of experimental outcomes emphasizing the biological relevance of histone variants and their central role in epigenetic control [53].

Regulating the architecture of chromatin involves complex and dynamic mechanisms. The structure of chromatin is controlled on multiple levels by distinct processes such as nucleosome remodeling, DNA methylation, histone post-translational modifications, incorporation of histone variants, and non-coding RNA. Aberrant activity within such epigenetic processes is likely to broadly affect protein expression as well as other biological events such as apoptosis and condensation and segregation of chromosomes.

Tumorigenesis is a graded process through which a succession of genetic aberrations leads to the progressive transformation of healthy cells. While modifications in genetic sequence certainly account for many of these aberrations, an increasing number of modifications in gene expression observed in tumorigenesis have been found to be the result by epigenetic aberrations. These observations point to the relevance of epigenetic mechanisms in the maintenance of proper cell function. Aberrant events related to such mechanisms often act in concert with genetic mutations thereby contributing to the development and progression of cancer.

Over the last two decades, an increasing number of investigations have highlighted the aberrant gain or loss of histone methyltransferase activity in carcinogenesis. At one end of the spectrum, it has been shown that mice which fail to express the H3K9-specific histone methyltransferase, SUV39H1, are subject to increased incidence of chromosomal instability and subsequent tumorigenic potential [106]. At the opposite end of the spectrum, it is overexpression of Smyd3, another histone methyltransferase that is specific for H3K4, that has been shown to be responsible for unrestrained proliferation of many cancer cells [107]. A transcription factor binding element polymorphism in the upstream regulatory sequence for Smyd3 has been associated with an increased risk for cancer [108, 109].

In addition to histone targets, some SET domain-containing methyltransferases have been shown to methylate other proteins including tumor suppressors. Smyd2, which methylates H3K36 [6, 110], has also been directly linked to the regulation of p53 [111, 112]. Methylating lysine 370 of p53, Smyd2 has been shown to inhibit the transcriptional regulatory activity of p53. Smyd2 regulation of the retinoblastoma tumor suppressor (RB) has also been observed by its capacity to methylate of RB at K860 [113]. In a second example, Set9, which methylates

H3K4 [114, 115], has also been linked to the regulation of p53 by its capacity to methylate that protein at lysine 372 [116, 117]. Methylation of that site stabilizes p53 and limits its localization to the nucleus [116].

The broad roles of aberrant lysine methylation in the induction of carcinogenesis have paved the way for a novel line of cancer therapeutics. [118]. Those therapeutics bank on the potential to manipulate of the demethylating activity of a host of demethylases. The fact that many demethylases target highly specific substrates heightens their potential utility as highly effective therapeutics with lower likelihood of instigating adverse effects.

## 4. Conclusion

While it is true that chromatin architecture has the capacity to be epigenetically maintained and inherited via modified states of methylation, recent studies have highlighted the fact that methylation-induced control of gene expression may be altered by environmental stressors and toxicants. Such modifications may, in consequence, induce aberrations toward genome integrity and stability. Distinct from genetic mutations, these epigenetic aberrations have been termed epimutations. In contrast to genetic mutations, which may be passively inherited, epimutations require active maintenance [119]. That epimutations rare appearance in normal tissues highlights the potential for epigenetic therapies based on high tumor specificity. Likewise, while therapeutics based on genetic deletions commonly induce an irreversible loss of gene function, epigenetic alterations are reversible, further enhancing their potential utility for therapeutic intervention [120]. Reversal of epimutations to restore normal expression of tumor suppressors has become the holy grail in epigenetic cancer therapeutics. Already, numerous studies have proven that aberrant gene silencing mediated by DNA methylation can be easily reversed by the incorporation of DNA methyltransferase inhibitors [121]. Positive results have been observed after treating tumor cells with such pharmacological agents [122, 123].

In the last two decades, our knowledge of chromatin methylation patterns and their role in the regulation of nuclear processes have been broadly elucidated. Understanding those patterns of histone changes, decoding the association between those alterations and DNA methylation, and characterizing their relevance in tumorigenesis comprise the next hurdles in the etiology of the role of methylation in cancer.

## Acknowledgements

This work was supported by funding to Mark A. Brown from the National Science Foundation (1060548).

## Author details

Melissa A. Edwards[1], Pashayar P. Lookian[2], Drew R. Neavin[3] and Mark A. Brown[4*]

*Address all correspondence to: M.Brown@colostate.edu

1 Cell and Molecular Biology Program at Colorado State University, USA

2 Department of Biology at Colorado State University, USA

3 Department of Biology at Colorado State University, USA

4 Flint Cancer Center and Department of Clinical Sciences at Colorado State University, USA

## References

[1] Natoli G: Maintaining Cell Identity through Global Control of Genomic Organization. Immunity 2010, 33(1):12-24.

[2] Müller C, Leutz A: Chromatin remodeling in development and differentiation. Current Opinion in Genetics & Development 2001, 11(2):167-174.

[3] Cavalli G: Chromatin and epigenetics in development: blending cellular memory with cell fate plasticity. Development 2006, 133(11):2089-2094.

[4] Vasanthi D, Mishra RK: Epigenetic regulation of genes during development: A conserved theme from flies to mammals. Journal of Genetics and Genomics 2008, 35(7): 413-429.

[5] Kiefer JC: Epigenetics in development. Developmental Dynamics 2007, 236(4): 1144-1156.

[6] Brown M, Sims R, Gottlieb P, Tucker P: Identification and characterization of Smyd2: a split SET/MYND domain-containing histone H3 lysine 36-specific methyltransferase that interacts with the Sin3 histone deacetylase complex. Molecular Cancer 2006, 5(1):26.

[7] Jenuwein T, Allis CD: Translating the Histone Code. Science 2001, 293(5532): 1074-1080.

[8] Jenuwein T: The epigenetic magic of histone lysine methylation. FEBS Journal 2006, 273(14):3121-3135.

[9] Festenstein R, Aragon L: Decoding the epigenetic effects of chromatin. Genome Biology 2003, 4(10):342.

[10] Imhof A: Epigenetic regulators and histone modification. Briefings in Functional Genomics & Proteomics 2006, 5(3):222-227.

[11] Mito Y, Henikoff JG, Henikoff S: Genome-scale profiling of histone H3.3 replacement patterns. Nat Genet 2005, 37(10):1090-1097.

[12] Zhang Y, Fatima N, Dufau ML: Coordinated Changes in DNA Methylation and Histone Modifications Regulate Silencing/Derepression of Luteinizing Hormone Receptor Gene Transcription. Molecular and Cellular Biology 2005, 25(18):7929-7939.

[13] Misteli T: Beyond the Sequence: Cellular Organization of Genome Function. Cell 2007, 128(4):787-800.

[14] Barkess G: Chromatin remodeling and genome stability. Genome Biology 2006, 7(6): 319.

[15] Turner BM: Cellular Memory and the Histone Code. Cell 2002, 111(3):285-291.

[16] Turner BM: Reading signals on the nucleosome with a new nomenclature for modified histones. Nat Struct Mol Biol 2005, 12(2):110-112.

[17] Staub E, Grone J, Mennerich D, Ropcke S, Klamann I, Hinzmann B, Castanos-Velez E, Mann B, Pilarsky C, Brummendorf T et al: A genome-wide map of aberrantly expressed chromosomal islands in colorectal cancer. Molecular Cancer 2006, 5(1):37.

[18] Ducasse M, Brown M: Epigenetic aberrations and cancer. Molecular Cancer 2006, 5(1):60.

[19] Ballestar E, Esteller M: Chapter 9 Epigenetic Gene Regulation in Cancer. In: Advances in Genetics. Edited by Veronica van H, Robert EH, vol. Volume 61: Academic Press; 2008: 247-267.

[20] Sandoval J, Esteller M: Cancer epigenomics: beyond genomics. Current Opinion in Genetics & Development 2012, 22(1):50-55.

[21] Shenker N, Flanagan JM: Intragenic DNA methylation: implications of this epigenetic mechanism for cancer research. Br J Cancer 2012, 106(2):248-253.

[22] Baylin SB, Jones PA: A decade of exploring the cancer epigenome — biological and translational implications. Nat Rev Cancer 2011, 11(10):726-734.

[23] Fullgrabe J, Kavanagh E, Joseph B: Histone onco-modifications. Oncogene 2011, 30(31):3391-3403.

[24] Alabert C, Groth A: Chromatin replication and epigenome maintenance. Nat Rev Mol Cell Biol 2012, 13(3):153-167.

[25] Bell O, Tiwari VK, Thomä NH, Schübeler D: Determinants and dynamics of genome accessibility. Nat Rev Genet 2011, 12(8):554-564.

[26] Varga-Weisz PD, Becker PB: Regulation of higher-order chromatin structures by nucleosome-remodelling factors. Current Opinion in Genetics & Development 2006, 16(2):151-156.

[27] Svaren J, Hörz W: Regulation of gene expression by nucleosomes. Current Opinion in Genetics & Development 1996, 6(2):164-170.

[28] Fransz P, de Jong H: From nucleosome to chromosome: a dynamic organization of genetic information. The Plant Journal 2011, 66(1):4-17.

[29] Luger K, Mader AW, Richmond RK, Sargent DF, Richmond TJ: Crystal structure of the nucleosome core particle at 2.8[thinsp]A resolution. Nature 1997, 389(6648): 251-260.

[30] Richmond TJ, Davey CA: The structure of DNA in the nucleosome core. Nature 2003, 423(6936):145-150.

[31] Luger K: Dynamic nucleosomes. Chromosome Research 2006, 14(1):5-16.

[32] Khorasanizadeh S: The Nucleosome: From Genomic Organization to Genomic Regulation. Cell 2004, 116(2):259-272.

[33] Bassett A, Cooper S, Wu C, Travers A: The folding and unfolding of eukaryotic chromatin. Current Opinion in Genetics & Development 2009, 19(2):159-165.

[34] Vitolo JM, Thiriet C, Hayes JJ: The H3-H4 N-Terminal Tail Domains Are the Primary Mediators of Transcription Factor IIIA Access to 5S DNA within a Nucleosome. Molecular and Cellular Biology 2000, 20(6):2167-2175.

[35] Davey CA, Sargent DF, Luger K, Maeder AW, Richmond TJ: Solvent Mediated Interactions in the Structure of the Nucleosome Core Particle at 1.9 Å Resolution. Journal of Molecular Biology 2002, 319(5):1097-1113.

[36] Kaplan N, Moore IK, Fondufe-Mittendorf Y, Gossett AJ, Tillo D, Field Y, LeProust EM, Hughes TR, Lieb JD, Widom J et al: The DNA-encoded nucleosome organization of a eukaryotic genome. Nature 2009, 458(7236):362-366.

[37] Vicent GP, Nacht AS, Smith CL, Peterson CL, Dimitrov S, Beato M: DNA Instructed Displacement of Histones H2A and H2B at an Inducible Promoter. Molecular Cell 2004, 16(3):439-452.

[38] Robinson PJJ, Rhodes D: Structure of the '30 nm' chromatin fibre: A key role for the linker histone. Current Opinion in Structural Biology 2006, 16(3):336-343.

[39] Oudet P, Gross-Bellard M, Chambon P: Electron microscopic and biochemical evidence that chromatin structure is a repeating unit. Cell 1975, 4(4):281-300.

[40] Schalch T, Duda S, Sargent DF, Richmond TJ: X-ray structure of a tetranucleosome and its implications for the chromatin fibre. Nature 2005, 436(7047):138-141.

[41] Bharath MMS, Chandra NR, Rao MRS: Molecular modeling of the chromatosome particle. Nucleic Acids Research 2003, 31(14):4264-4274.

[42] Bednar J, Horowitz RA, Grigoryev SA, Carruthers LM, Hansen JC, Koster AJ, Woodcock CL: Nucleosomes, linker DNA, and linker histone form a unique structural motif that directs the higher-order folding and compaction of chromatin. Proceedings of the National Academy of Sciences 1998, 95(24):14173-14178.

[43] Bednar J, Dimitrov S: Chromatin under mechanical stress: from single 30 nm fibers to single nucleosomes. FEBS Journal 2011, 278(13):2231-2243.

[44] Cui Y, Bustamante C: Pulling a single chromatin fiber reveals the forces that maintain its higher-order structure. Proceedings of the National Academy of Sciences 2000, 97(1):127-132.

[45] Staynov D, Proykova Y: Topological constraints on the possible structures of the 30 nm chromatin fibre. Chromosoma 2008, 117(1):67-76.

[46] Adkins NL, Watts M, Georgel PT: To the 30-nm chromatin fiber and beyond. Biochimica et Biophysica Acta (BBA) - Gene Structure and Expression 2004, 1677(1–3): 12-23.

[47] McBryant S, Adams V, Hansen J: Chromatin architectural proteins. Chromosome Research 2006, 14(1):39-51.

[48] Reiner SL: Epigenetic control in the immune response. Human Molecular Genetics 2005, 14(suppl 1):R41-R46.

[49] Turner BM: Defining an epigenetic code. Nat Cell Biol 2007, 9(1):2-6.

[50] Margueron R, Trojer P, Reinberg D: The key to development: interpreting the histone code? Current Opinion in Genetics & Development 2005, 15(2):163-176.

[51] Lin W, Dent SYR: Functions of histone-modifying enzymes in development. Current Opinion in Genetics & Development 2006, 16(2):137-142.

[52] Martin C, Zhang Y: The diverse functions of histone lysine methylation. Nat Rev Mol Cell Biol 2005, 6(11):838-849.

[53] Bernstein E, Hake SB: The nucleosome: a little variation goes a long wayThis paper is one of a selection of papers published in this Special Issue, entitled 27th International West Coast Chromatin and Chromosome Conference, and has undergone the Journal's usual peer review process. Biochemistry and Cell Biology 2006, 84(4):505-507.

[54] Barakat TS, Gribnau J: X chromosome inactivation in the cycle of life. Development 2012, 139(12):2085-2089.

[55] Hassa PO, Hottiger MO: An epigenetic code for DNA damage repair pathways? Biochemistry and Cell Biology 2005, 83(3):270-285.

[56] Méndez-Acuña L, Di Tomaso MV, Palitti F, Martínez-López W: Histone Post-Translational Modifications in DNA Damage Response. Cytogenetic and Genome Research 2010, 128(1-3):28-36.

[57] GrØNbÆK K, Hother C, Jones PA: Epigenetic changes in cancer. APMIS 2007, 115(10):1039-1059.

[58] Fraga MF, Esteller M: Towards the Human Cancer Epigenome: A First Draft of Histone Modifications. Cell Cycle 2005, 4(10):1377-1381.

[59] Agrelo R, Cheng W-H, Setien F, Ropero S, Espada J, Fraga MF, Herranz M, Paz MF, Sanchez-Cespedes M, Artiga MJ et al: Epigenetic inactivation of the premature aging Werner syndrome gene in human cancer. Proceedings of the National Academy of Sciences 2006, 103(23):8822-8827.

[60] Popovic R, Licht JD: Emerging Epigenetic Targets and Therapies in Cancer Medicine. Cancer Discovery 2012, 2(5):405-413.

[61] Bogdanović O, Veenstra G: DNA methylation and methyl-CpG binding proteins: developmental requirements and function. Chromosoma 2009, 118(5):549-565.

[62] Klose RJ, Bird AP: Genomic DNA methylation: the mark and its mediators. Trends in Biochemical Sciences 2006, 31(2):89-97.

[63] Wade PA: Methyl CpG-binding proteins and transcriptional repression*. BioEssays 2001, 23(12):1131-1137.

[64] Vaissière T, Sawan C, Herceg Z: Epigenetic interplay between histone modifications and DNA methylation in gene silencing. Mutation Research/Reviews in Mutation Research 2008, 659(1–2):40-48.

[65] Kanwal R, Gupta S: Epigenetic modifications in cancer. Clinical Genetics 2012, 81(4): 303-311.

[66] Hendrich B, Tweedie S: The methyl-CpG binding domain and the evolving role of DNA methylation in animals. Trends in Genetics 2003, 19(5):269-277.

[67] Jones PA, Baylin SB: The fundamental role of epigenetic events in cancer. Nat Rev Genet 2002, 3(6):415-428.

[68] Tryndyak V, Kovalchuk O, Pogribny IP: Identification of differentially methylated sites within unmethylated DNA domains in normal and cancer cells. Analytical Biochemistry 2006, 356(2):202-207.

[69] Tryndyak VP, Kovalchuk O, Pogribny IP: Loss of DNA methylation and histone H4 lysine 20 trimethylation in human breast cancer cells is associated with aberrant expression of DNA methyltransferase 1, Suv4-20h2 histone methyltransferase and methyl-binding proteins. Cancer Biology & Therapy 2006, 5(1):65-70.

[70] Jones PA, Baylin SB: The Epigenomics of Cancer. Cell 2007, 128(4):683-692.

[71] Baylin SB, Herman JG: DNA hypermethylation in tumorigenesis: epigenetics joins genetics. Trends in Genetics 2000, 16(4):168-174.

[72] Lyko F, Stach D, Brenner A, Stilgenbauer S, Döhner H, Wirtz M, Wiessler M, Schmitz OJ: Quantitative analysis of DNA methylation in chronic lymphocytic leukemia patients. ELECTROPHORESIS 2004, 25(10-11):1530-1535.

[73] Teodoridis JM, Strathdee G, Brown R: Epigenetic silencing mediated by CpG island methylation: potential as a therapeutic target and as a biomarker. Drug Resistance Updates 2004, 7(4–5):267-278.

[74] Omenn GS: Strategies for plasma proteomic profiling of cancers. PROTEOMICS 2006, 6(20):5662-5673.

[75] Patai ÁV, Molnár B, Kalmár A, Schöller A, Tóth K, Tulassay Z: Role of DNA Methylation in Colorectal Carcinogenesis. Digestive Diseases 2012, 30(3):310-315.

[76] Meiers I, Shanks JH, Bostwick DG: Glutathione S-transferase pi (GSTP1) hypermethylation in prostate cancer: review 2007. Pathology Journal of the RCPA 2007, 39(3):299-304 210.1080/00313020701329906.

[77] Yamanaka M, Watanabe M, Yamada Y, Takagi A, Murata T, Takahashi H, Suzuki H, Ito H, Tsukino H, Katoh T et al: Altered methylation of multiple genes in carcinogenesis of the prostate. International Journal of Cancer 2003, 106(3):382-387.

[78] Brooks JD, Weinstein M, Lin X, Sun Y, Pin SS, Bova GS, Epstein JI, Isaacs WB, Nelson WG: CG island methylation changes near the GSTP1 gene in prostatic intraepithelial neoplasia. Cancer Epidemiology Biomarkers & Prevention 1998, 7(6):531-536.

[79] Wolff DW, Xie Y, Deng C, Gatalica Z, Yang M, Wang B, Wang J, Lin M-F, Abel PW, Tu Y: Epigenetic repression of regulator of G-protein signaling 2 promotes androgen-independent prostate cancer cell growth. International Journal of Cancer 2012, 130(7): 1521-1531.

[80] Nakayama M, Gonzalgo ML, Yegnasubramanian S, Lin X, De Marzo AM, Nelson WG: GSTP1 CpG island hypermethylation as a molecular biomarker for prostate cancer. Journal of Cellular Biochemistry 2004, 91(3):540-552.

[81] Cho NY, Kim BH, Choi M, Yoo EJ, Moon KC, Cho YM, Kim D, Kang GH: Hypermethylation of CpG island loci and hypomethylation of LINE-1 and Alu repeats in prostate adenocarcinoma and their relationship to clinicopathological features. The Journal of Pathology 2007, 211(3):269-277.

[82] Cho N-Y, Kim J, Moon K, Kang G: Genomic hypomethylation and CpG island hypermethylation in prostatic intraepithelial neoplasm. Virchows Archiv 2009, 454(1): 17-23.

[83] Ogishima T, Shiina H, Breault JE, Tabatabai L, Bassett WW, Enokida H, Li L-C, Kawakami T, Urakami S, Ribeiro-Filho LA et al: Increased Heparanase Expression Is Caused by Promoter Hypomethylation and Up-Regulation of Transcriptional Factor Early Growth Response-1 in Human Prostate Cancer. Clinical Cancer Research 2005, 11(3):1028-1036.

[84] Hansen KD, Timp W, Bravo HC, Sabunciyan S, Langmead B, McDonald OG, Wen B, Wu H, Liu Y, Diep D et al: Increased methylation variation in epigenetic domains across cancer types. Nat Genet 2011, 43(8):768-775.

[85] Shames DS, Girard L, Gao B, Sato M, Lewis CM, Shivapurkar N, Jiang A, Perou CM, Kim YH, Pollack JR et al: A Genome-Wide Screen for Promoter Methylation in Lung Cancer Identifies Novel Methylation Markers for Multiple Malignancies. PLoS Med 2006, 3(12):e486.

[86] Colacino JA, Arthur AE, Dolinoy DC, Sartor MA, Duffy SA, Chepeha DB, Bradford CR, Walline HM, McHugh JB, D'Silva N et al: Pretreatment dietary intake is associated with tumor suppressor DNA methylation in head and neck squamous cell carcinomas. Epigenetics 2012, 7(8):4-12.

[87] Lee J-S, Smith E, Shilatifard A: The Language of Histone Crosstalk. Cell 2010, 142(5): 682-685.

[88] Hayes JJ, Clark DJ, Wolffe AP: Histone contributions to the structure of DNA in the nucleosome. Proceedings of the National Academy of Sciences 1991, 88(15): 6829-6833.

[89] Strahl BD, Allis CD: The language of covalent histone modifications. Nature 2000, 403(6765):41-45.

[90] Greer EL, Shi Y: Histone methylation: a dynamic mark in health, disease and inheritance. Nat Rev Genet 2012, 13(5):343-357.

[91] Lachner M, Jenuwein T: The many faces of histone lysine methylation. Current Opinion in Cell Biology 2002, 14(3):286-298.

[92] Kouzarides T: Histone methylation in transcriptional control. Current Opinion in Genetics & Development 2002, 12(2):198-209.

[93] Wang H, An W, Cao R, Xia L, Erdjument-Bromage H, Chatton B, Tempst P, Roeder RG, Zhang Y: mAM Facilitates Conversion by ESET of Dimethyl to Trimethyl Lysine 9 of Histone H3 to Cause Transcriptional Repression. Molecular Cell 2003, 12(2): 475-487.

[94] Santos-Rosa H, Schneider R, Bannister AJ, Sherriff J, Bernstein BE, Emre NCT, Schreiber SL, Mellor J, Kouzarides T: Active genes are tri-methylated at K4 of histone H3. Nature 2002, 419(6905):407-411.

[95] Khorasanizadeh S: Recognition of methylated histones: new twists and variations. Current Opinion in Structural Biology 2011, 21(6):744-749.

[96] Sims Iii RJ, Nishioka K, Reinberg D: Histone lysine methylation: a signature for chromatin function. Trends in Genetics 2003, 19(11):629-639.

[97] Sims RJ, Chen C-F, Santos-Rosa H, Kouzarides T, Patel SS, Reinberg D: Human but Not Yeast CHD1 Binds Directly and Selectively to Histone H3 Methylated at Lysine 4

via Its Tandem Chromodomains. Journal of Biological Chemistry 2005, 280(51): 41789-41792.

[98] Verrier L, Vandromme M, Trouche D: Histone demethylases in chromatin cross-talks. Biology of the Cell 2011, 103(8):381-401.

[99] Tsukada Y-i, Fang J, Erdjument-Bromage H, Warren ME, Borchers CH, Tempst P, Zhang Y: Histone demethylation by a family of JmjC domain-containing proteins. Nature 2006, 439(7078):811-816.

[100] Shi Y, Lan F, Matson C, Mulligan P, Whetstine JR, Cole PA, Casero RA, Shi Y: Histone Demethylation Mediated by the Nuclear Amine Oxidase Homolog LSD1. Cell 2004, 119(7):941-953.

[101] Ahmad K, Henikoff S: The Histone Variant H3.3 Marks Active Chromatin by Replication-Independent Nucleosome Assembly. Molecular Cell 2002, 9(6):1191-1200.

[102] Meneghini MD, Wu M, Madhani HD: Conserved Histone Variant H2A.Z Protects Euchromatin from the Ectopic Spread of Silent Heterochromatin. Cell 2003, 112(5): 725-736.

[103] Chakravarthy S, Gundimella SKY, Caron C, Perche P-Y, Pehrson JR, Khochbin S, Luger K: Structural Characterization of the Histone Variant macroH2A. Molecular and Cellular Biology 2005, 25(17):7616-7624.

[104] Ausió J: Histone variants—the structure behind the function. Briefings in Functional Genomics & Proteomics 2006, 5(3):228-243.

[105] Régnier V, Vagnarelli P, Fukagawa T, Zerjal T, Burns E, Trouche D, Earnshaw W, Brown W: CENP-A Is Required for Accurate Chromosome Segregation and Sustained Kinetochore Association of BubR1. Molecular and Cellular Biology 2005, 25(10):3967-3981.

[106] Peters AHFM, O'Carroll D, Scherthan H, Mechtler K, Sauer S, Schöfer C, Weipoltshammer K, Pagani M, Lachner M, Kohlmaier A et al: Loss of the Suv39h Histone Methyltransferases Impairs Mammalian Heterochromatin and Genome Stability. Cell 2001, 107(3):323-337.

[107] Hamamoto R, Furukawa Y, Morita M, Iimura Y, Silva FP, Li M, Yagyu R, Nakamura Y: SMYD3 encodes a histone methyltransferase involved in the proliferation of cancer cells. Nat Cell Biol 2004, 6(8):731-740.

[108] Tsuge M, Hamamoto R, Silva FP, Ohnishi Y, Chayama K, Kamatani N, Furukawa Y, Nakamura Y: A variable number of tandem repeats polymorphism in an E2F-1 binding element in the 5[prime] flanking region of SMYD3 is a risk factor for human cancers. Nat Genet 2005, 37(10):1104-1107.

[109] Frank B, Hemminki K, Wappenschmidt B, Klaes R, Meindl A, Schmutzler RK, Bugert P, Untch M, Bartram CR, Burwinkel B: Variable number of tandem repeats polymor-

phism in the SMYD3 promoter region and the risk of familial breast cancer. International Journal of Cancer 2006, 118(11):2917-2918.

[110] Diehl F, Brown MA, van Amerongen MJ, Novoyatleva T, Wietelmann A, Harriss J, Ferrazzi F, Böttger T, Harvey RP, Tucker PW et al: Cardiac Deletion of Smyd2 Is Dispensable for Mouse Heart Development. PLoS ONE 2010, 5(3):e9748.

[111] Wang L, Li L, Zhang H, Luo X, Dai J, Zhou S, Gu J, Zhu J, Atadja P, Lu C et al: Structure of Human SMYD2 Protein Reveals the Basis of p53 Tumor Suppressor Methylation. Journal of Biological Chemistry 2011, 286(44):38725-38737.

[112] Huang J, Perez-Burgos L, Placek BJ, Sengupta R, Richter M, Dorsey JA, Kubicek S, Opravil S, Jenuwein T, Berger SL: Repression of p53 activity by Smyd2-mediated methylation. Nature 2006, 444(7119):629-632.

[113] Saddic LA, West LE, Aslanian A, Yates JR, Rubin SM, Gozani O, Sage J: Methylation of the Retinoblastoma Tumor Suppressor by SMYD2. Journal of Biological Chemistry 2010, 285(48):37733-37740.

[114] Wang H, Cao R, Xia L, Erdjument-Bromage H, Borchers C, Tempst P, Zhang Y: Purification and Functional Characterization of a Histone H3-Lysine 4-Specific Methyltransferase. Molecular Cell 2001, 8(6):1207-1217.

[115] Kouskouti A, Scheer E, Staub A, Tora L, Talianidis I: Gene-Specific Modulation of TAF10 Function by SET9-Mediated Methylation. Molecular Cell 2004, 14(2):175-182.

[116] Chuikov S, Kurash JK, Wilson JR, Xiao B, Justin N, Ivanov GS, McKinney K, Tempst P, Prives C, Gamblin SJ et al: Regulation of p53 activity through lysine methylation. Nature 2004, 432(7015):353-360.

[117] Yoshida K, Miki Y: The cell death machinery governed by the p53 tumor suppressor in response to DNA damage. Cancer Science 2010, 101(4):831-835.

[118] He Y, Korboukh I, Jin J, Huang J: Targeting protein lysine methylation and demethylation in cancers. Acta Biochimica et Biophysica Sinica 2012, 44(1):70-79.

[119] Jiang Y-h, Bressler J, Beaudet AL: EPIGENETICS AND HUMAN DISEASE. Annual Review of Genomics and Human Genetics 2004, 5(1):479-510.

[120] Brown R, Strathdee G: Epigenomics and epigenetic therapy of cancer. Trends in Molecular Medicine 2002, 8(4):S43-S48.

[121] Lyko F, Brown R: DNA Methyltransferase Inhibitors and the Development of Epigenetic Cancer Therapies. Journal of the National Cancer Institute 2005, 97(20): 1498-1506.

[122] Lind G, Thorstensen L, Lovig T, Meling G, Hamelin R, Rognum T, Esteller M, Lothe R: A CpG island hypermethylation profile of primary colorectal carcinomas and colon cancer cell lines. Molecular Cancer 2004, 3(1):28.

[123] Claus R, Fliegauf M, Stock M, Duque JA, Kolanczyk M, Lübbert M: Inhibitors of DNA methylation and histone deacetylation independently relieve AML1/ETO-mediated lysozyme repression. Journal of Leukocyte Biology 2006, 80(6):1462-1472.

Chapter 6

# Circulating Methylated DNA as Biomarkers for Cancer Detection

Hongchuan Jin, Yanning Ma, Qi Shen and Xian Wang

Additional information is available at the end of the chapter

http://dx.doi.org/10.5772/51419

## 1. Introduction

In addition to genetic alterations including deletion or point mutations, epigenetic changes such as DNA methylation play an important role in silencing tumor suppressor genes during cancer development. By adding a methyl group from S-adenosyl-L-methionine to the cytosine pyrimidine or adenine purine ring, DNA methylation is important to maintain genome structure and regulate gene expression. In mammalian adult tissues, DNA methylation occurs in CpG dinucleotides that often cluster in the genome as CpG islands in the 5′ regulatory regions of the genes. Through recruiting transcriptional co-repressors including methyl-CpG-binding domain proteins (MBDs) and chromatin remodeling proteins like histone deacetylases (HDACs) or impeding the binding of transcriptional activators, DNA methylation could suppress the transcription of many tumor suppressor genes critical to cancer initiation and progression [1-3].

More and more results confirmed that cancer is a multi-stage process fuelled by many epigenetic changes in addition to genetic changes in DNA sequence [4]. Chemical molecules like Trichostatin A (TSA) and 5-aza-2'-deoxycytidine (5-Aza-CdR) targeting epigenetic regulators such as histone modifications and DNMTs (DNA methyltransferases) have been found to inhibit tumor growth both in vitro and in vivo. By reversing the epigenetic silencing of important tumor suppressor genes, an increasing number of epigenetic drugs such as 5-Aza-CdR, 5-Aza-CR and Vorinostat (SAHA) are currently investigated in the clinical trials for cancer treatment as a single drug or in combination with other epigenetic drugs or other approaches such as chemotherapy and showed very promising activities by offering significant clinical benefits to cancer patients [5-13].

As one of the major epigenetic changes to inactivate tumor suppressor genes critical to human cancer development, DNA methylation was recognized as the biomarker for cancer detection or outcome prediction in addition to the identification of novel tumor suppressor genes. DNA mutations will occur randomly in any nucleotides of one particular gene and the comprehensive determination of DNA mutations is thus very difficult and time-consuming. In contrast, aberrant DNA hypermethylation usually takes place in defined CpG Islands within the regulatory region of the genes and it is much more convenient to detect DNA methylation in a quantitatively manner. In addition, DNA methylation can be amplified and is thus easily detectable using PCR-based approaches even when the DNA concentration after sample extraction is relatively low. Due to such advantages over DNA mutation- or protein-based biomarkers, DNA methylation-based biomarkers have been intensively investigated in the recent years. A large body of research reports has proved the value of DNA methylations in the prognosis prediction and detection of various cancers. DNAs used for such methylation analyses are usually extracted from tumor tissues harvested after surgical operation or biopsy, thus limiting its wide application as the biomarkers for the early detection or screening of human cancers. Recently, it has been reported that there are certain amount of circulating DNAs in the peripheral blood of cancer patients, providing an ideal source to identify novel biomarkers for non-invasive detection of cancers. Both genetic and epigenetic changes found in the genomic DNAs extracted from primary tumor cells could be detected in the circulating DNAs, indicating that the detection of methylated DNAs in the circulation represents a new direction to develop novel biomarkers for cancer detection or screening in a non-invasive manner.

## 2. Cell free DNA in the circulation

According to the origin of circulating tumor-related DNA, it could be grouped into circulating cell free DNA or DNA from cells in the blood such as circulating tumor cells (CTC) in cancer patients (Figure 1).

In 1869, the Australian physician Thomas Ashworth observed CTCs in the blood of a cancer patient. Therefore, it was postulated that CTCs were responsible for the tumor metastases in distal sites and should have important prognostic and therapeutic implications [14-16]. However, the number of CTCs is very small compared with blood cells. Usually around 1-10 CTCs together with several million blood cells could be found in 1 ml of whole blood, making the specific and sensitive detection of CTCs very difficult [17-18]. Until recently, technologies with the requisite sensitivity and reproducibility for CTC detection have been developed to precisely analyze its biological and clinical relevance. The US Food and Drug Administration (FDA) approved the test for determining CTC levels in patients with metastatic breast cancer in 2004. Currently, it has been expanded to other cancer types such as advanced colorectal cancer and prostate cancer. Although CTCs-counting based test have proven its value in predicting prognosis and monitoring therapeutic effects, the number of CTCs per ml of blood limited its sensitivity greatly [19]. With the development of high-sensitive PCR-based methods, the detection of gene mutations or epigenetic changes such as

DNA methylation within small amount of CTCs could be the next generation of CTC-based test for cancer detection. However, the cost of such tests will be greatly exacerbated, thus limiting its wide application in the clinic [20-22].

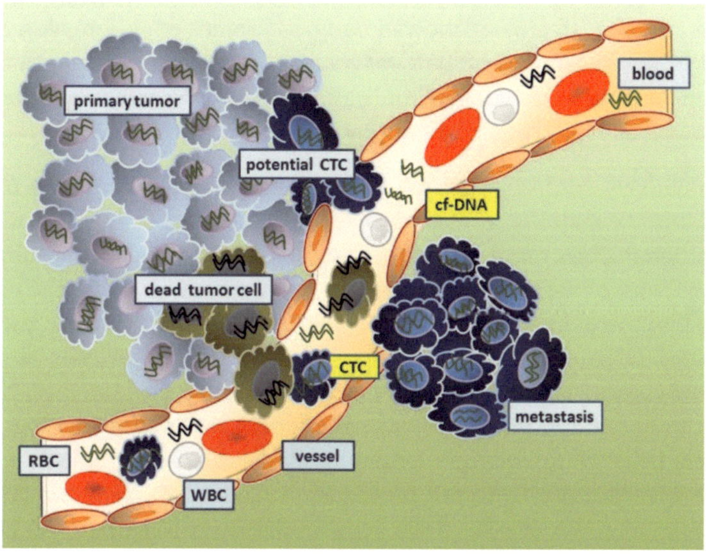


**Figure 1.** Circulating tumor cells and cell free DNA. Circulating Tumor cells (CTC) escape from primary sites and spread into the vessel to form metastases in the distal organs with. Cell free DNAs (cf-DNAs) are released into the circulation from dead cancer cells or proliferating tumor cells. RBC: red blood cell; WBC: white blood cell.

Although its origin and biological relevance remains unknown, circulating cell free DNA (cf-DNA) is supposed to be valuable source to identify cancer markers with ideal sensitivity and specificity for non-invasive detection of cancer [23-24]. Early in 1948, two French scientists Mandel and Metais firstly reported the presence of cf-DNAs in human plasma [25]. Such an important discovery has been unnoticed for a long time until cell-free circulating nucleic acid was found to promote the spread and metastasis of crown gall tumor in plants [26]. Subsequently, increased level of cf-DNAs was found in patients with various diseases such as lupus erythematosus and rheumatoid arthritis cancer [27-28]. In 1977, Leon et al. reported that higher level of circulating DNA in the plasma of cancer patients when compared to healthy controls. Moreover, greater amounts of cf-DNA were found in the peripheral blood of cancer patients with tumor metastases and cf-DNA levels decreased dramatically after radiotherapy while persistently high or increasing DNA concentrations were associated with a lack of response to treatment [29], clearly revealing the potential value of cf-DNA as biomarker for cancer detection. Following studies confirmed that cf-DNAs in the plasma contains genetic and epigenetic changes specific to DNAs within the tumor cells from primary tissues, indicating that tumor specific cf-DNAs are originated from tumor cells rather than lymphocytes reacting towards the disease [30-31]. For example, K-Ras mutation was found in cf-DNA from 17 out of 21 patients with pancreatic adenocarcinoma and mutations were similar in corresponding plasma and tissues samples. Importantly, such DNA alterations were found in patients with pancreatitis who were diagnosed as pancreatic cancer 5-14 months later, indicating that release of tumor-specific DNA into the circulation is an early event in cancer development and cf-DNA could be used as the biomarkers for early cancer detection [32]. Treatment resulted in disappearance of K-Ras mutations in plasma DNA in six of nine patients. Three patients with a persistently positive K-Ras gene mutation in plasma samples from patients before and after treatment showed early recurrence or progression and pancreatic carcinoma patients with the mutant-type K-ras gene in plasma DNA exhibited a shorter survival time than patients with the wild-type gene, indicating the cf-DNA could be of value in monitoring disease progression or evaluating treatment response [31, 33].

Through quantitatively analyzing plasma DNAs from patients with organ transplantation, Lo et al found that the majority of plasma DNAs was released from the hematopoietic system. However, donor DNA could be detected in the plasma of recipients suffering from the graft rejection because of the large amount of cell death which promotes the release of donor DNAs into the peripheral blood of the recipients [34]. Therefore, it was postulated that cell-free tumor related DNA could originate from the apoptotic tumor cells since high-rate of apoptosis indeed occurs in primary and metastatic tumor tissues. However, cf-DNA quantities are significantly reduced in cancer patients after radiotherapy when a great number of tumor cells were believed to undergo apoptotic cell death and cf-DNAs in supernatants of cultured cancer cells increases with cell proliferation rather than apoptosis or necrosis, indicating that proliferating tumor cells could actively release cf-DNA into the tumor microenvironment and circulation.

In contrast to labile RNAs that were included into the actively secreted exosomes, the nature of cf-DNAs remains to be clarified. As negatively charged molecules, cf-DNA was bound by plasma proteins to escape from endonuclease-mediated degradation. Unfortunately, plasma proteins bound to cf-DNAs was not well characterized yet. Meanwhile, secreted exosomes could remodel microenviroments and promote tumor metastasis since RNAs within exosomes especially microRNA with high stability may influence gene expression in neighbor cells. The biological relevance of cf-DNAs remains unknown. DNA was believed to be more structural rather than functional. However, it was supposed that cf-DNA could play a role as vaccine in tumor microenvironment.

## 3. Methods for the detection of methylated DNA

It is unclear so far whether serum or plasma is better for cf-DNA extraction. Although the DNA amount is significantly higher in the serum, the majority of the increase was due to the release of nuclear acids from destroyed blood cells during blood clotting [35]. In addition, the time gap between blooding drawing and DNA extraction as well as the methodologies used for DNA isolation contribute greatly to the amount of cf-DNA harvested. On an average, around 30 ng cf-DNA could be extracted from one ml of blood sample [36]. Therefore, in order to determine the quantity of potential cf-DNA-based biomarkers precisely and promote its wide application for cancer detection, it is very important to unify the source as well as the methodologies for cf-DNA extraction and use various internal controls to adjust possible inter-laboratory variations.

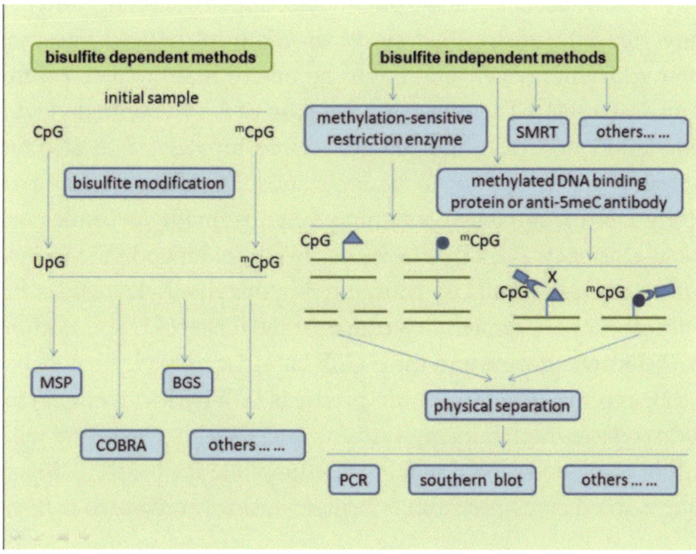


**Figure 2.** Schematic introductions of various methods for methylation analyses. MSP, BGS and COBRA are based on bisulfite-mediated conversion of unmethylated cytosines into uracils. CpG methylation could block DNA digestion by some restriction enzymes, making it possible to determine methylation status independent of bisulfite treatment by analyzing digestion products. Alternatively, DNA fragments containing methylated CpG sites could be enriched by anti-methylcytosine antibody or methylation binding proteins. Advances in next generation genome sequencing technology led to the development of noel techniques such as SMRT which can specially analyze 5-methylcytosines with genome wide coverage.

In general, the detection of DNA methylation could be bisulfite-dependent or -independent (Figure 2).

The chemical reaction of sodium bisulfite with DNA could convert unmethylated cytosine of CpG into uracil or UpG but leave methylated cytosine of CpG unchanged. The following analyses such as methylation-and unmethylation specific polymerase chain reaction (M- and U-SP), bisulfite genome sequencing (BGS) or combined bisulfite restriction analysis (COBRA) could determine the conversion of CpG sites of interest, thus reflecting their methylation status as methylated or unmethylated [37]. With varied resolution levels, different bisulfite-dependent DNA methylation analysis methods detect the conversion after bisulfite treatment of genomic DNA, which could have certain artificial effects such as incomplete conversion of unmethylated CpG into UpG, leading to high rate of false negative conclusion of DNA methylation status.

Recently, some new modifications of cytosine in CpG dinucleotides have been discovered such as 5-hydoxymethylcytosine which was called the sixth base since 5-methylcytosine was named as the fifth base [38]. Generated from the oxidation of 5-methylcytosine by the Tet family of enzymes, 5-hydoxymethylcytosine was first found in bacteriophages and recently shown to be abundant in human and mouse brains as well as in embryonic stem cells [39-40]. Although the exact relevance of 5-hydoxymethylcytosine in the genome is still not fully clarified, it has been found to regulate gene expression or promote DNA demethylation. The in vitro synthesized artificial oligonucleotides containing 5-hydoxymethylcytosines can be converted into unmodified cytosines when introduced into mammalian cells, indicating that 5-hydoxymethylcytosine might be one of intermediate products during active DNA demethylation [41]. Therefore, the increase of 5-hydoxymethylcytosine might reflect the demethylation of CpG dinucleotides. Unfortunately, 5-hydoxymethylcytosines, similar to 5-methylcytosines, appear to be resistant to bisulfite-mediated conversion and PCR could amplify DNA fragments containing 5-hydoxymethylcytosines or 5-methylcytosines with similar efficiency [42-43]. Therefore, bisulfite-dependent methylation analyses could produce false positive results by counting 5-hydoxymethylcytosines into 5-methylcytosines. In addition to 5-hydroxymethylcytosines, some forms of DNA modifications such as the seventh base, 5-formylcytosine and the eighth base, 5-carboxylcytosine, have been found in mammalian cells recently [44-47]. As the products of 5-hydoxymethylcytosine oxidation through TET hydroxylases, both 5-formylcytosine and 5-carboxylcytosine will be read as the uracil after bisulfite conversion, thus making it impossible for bisulfite-dependent analyses to distinguish unmodified cytosines from 5-formylcytosines and 5-carboxylcytosines.

Bisulfite independent analyses such as MedIP (methylated DNA immunoprecipitation) could more or less detect DNA methylation specifically. In bisulfite independent analyses, 5-methylcytosines are differentiated from unmethylated cytosine by either enzyme digestion or affinity enrichment. DNA methylation analysis using restriction enzyme digestion is based on the property of some methylation-sensitive and -resistant restriction enzymes such as HpaII and MspI that target CCGG for digestion. HpaII fails to cut it once the second cytosine was methylated while MspI-mediated digestion is not affected by DNA methylation, thus making it possible to determine the methylation status of CpG in the context of CCGG tetranucleotides by analyzing the products of DNAs digested by HpaII and MspI respectively. As a primary method to analyze DNA methylation, it can only determine the methylation of CpG in the context of CCGG tetranucleotides and will overlook the majority of CpG dinucleotides in the genome.

The development of monoclonal antibody specific to 5-methylcytosines revolutionized the analyses of DNA methylation [48-49]. Immunoprecipitated DNA by this antibody could be subject to DNA microarray or even deep sequencing to reveal novel sequences or sites containing 5-methylcytosines [50]. This antibody specifically recognizes 5-methylcytosines but not 5-hydoxymethylcytosines. However, 5-methylcytosines could present not only in CpG dinucleotides but also in CHH or CHG trinucleotides, especially in plants, human embryonic stem cells and probably cancer cells as well. CHH methylation indicates a 5-methylcytosine followed by two nucleotides that may not be guanine and CHG methylation refers to a 5-methylcytosine preceding an adenine, thymine or cytosine base followed by guanine. Such non-CpG DNA methylations were enriched at transposons and repetitive regions, although the exact biological relevance remains unknown. However, antibody against 5-methylcyto-

http://dx.doi.org/10.5772/51419

sine may precipitate methylated CHH and CHG trinucleotide containing DNA fragments in addition to DNA sequences with methylated CpG sites.

DNA methylation functions as the signal for DNA-interacting proteins to maintain genome structure or regulate gene expression. The proteins such as MBD1 (methyl-CpG binding domain protein 1), MeCP2 (methyl CpG binding protein 2) and MBD4 (methyl-CpG binding domain protein 4) bind methylated CpG specifically to regulate gene expression [51-52]. Therefore, methyl-CpG binding domain could specifically enrich differentially methylated regions (DMRs) of physiological relevance [53]. Similar to MeDIP, MBD capture specifically enrich methylated CpG sites rather than hydroxymethlated CpG sites. The detailed analysis to compare MeDIP and MBD capture revealed that both enrichment techniques are sensitive enough to identify DMRs in human cancer cells. However, MeDIP enriched more methylated regions with low CpG densities while MBD capture favors regions of high CpG densities and identifies the greater proportion of CpG islands [49].

Recently, the advance of next generation sequencing led to the development of several novel techniques, making it possible to quantitatively analyze DNA methylation at single nucleotide resolution with genome wide coverage. Both the single molecule real time sequencing technology (SMRT) and the single-molecule nanopore DNA sequencing platform could discriminate 5-methylcytosines from other DNA bases including 5-hydroxymethylcytosines even methyladenine independent of bisulfite conversion [54-55]. With many advantages such as less bias during template preparation, lower cost and better accuracy, such new techniques could offer more methods to detect DNA methylation with high specificity and sensitivity in addition to more potential DNA methylation based biomarkers for cancer detection and screening.

## 4. Potential DNA methylation biomarkers for cancer detection

It has been questioned whether the methylated DNA in the circulation is sensitive to detect cancers early enough for curative resection. However, the development of sensitive detection methods confirmed the potential value of DNA methylation in cancer detection (Table 1).

Most of DNA methylation biomarkers are well-known tumor suppressor genes silenced in primary tumor tissues. However, the biomarks do not have to be functional relevant. For example, currently well-used biomarkers such as AFP (Alpha-Fetal Protein), PSA (Prostate-specific antigen) and CEA (Carcinoembryonic antigen) are not tumor suppressor genes with important biological functions. Profiling of methylated DNA in the circulation instead of primary tumor tissues with MeDIP or MBD capture or other methylation specific analyses methods would identify more potential biomarks rather than functional important tumor suppressor genes.

| Cancer | Markers | Sensitivity | Specificity | Methods | Ref. |
|---|---|---|---|---|---|
| Bladder cancer | CDKN2A (ARF) CDKN2A | 13/27 (48%) | N/A | MSP | [58] |
| | (INK4A) | 2/27 (7%) | N/A | MSP | |
| | CDKN2A (INK4A) | 19/86 (22%) | 31/31 (100%) | MSP | [59] |
| Breast cancer | CDKN2A (INK4A) | 5/35 (14%) | N/A | MS-AP-PCR | [56] |
| | CDKN2A (INK4A) | 6/43 (14%) | N/A | MS-AP-PCR | [57] |
| Colorectal cancer | MLH1 | 3/18 (17%) | N/A | MSP | [60] |
| | CDKN2A (INK4A) CDKN2A | 14/52 (27%) | 44/44 (100%) | MSP | [61] |
| | (INK4A) CDKN2A (INK4A) | 13/94 (11%) | N/A | MSP | [62] |
| | ALX4 | 21/58 (36%) | N/A | MSP | [63] |
| | CDH4 | 25/30 (83%) | 36/52 (70%) | MSP | [64] |
| | NGFR | 32/46 (70%) | 17/17 (100%) | MSP | [65] |
| | RUNX3 | 68/133 (51%) | 150/179 (84%) | MSP | [66] |
| | SEPT9 | 11/17 (65%) | 10/10 (100%) | MSP | [67] |
| | TMEFF2 | 92/133 (69%) | 154/179 (86%) | MSP | [66] |
| | | 87/133 (65%) | 123/179 (69%) | MSP | |
| Esophageal cancer | APC | 13/52 (25%) | 54/54 (100%) | MSP | [68] |
| | APC | 2/32 (6%) | 54/54 (100%) | MSP | |
| | CDKN2A (INK4A) | 7/38 (18%) | N/A | MSP | [69] |
| Gastric cancer | CDH1 | 31/54 (57%) | 30/30 (100%) | MSP | [70] |
| | CDKN2A (INK4A) | 28/54 (52%) | 30/30 (100%) | MSP | |
| | CDKN2B (INK4B) | 30/54 (56%) | 30/30 (100%) | MSP | |
| | DAPK1 | 26/54 (48%) | 30/30 (100%) | MSP | |
| | GSTP1 | 18/54 (15%) | 30/30 (100%) | MSP | |
| | Panel of five | 45/54 (83%) | 30/30 (100%) | MSP | |
| Head and neck cancer | CDKN2A (INK4A) | 8/95 (8%) | N/A | MSP | [71] |
| | DAPK1 | 3/95 (3%) | N/A | MSP | |
| | MGMT | 14/95 (15%) | N/A | MSP | |
| | Panel of three | 21/95 (22%) | N/A | MSP | |
| | DAPK1 | N/A | N/A | MSP | [72] |
| Liver cancer | CDKN2A (INK4A) CDKN2B | 13/22 (45%) | 48/48 (100%) | MSP | [73] |
| | (INK4B) | 4/25 (16%) | 35/35 (100%) | MSP | [74] |
| Lung cancer | CDKN2A (INK4A) | 3/22 (14%) | N/A | MSP | [75] |
| | DAPK1 | 4/22 (18%) | N/A | MSP | |
| | GSTP1 | 1/22 (5%) | N/A | MSP | |
| | MGMT | 4/22 (18%) | N/A | MSP | |
| | Panel of four | 11/22 (50%) | N/A | MSP | |
| | CDKN2A (INK4A) | N/A | N/A | MSP | [76] |
| | APC | 42/89 (47%) | 50/50 (100%) | MSP | [77] |

| Cancer | Markers | Sensitivity | Specificity | Methods | Ref. |
|---|---|---|---|---|---|
| | CDKN2A (INK4A) | 77/105 (73%) | N/A | MSP | [78] |
| | CDKN2A (INK4A) | 12/35 (34%) | 15/15 (100%) | MSP | [79] |
| Prostate cancer | GSTP1 | 23/33 (70%) | 22/22 (100%) | MSP | [80] |
| | GSTP1 | 25/69 (36%) | 31/31 (100%) | MSP | [81] |

**Table 1.** Methylated DNA biomarkers in the literature.

Most of the methods used for methylation biomarkers analyses are still bisulfite dependent. Few reports used MS-AP-PCR (methylation-sensitive arbitrarily primed PCR) which takes the advantage of methylation sensitive restriction endonucleases to distinguish methylated CpG from unmethylated form, although the sensitivity seems to be lower than MSP [56-57]. Interestingly, combination of more than one methylated DNA as a methylation panel could great increase the sensitivity for cancer detection without significant reduction of specificity. Unfortunately, most of studies were performed in a retrospective manner. More prospective studies with large sample sizes will be warranted to compare different approaches especially bisulfite-independent methods in addition to confirm the value of DNA methylation for cancer detection.

## 5. Conclusion and Perspectives

With the development of the next generation genome sequencing as well as single molecular PCR, it became possible to analyze trace amount of DNAs including circulating cell-free DNA. Circulating tumor cells have been proven its value in prognosis predication even early detection of various cancers. The analyses of methylated DNAs in the circulating will be the next promising epigenetic biomarkers for cancer detection. As one of the intermediate products of DNA demethylation, 5-hydroxymethlcytosines are resistant to bisulfite conversion. Therefore, it should be carefully to interpret the data of methylation analyses based on bisulfite treatment due to potentially high rate of false positive results. Although some methylated DNAs were found to valuable as a single biomarker for cancer detection, more potential DNA methylations will be found after the wide application of SMRT and other sequencing platforms with high speed, depth and accuracy. DNA methylation signatures including a panel of methylated DNAs will show the potential in the early diagnosis or screening and prognosis or therapy response prediction of many cancers. In addition, such DNA methylation biomarkers could be more sensitive and specific for cancer detection when combined with well-used biochemical biomarkers. However, unified methods with gold standards will be warranted to promote the development and clinical application of DNA methylation biomarkers.

## Acknowledgements

This work was supported by the National Natural Science Foundation of China (81071963; 81071652), Program for Innovative Research Team in Science and technology of Zhejiang Province (2010R50046) and Program for Qianjiang Scholarship in Zhejiang Province (2011R10061; 2011R10073).

## Author details

Hongchuan Jin, Yanning Ma, Qi Shen and Xian Wang*

*Address all correspondence to: wangx118@yahoo.com

Department of Medical Oncology, Laboratory of Cancer Epigenetics, Biomedical Research Center, Sir Runrun Shaw Hospital, Zhejiang University, China

## References

[1] Jones, P. A., & Baylin, S. B. (2007). The epigenomics of cancer. *Cell*, 128, 683-692.

[2] Jones, P. A., & Baylin, S. B. (2002). The fundamental role of epigenetic events in cancer. *Nat Rev Genet*, 3, 415-428.

[3] Baylin, S. B., Esteller, M., Rountree, M. R., Bachman, K. E., Schuebel, K., & Herman, J. G. (2001). Aberrant patterns of DNA methylation, chromatin formation and gene expression in cancer. *Hum Mol Genet*, 10, 687-692.

[4] Baylin, S. B., & Herman, J. G. (2000). DNA hypermethylation in tumorigenesis: epigenetics joins genetics. *Trends Genet*, 16, 168-174.

[5] Oki, Y., & Issa, J. P. (2006). Review: recent clinical trials in epigenetic therapy. *Rev Recent Clin Trials*, 1, 169-182.

[6] Kelly, T. K., De Carvalho, D. D., & Jones, P. A. (2010). Epigenetic modifications as therapeutic targets. *Nat Biotechnol*, 28, 1069-1078.

[7] Ramalingam, S. S., Maitland, M. L., Frankel, P., Argiris, A. E., Koczywas, M., Gitlitz, B., Thomas, S., Espinoza-Delgado, I., Vokes, E. E, Gandara, D. R., & Belani, C. P. (2010). Carboplatin and Paclitaxel in combination with either vorinostat or placebo for first-line therapy of advanced non-small-cell lung cancer. *J Clin Oncol*, 28, 56-62.

[8] Braiteh, F., Soriano, A. O., Garcia-Manero, G., Hong, D., Johnson, MM, Silva Lde, P., Yang, H., Alexander, S., Wolff, J., & Kurzrock, R. (2008). Phase I study of epigenetic modulation with 5-azacytidine and valproic acid in patients with advanced cancers. *Clin Cancer Res*, 14, 6296-6301.

[9] Font, P. (2011). Azacitidine for the treatment of patients with acute myeloid leukemia with 20%-30% blasts and multilineage dysplasia. *Adv Ther*, 3(28), 1-9.

[10] Fu, S., Hu, W., Iyer, R., Kavanagh, J. J., Coleman, R. L., Levenback, C. F., Sood, A. K., Wolf, J. K., Gershenson, D. M., Markman, M., Hennessy, B. T., Kurzrock, R., & Bast, R. C., Jr. (2011). Phase 1b-2a study to reverse platinum resistance through use of a hypomethylating agent, azacitidine, in patients with platinum-resistant or platinum-refractory epithelial ovarian cancer. *Cancer*, 117, 1661-1669.

[11] Silverman, L. R., Fenaux, P., Mufti, G. J., Santini, V., Hellstrom-Lindberg, E., Gattermann, N., Sanz, G., List, A. F., Gore, S. D., & Seymour, J. F. (2011). Continued azacitidine therapy beyond time of first response improves quality of response in patients with higher-risk myelodysplastic syndromes. *Cancer*.

[12] Sonpavde, G., Aparicio, A. M., Zhan, F., North, B., Delaune, R., Garbo, L. E., Rousey, S. R., Weinstein, R. E., Xiao, L., Boehm, K. A., Asmar, L., Fleming, M. T., Galsky, M. D., Berry, W. R., & Von Hoff, D. D. (2011). Azacitidine favorably modulates PSA kinetics correlating with plasma DNA LINE-1 hypomethylation in men with chemo-naive castration-resistant prostate cancer. *Urol Oncol*, 29, 682-689.

[13] Keating, G. M. (2012). Azacitidine: a review of its use in the management of myelodysplastic syndromes/acute myeloid leukaemia. *Drugs*, 72, 1111-1136.

[14] Alix-Panabieres, C., Schwarzenbach, H., & Pantel, K. (2012). Circulating tumor cells and circulating tumor DNA. *Annu Rev Med*, 63, 199-215.

[15] Zhe, X., Cher, M. L., & Bonfil, R. D. (2011). Circulating tumor cells: finding the needle in the haystack. *Am J Cancer Res*, 1, 740-751.

[16] Fidler, I. J. (2003). The pathogenesis of cancer metastasis: the 'seed and soil' hypothesis revisited. *Nat Rev Cancer*, 3, 453-458.

[17] Ghossein, RA, Bhattacharya, S, & Rosai, J. (1999). Molecular detection of micrometastases and circulating tumor cells in solid tumors. *Clin Cancer Res*, 5, 1950-1960.

[18] Pelkey, TJ, Frierson, H. F., Jr, & Bruns, D. E. (1996). Molecular and immunological detection of circulating tumor cells and micrometastases from solid tumors. *Clin Chem*, 42, 1369-1381.

[19] Mocellin, S., Keilholz, U., Rossi, C. R., & Nitti, D. (2006). Circulating tumor cells: the 'leukemic phase' of solid cancers. *Trends Mol Med*, 12, 130-139.

[20] Chimonidou, M., Strati, A., Tzitzira, A., Sotiropoulou, G., Malamos, N., Georgoulias, V., & Lianidou, E. S. (2011). DNA methylation of tumor suppressor and metastasis suppressor genes in circulating tumor cells. *Clin Chem*, 57, 1169-1177.

[21] Garcia-Olmo, D. C., Gutierrez-Gonzalez, L., Ruiz-Piqueras, R., Picazo, M. G., & Garcia-Olmo, D. (2005). Detection of circulating tumor cells and of tumor DNA in plasma during tumor progression in rats. *Cancer Lett*, 217, 115-123.

[22] Matuschek, C., Bolke, E., Lammering, G., Gerber, P. A., Peiper, M., Budach, W., Taskin, H., Prisack, H. B., Schieren, G., Orth, K., & Bojar, H. (2010). Methylated APC and GSTP1 Genes in Serum DNA Correlate with the Presence of Circulating Blood Tumor Cells and are Associated with a More Aggressive and Advanced Breast Cancer Disease. *Eur J Med Res*, 15, 277-286.

[23] Kohler, C., Barekati, Z., Radpour, R., & Zhong, X. Y. (2011). Cell-free DNA in the circulation as a potential cancer biomarker. *Anticancer Res*, 31, 2623-2628.

[24] Mittra, I., Nair, N. K., & Mishra, P. K. (2012). Nucleic acids in circulation: Are they harmful to the host? *J Biosci*, 37, 301-312.

[25] Hung, EC, Chiu, RW, & Lo, YM. (2009). Detection of circulating fetal nucleic acids: a review of methods and applications. *J Clin Pathol*, 62, 308-313.

[26] Stroun, M., & Anker, P. (2005). Circulating DNA in higher organisms cancer detection brings back to life an ignored phenomenon. *Cell Mol Biol (Noisy-le-grand)*, 51, 767-774.

[27] Koffler, D., Agnello, V., Winchester, R., & Kunkel, H. G. (1973). The occurrence of single-stranded DNA in the serum of patients with systemic lupus erythematosus and other diseases. *J Clin Invest*, 52, 198-204.

[28] Leon, S. A., Ehrlich, G. E., Shapiro, B., & Labbate, V. A. (1977). Free DNA in the serum of rheumatoid arthritis patients. *J Rheumatol*, 4, 139-143.

[29] Leon, S. A., Shapiro, B., Sklaroff, D. M., & Yaros, M. J. (1977). Free DNA in the serum of cancer patients and the effect of therapy. *Cancer Res*, 37, 646-650.

[30] Lo, Y. M. (2001). Circulating nucleic acids in plasma and serum: an overview. *Ann N Y Acad Sci*, 945, 1-7.

[31] Anker, P., Lyautey, J., Lederrey, C., & Stroun, M. (2001). Circulating nucleic acids in plasma or serum. Clin Chim Acta ., 313, 143-146.

[32] Yamada, T., Nakamori, S., Ohzato, H., Oshima, S., Aoki, T., Higaki, N., Sugimoto, K., Akagi, K., Fujiwara, Y., Nishisho, I., Sakon, M., Gotoh, M., & Monden, M. (1998). Detection of K-ras gene mutations in plasma DNA of patients with pancreatic adenocarcinoma: correlation with clinicopathological features. *Clin Cancer Res*, 4, 1527-1532.

[33] Castells, A., Puig, P., Mora, J., Boadas, J., Boix, L., Urgell, E., Sole, M., Capella, G., Lluis, F., Fernandez-Cruz, L., Navarro, S., & Farre, A. (1999 ). Kras mutations in DNA extracted from the plasma of patients with pancreatic carcinoma: diagnostic utility and prognostic significance. *J Clin Oncol*, 17, 578-584.

[34] Lui, Y. Y., Woo, K. S., Wang, A. Y., Yeung, C. K., Li, P. K., Chau, E., Ruygrok, P., & Lo, Y. M. (2003). Origin of plasma cell-free DNA after solid organ transplantation. *Clin Chem*, 49, 495-496.

[35] Chan, K. C., Yeung, S. W., Lui, W. B., Rainer, T. H., & Lo, Y. M. (2005). Effects of pre-analytical factors on the molecular size of cell-free DNA in blood. *Clin Chem*, 51, 781-784.

[36] Board, R. E., Knight, L., Greystoke, A., Blackhall, F. H., Hughes, A., Dive, C., & Ranson, M. (2008). DNA methylation in circulating tumour DNA as a biomarker for cancer. *Biomark Insights*, 2, 307-319.

[37] Herman, J. G., Graff, J. R., Myohanen, S., Nelkin, B. D., & Baylin, S. B. (1996). Methylation-specific PCR: a novel PCR assay for methylation status of CpG islands. *Proc Natl Acad Sci U S A*, 93, 9821-9826.

[38] Branco, M. R., Ficz, G., & Reik, W. (2012). Uncovering the role of 5-hydroxymethylcytosine in the epigenome. *Nat Rev Genet*, 13, 7-13.

[39] Tahiliani, M., Koh, K. P., Shen, Y., Pastor, W. A., Bandukwala, H., Brudno, Y., Agarwal, S., Iyer, L. M., Liu, D. R., Aravind, L., & Rao, A. (2009). Conversion of 5-methylcytosine to 5-hydroxymethylcytosine in mammalian DNA by MLL partner TET1. *Science*, 324, 930-935.

[40] Wyatt, G. R., & Cohen, SS. (1952). A new pyrimidine base from bacteriophage nucleic acids. *Nature*, 170, 1072-1073.

[41] Guo, J. U., Su, Y., Zhong, C., Ming, G. L., & Song, H. (2011). Hydroxylation of 5-methylcytosine by TET1 promotes active DNA demethylation in the adult brain. *Cell*, 145, 423-434.

[42] Nestor, C., Ruzov, A., Meehan, R., & Dunican, D. (2010). Enzymatic approaches and bisulfite sequencing cannot distinguish between 5-methylcytosine and 5-hydroxymethylcytosine in DNA. *Biotechniques*, 48, 317-319.

[43] Huang, Y., Pastor, W. A., Shen, Y., Tahiliani, M., Liu, D. R., & Rao, A. (2010). The behaviour of 5-hydroxymethylcytosine in bisulfite sequencing. *PLoS One*, 5, e8888.

[44] Pfaffeneder, T., Hackner, B., Truss, M., Munzel, M., Muller, M., Deiml, C. A., Hagemeier, C., & Carell, T. (2011). The discovery of 5-formylcytosine in embryonic stem cell DNA. *Angew Chem Int Ed Engl*, 50, 7008-7012.

[45] Zhang, L., Lu, X., Lu, J., Liang, H., Dai, Q., Xu, G. L., Luo, C., Jiang, H., & He, C. (2012). Thymine DNA glycosylase specifically recognizes 5-carboxylcytosine-modified DNA. *Nat Chem Biol*, 8, 328-330.

[46] Maiti, A., & Drohat, A. C. (2011). Thymine DNA glycosylase can rapidly excise 5-formylcytosine and 5-carboxylcytosine: potential implications for active demethylation of CpG sites. *J Biol Chem*, 286, 35334-35338.

[47] Ito, S., Shen, L., Dai, Q., Wu, S. C., Collins, L. B., Swenberg, J. A., He, C., & Zhang, Y. (2011). Tet proteins can convert 5-methylcytosine to 5-formylcytosine and 5-carboxylcytosine. *Science*, 333, 1300-1303.

[48] Jacinto, F. V., Ballestar, E., & Esteller, M. (2008). Methyl-DNA immunoprecipitation (MeDIP): hunting down the DNA methylome. *Biotechniques*, 44, 35, 37,39passim.

[49] Nair, S. S., Coolen, M. W., Stirzaker, C., Song, J. Z., Statham, A. L., Strbenac, D., Robinson, M. D., & Clark, S. J. (2011). Comparison of methyl-DNA immunoprecipitation (MeDIP) and methyl-CpG binding domain (MBD) protein capture for genome-wide DNA methylation analysis reveal CpG sequence coverage bias. *Epigenetics*, 6, 34-44.

[50] Gupta, R., Nagarajan, A., & Wajapeyee, N. (2010). Advances in genome-wide DNA methylation analysis. *Biotechniques*, 49, 3-11.

[51] Bogdanovic, O., & Veenstra, G. J. (2009). DNA methylation and methyl-CpG binding proteins: developmental requirements and function. *Chromosoma*, 118, 549-565.

[52] Ballestar, E., & Esteller, M. (2005). Methyl-CpG-binding proteins in cancer: blaming the DNA methylation messenger. *Biochem Cell Biol*, 83, 374-384.

[53] Fraga, M. F., Ballestar, E., Montoya, G., Taysavang, P., Wade, P. A., & Esteller, M. (2003). The affinity of different MBD proteins for a specific methylated locus depends on their intrinsic binding properties. *Nucleic Acids Res*, 31, 1765-1774.

[54] Flusberg, BA, Webster, D. R., Lee, J. H., Travers, K. J., Olivares, E. C., Clark, T. A., Korlach, J., & Turner, S. W. (2010). Direct detection of DNA methylation during single-molecule, real-time sequencing. *Nat Methods*, 7, 461-465.

[55] Clarke, J., Wu, H. C., Jayasinghe, L., Patel, A., Reid, S., & Bayley, H. (2009). Continuous base identification for single-molecule nanopore DNA sequencing. *Nat Nanotechnol*, 4, 265-270.

[56] Silva, J. M., Dominguez, G., Villanueva, Gonzalez. R., Garcia, J. M., Corbacho, C., Provencio, M., Espana, P., & Bonilla, F. (1999). Aberrant DNA methylation of the p16INK4a gene in plasma DNA of breast cancer patients. *Br J Cancer*, 80, 1262-1264.

[57] Silva, J. M., Dominguez, G., Garcia, J. M., Gonzalez, R., Villanueva, M. J., Navarro, F., Provencio, M., San Martin, S., Espana, P., & Bonilla, F. (1999). Presence of tumor DNA in plasma of breast cancer patients: clinicopathological correlations. *Cancer Res*, 59, 3251-3256.

[58] Domínguez, G., Carballido, J., Silva, J., Silva, J. M., García, J. M., Menéndez, J., Provencio, M., España, P., & Bonilla, F. (2002). p14ARF Promoter Hypermethylation in Plasma DNA as an Indicator of Disease Recurrence in Bladder Cancer Patients. *Clinical Cancer Research*, 8, 980-985.

[59] Valenzuela, M. T., Galisteo, R., Zuluaga, A., Villalobos, M., Núñez, M. I., Oliver, F. J., & Ruiz de, Almodóvar. J. M. (2002). Assessing the Use of p16INK4a Promoter Gene Methylation in Serum for Detection of Bladder Cancer. *European Urology*, 42, 622-630.

[60] Grady, W. M., Rajput, A., Lutterbaugh, J. D., & Markowitz, S. D. (2001). Detection of aberrantly methylated hMLH1 promoter DNA in the serum of patients with microsatellite unstable colon cancer. *Cancer Res*, 61, 900-902.

[61] Zou, H. Z., Yu, B. M., Wang, Z. W., Sun, J. Y., Cang, H., Gao, F., Li, D. H., Zhao, R., Feng, G. G., & Yi, J. (2002). Detection of aberrant 16-methylation in the serum of colorectal cancer patients. *Clinical Cancer Research*, 8, 188-191.

[62] Nakayama, H., Hibi, K., Taguchi, M., Takase, T., Yamazaki, T., Kasai, Y., Ito, K., Akiyama, S., & Nakao, A. (2002). Molecular detection of p16 promoter methylation in the serum of colorectal cancer patients. *Cancer letters*, 188, 115-119.

[63] Lecomte, T., Berger, A., Zinzindohoué, F., Micard, S., Landi, B., Blons, H., Beaune, P., Cugnenc, P. H., & Laurent-Puig, P. (2002). Detection of free-circulating tumor-associated DNA in plasma of colorectal cancer patients and its association with prognosis. *International journal of cancer*, 100, 542-548.

[64] Ebert, M., Model, F., Mooney, S., Hale, K., Lograsso, J., Tonnes-Priddy, L., Hoffmann, J., Csepregi, A., Röcken, C., & Molnar, B. (2006). Aristaless-like Homeobox-4 Gene Methylation Is a Potential Marker for Colorectal Adenocarcinomas. *Gastroenterology*, 131, 1418-1430.

[65] Miotto, E., Sabbioni, S., Veronese, A., Calin, G. A., Gullini, S., Liboni, A., Gramantieri, L., Bolondi, L., Ferrazzi, E., & Gafà, R. (2004). Frequent aberrant methylation of the CDH4 gene promoter in human colorectal and gastric cancer. *Cancer research*, 64, 8156.

[66] Lofton-Day, C., Model, F., De Vos, T., Tetzner, R., Distler, J., Schuster, M., Song, X., Lesche, R., Liebenberg, V., & Ebert, M. (2008). DNA methylation biomarkers for blood-based colorectal cancer screening. *Clinical chemistry*, 54, 414-423.

[67] Tan, S. H., Ida, H., Lau, Q. C., Goh, B. C., Chieng, W. S., Loh, M., & Ito, Y. (2007). Detection of promoter hypermethylation in serum samples of cancer patients by methylation-specific polymerase chain reaction for tumour suppressor genes including RUNX3. *Oncology reports*, 18, 1225-1230.

[68] Kawakami, K, Brabender, J, Lord, RV, Groshen, S, Greenwald, BD, Krasna, MJ, Yin, J, Fleisher, AS, Abraham, J. M., & Beer, D. G. (2000). Hypermethylated APC DNA in plasma and prognosis of patients with esophageal adenocarcinoma. *Journal of the National Cancer Institute*, 92, 1805-1811.

[69] Hibi, K., Taguchi, M., Nakayama, H., Takase, T., Kasai, Y., Ito, K., Akiyama, S., & Nakao, A. (2001). Molecular detection of p16 promoter methylation in the serum of patients with esophageal squamous cell carcinoma. *Clinical Cancer Research*, 7, 3135-3138.

[70] Lee, T. L., Leung, W. K., Chan, M. W. Y., Ng, E. K. W., Tong, J. H. M., Lo., K. W., Chung, S. C. S., Sung, J. J. Y., & To, K. F. (2002). Detection of gene promoter hypermethylation in the tumor and serum of patients with gastric carcinoma. *Clinical Cancer Research*, 8, 1761-1766.

[71] Sanchez-Cespedes, M., Esteller, M., Wu, L., Nawroz-Danish, H., Yoo, G. H., Koch, W. M., Jen, J., Herman, J. G., & Sidransky, D. (2000). Gene promoter hypermethylation in tumors and serum of head and neck cancer patients. *Cancer research*, 60, 892.

[72] Wong, T. S., Chang, H. W., Tang, K. C., Wei, W. I., Kwong, D. L. W., Jen, J., Sham, J. S. T., Yuen, A. P. W., & Kwong, Y. L. (2002). High frequency of promoter hypermethylation of the death-associated protein-kinase gene in nasopharyngeal carcinoma and its detection in the peripheral blood of patients. *Clinical Cancer Research*, 8, 433-437.

[73] Wong, I. H. N., Dennis, Lo. Y., Zhang, J., Liew, C. T., Ng, M. H. L., Wong, N., Lai, P., Lau, W. Y., Hjelm, N. M., & Johnson, P. J. (1999). Detection of aberrant p16methylation in the plasma and serum of liver cancer patients. *Cancer research*, 59, 71.

[74] Wong, I. H. N., Lo, Y. M. D., Yeo, W., Lau, W. Y., & Johnson, P. J. (2000). Frequent p15 promoter methylation in tumor and peripheral blood from hepatocellular carcinoma patients. *Clinical Cancer Research*, 6, 3516-3521.

[75] Esteller, M., Sanchez-Cespedes, M., Rosell, R., Sidransky, D., Baylin, S. B., & Herman, J. G. (1999). Detection of aberrant promoter hypermethylation of tumor suppressor genes in serum DNA from non-small cell lung cancer patients. *Cancer research*, 59, 67.

[76] Kurakawa, E., Shimamoto, T., Utsumi, K., Hirano, T., Kato, H., & Ohyashiki, K. (2001). Hypermethylation of p16INK4 a) and p15 (INK4b) genes in non-small cell lung cancer. *International journal of oncology*, 19, 277.

[77] Usadel, H., Brabender, J., Danenberg, K. D., Jerónimo, C., Harden, S., Engles, J., Danenberg, P. V., Yang, S., & Sidransky, D. (2002). Quantitative adenomatous polyposis coli promoter methylation analysis in tumor tissue, serum, and plasma DNA of patients with lung cancer. *Cancer research*, 62, 371-375.

[78] An, Q., Liu, Y., Gao, Y., Huang, J., Fong, X., Li, L., Zhang, D., & Cheng, S. (2002). Detection of p16 hypermethylation in circulating plasma DNA of non-small cell lung cancer patients. *Cancer letters*, 188, 109-114.

[79] Bearzatto, A., Conte, D., Frattini, M., Zaffaroni, N., Andriani, F., Balestra, D., Tavecchio, L., Daidone, M. G., & Sozzi, G. (2002). p16INK4ahypermethylation detected by fluorescent methylation-specific PCR in plasmas from non-small cell lung cancer. *Clinical Cancer Research*, 8, 3782-3787.

[80] Goessl, C., Krause, H., Müller, M., Heicappell, R., Schrader, M., Sachsinger, J., & Miller, K. (2000). Fluorescent methylation-specific polymerase chain reaction for DNA-based detection of prostate cancer in bodily fluids. *Cancer research*, 60, 5941-5945.

[81] Jeronimo, C., Usadel, H., Henrique, R., Silva, C., Oliveira, J., Lopes, C., & Sidransky, D. (2002). Quantitative GSTP1 hypermethylation in bodily fluids of patients with prostate cancer. *Urology*, 60, 1131-1135.

Chapter 7

# DNA Methylation, Stem Cells and Cancer

Anica Dricu, Stefana Oana Purcaru,
Alice Sandra Buteica, Daniela Elise Tache,
Oana Daianu, Bogdan Stoleru,
Amelia Mihaela Dobrescu, Tiberiu Daianu and
Ligia Gabriela Tataranu

Additional information is available at the end of the chapter

http://dx.doi.org/10.5772/53263

## 1. Introduction

Cancer has been traditionally seen as a disease characterized by many genetic alterations, but recent studies have proven the implications of epigenetic abnormalities along carcinogenesis [1, 2].

The fundamental base of carcinogenesis is described by two major models: clonal evolution and cancer stem cell (CSC) model [3-5].

In the past few years 'cancer stem cells' (CSCs) area has become an interesting field of cancer research. In $19^{th}$ century, Durante and Conheim [6] and after one hundred year Sell and Pierce [6, 7] issued the hypothesis that stem cells could induce cancer in all type of tissues. Unlike normal tissue stem cells, cancer stem cells are characterized by an abnormal differentiation rate, which can lead to tumor [8, 9].

The five principal factors, reported to be involved in carcinogenesis are:

- chemicals – John Hill, in 1761, was the first who showed that the chemicals agents produce cancer of the nasal cavity [6];
- infections – Francis Peyton Rous was the pathologist awarded the Nobel Prize in Medicine for his research that reported that the viral agents are involved in the origin of cancer [10];
- mutations – Theodor Heinrich Boveri and Von Hansemann argued the association between development of cancer and abnormal mitoses [11];

- teratocarcinomas – the field theory, which explains that in pathology of cancer are implicated a mixture of mature and differentiated cells and also embryonic tissue [12];
- epigenetic alterations – coerce to development of abnormal phenotypes, without any structural changes of DNA [13];

The term epigenetic was introduced by Conrad Waddington in 1942, to explain the relationship between environment and genome. Model of „cancer stem cells" indicates that epigenetic changes occurred in stem or precursor cell are the earliest events that take place in cancer [14].

There are two primary mechanisms involved in the epigenetic process: methylation of DNA and covalent modification of histones [15].

DNA methylation is an inheritance mechanism, fundamentally important in normal development and cellular differentiation in mammalian organisms. This is a post-replication DNA modification, by the addition of a methyl group to carbon 5 (C5] of the pyrimidine ring of cytosines, predominantly in cytosine-phospho-guanine (CpG) dinucleotides.

In the eukaryotic cells, the pattern of methylation is the result of complex interactions between three types of normal methylation processes: *de novo* methylation, the maintenance of existing methylation and demethylation. DNA-methylation is catalyzed by several DNA cytosine-5-methyltransferases (DNMTs), which can catalyse cytosine methylation in different sequence context. DNMT family include: DNMT1, which is responsible for methylation maintenance and DNMT3a and DNMT3b, which are responsible for the *de novo* DNA-methylation [16].

The decisive developmental effect of DNA-methylation on gene expression is the long-term silencing of gene expression. In human, the process of DNA-methylation is associated with transcriptional silencing imprinted genes and X-chromosome inactivation. Both genomic imprinting and X-chromosome inactivation are suggested to regulate gene expression in embryonic and fetal growth.

Dysregulated normal imprinting is supposed to induce embryonic death and to impair fetal growth. Defects in DNA-methylation process may also have major consequences for embryonic development and are associated with congenital defects, autoimmunity, aging and malignant transformation.

In recent years, the human methylation profile of the whole genome has been investigated by DNA methylomic studies and altered DNA methylation has been found in cancer DNA [2, 17] The transformation of normal cells into dysplastic and cancerous cells is due to a broad range of genetic and epigenetic changes. Some of the epigenetic mechanisms of initiation and progression of cancer are strongly related to post translational modifications of histones, among which the methylation process is highly involved. The resistance of various types of cancer to therapy led to the hypothesis that cancers present some cells, able to self renew and differentiate into all types of cells that compose a tumor, named cancer stem cells [8]. During embryonic development, characteristic patterns of CpG methylation are produced in the different cell lineages that are then well conserved in normal adult cells, while in tumor cells, DNA methylation patterns become altered. A family of germline-specific genes that use DNA methylation as a primary silencing mechanism, has been indicated as a stem cells signature. These germline-specific genes expression in tumors, has also been hypothesised to reflect the expansion of constitutively expressing cancer stem cells [8].

Post-translational modification of histone proteins is an important area of regulation epigenetic. The post-translational modifications of the N-terminal tail domains include: methylation, acetylation, phosphorylation, citrullination, ADP-ribosylation, sumoylation and ubiquitination [18-20]. The most studied of these modifications are methylation and acetylation. Modifications of histone N terminal ends by methylation and acetylation processes are closely related to cancer and are done by the competition of two families of enzymes: histone acetyltransferases (HAT) and histone acetylases (HDAC). Lysine residues acetylation in the histone H3 and H4 by (HAT and lysine 4 methylation in the histone H3 (H3K4me) by histone methyltransferase (HMT) are generally correlated with active transcription of chromatin. In contrast, methylation of lysine 9 and lysine 27 (H3K9, H3K27me) in the histone 3, have been considered as markers in transcriptionally silenced-chromatin [21, 22].

Dysregulation of epigenetic mechanisms in stem cells may induce alteration in stem cells function, (i.e. self-renewal and differentiation potential), leading to cancer initiation and progression. During the last years, a major challenge in cancer biology is to elucidate how the histone modifications in stem cells influence carcinogenesis.

Thus, epigenetic control of gene expression patterns in embryogenesis, stem cells and cancer stem cells is a very important aspect for our understanding of human cancer development, progression and therapy.

## 2. DNA methylation

According to the cancer stem cell theory, aberrant epigenetic changes may allow the transformation of stem cells in cancer stem cells [14].

Epigenetic regulation is realized by modifications that consist in four important mechanisms: DNA methylation, covalent modification of histone, nucleosome positioning and changes of microRNA expression [23].

The biological process of DNA methylation is found in both eukaryotic and prokaryotic cells and it can be involved in pathogenesis of several diseases, especially in cancer. This is the most studied mechanism of epigenetic regulation, consisting in addition of a methyl group to the carbon-5 position of the pyrimidine base cytosine (C) from the nucleotide structure cytidine-5'-monophosphate (CMP). S-adenosyl-L-methionine (SAM), the active form of amino acid methionine, is the donor of methyl group resulting S-adenosylhomocysteine (SAH) [23].

In the mammalian genome, cytosine is coupled to guanine (G) to form a base pair, commonly called cytosine-phosphate-guanine (CpG) dinucleotides. These dinucleotides are generally methylated (CpG-poor regions) with the exception of GC-rich regions known as the CpG islands [24, 25]. In human normal cells, it was observed that CpG islands are often hypomethylated. In oncogenesis CpG islands suffer a hypermethylation process whereas the entire pool CpG-poor regions are hypomethylated. DNA hypermethylation and hypomethylation coexist in cancer cells, both processes demonstrating the importance of DNA methylation in sustaining a normal gene expression pattern, genomic imprinting and silencing of genes involved in X-chromosome inactivation [1, 23, 26-29].

The DNA methylation process is catalyzed by specific DNA methyltransferase (DNMTs). In human cells, five types of DNMTs enzymes have been reported [23, 30-33]. DNMT1 - DNA (cytosine-5-)-methyltransferase 1, with role in regulation of normal tissue-specific methylation; unusual methylation is related to the appearance of human cancer. DNMT2 has an uncertain role in human health and illness [34]. Grant A Challen et al. have shown that DNMT3A and DNMT3B are implicated in embryonic stem cells differentiation [35] and DNMT3L was reported to stimulate the activity of both DNMT3A and DNMT3B [36].

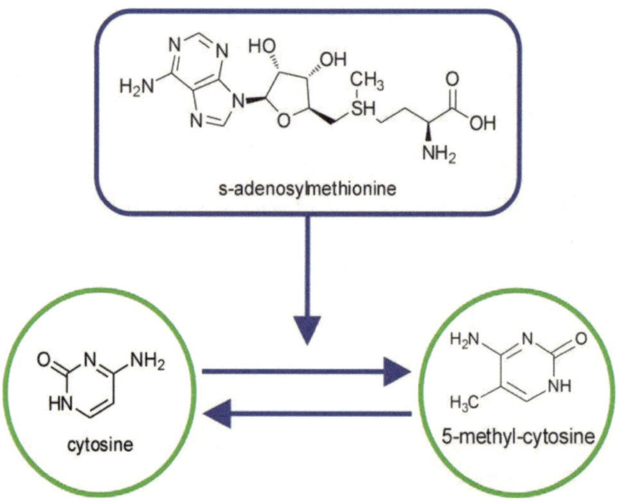


**Figure 1.** Methylation of cytosine. Cytosine methylation is one of the most extensive studied epigenetic processes. The donor of the methyl group is the active form of methionine, S-adenosyl-L-methionine (SAM) and its addition to cytosine is realised at the carbon-5 position.

Over the past two decades, it was shown that DNA methylation plays a major role in the regulation of the specific gene expression, during mitotic cell division, in the normal mammalian cell, as well as in the stem cell [13, 37, 38].

A new hypothesize about tumorigenesis consists in dysregulation of the stem cell self-renewal process. Dissemination of cancer stem cells is suggested to be induced by gene mutations and epigenetic modifications that may lead to metastasis [39].

DNA hypomethylation was found to activate cancer-germline (CG) genes or cancer-testis (CT) gene family in tumours. The promoter region of CG genes is demethylated in a several tumour types, inducing genes transcriptional activation. In their study, Costa et al. hypothesized that expression of CG genes may be indispensable for stem cell biology [40, 41].

In addition to DNA hypermethylation and hypomethylation, a DNA demethylation process was also described. While the active DNA demethylation process takes place in presence of enzymes that catalyzed specific reactions, passive DNA demethylation can occur during replication cycles and operates on DNA methyltransferases [42, 43]. Although the demethylation process is not fully elucidated, there are many studies showing transient involvement of this process in various types of tumors, especially in advanced stages of their development [44]. The mechanism of DNA demethylation in cancer has been relatively less studied. Until just a few years ago, scientists believed that the hypomethylation affects the whole genome, randomly [45]. Dysregulations in embryonic normal development and also in normal stem cells development, are generated by many signaling pathways, which can be associated with cancer. Pathways signaling implicated in regulation of normal stem cell evolution are also involved in stem cells self-renewal and carcinogenesis. The most common signaling pathways in all processes mentioned are: Wnt, Notch and Sonic hedgehog (Shh) [46, 47]. Other signaling pathways reported to be involved in stem cell maintenance and pluripotency are: TGF-beta, MET, MYC, EGF, p53, BMI, etc [5].

It is well-known that Wingless gene encodes the Wnt protein family that control the self–renewal and tumorigenesis processes. Wnt protein is well preserved from Drosophila melanogaster and has an essential role during normal embryonic development. Wnt protein is a part of a particularly signalling pathway, common to humans and Wnt protein dysregulation was reported to be involved in the development of tumors. It has been demonstrated that some genes implicated in the Wnt signaling pathway, are inactivated by promoter hypermethylation, generating lung metastasis from primary tumors [48].

The Notch signaling pathway was also suggested to have an important role in stem cell differentiation, proliferation and oncogenesis as well. Scientists have shown that in humans, exist four Notch paralogs (i.e. Notch 1, 2, 3, and 4) and five ligands (i.e. Delta-like 1, 3, 4 and Jagged 1 and 2). Activation of these Notch paralogs are found in stem cell self-renewal but also in many types of cancers [49].

Some epigenetic changes like histone methylation and downregulation of gene expression, which collaborate with the Notch developmental pathway during oncogenesis, were also described [50].

## 3. Chromatin dynamic and histones modifications

Chromatin is represented by the mandatory association between nuclear DNA and proteins. Chromatin presents different compression degrees during to cell cycles. It exists in two different types: euchromatin and heterochromatin.

Euchromatin has more non repetitive DNA with prevailing of guanine and cytosine bases and nonhistonic proteins; it is also less condensed and represents the active and transcriptional part of the chromatin; it replicates early at the beginning of S faze, being R positive bands from bands marked chromosomes [51].

Heterochromatin has more repetitive DNA with predominating adenine and thymine bases and histones; it is very compact, genetically inactive, with late replication. Heterochromatin functions are to stabilize the centromere and the telomeres of the chromosome, playing an important role in meiosis and in cellular differentiation [52]. Heterochromatin is expressed as constitutive or facultative chromatin. Constitutive heterochromatin is constantly found in a condensed form. It doesn't have functional genes and it is made of highly repetitive DNA (satellite DNA).

Facultative heterochromatin is a chromosome region, densely packed and inactive in a particular cells, having lost gene expression [53]. Both constitutive and facultative heterochromatin, are regulated by the DNA silencing in the mammalian cells. Constitutive heterochromatin is mandatory transcriptional silenced while facultative heterochromatin is conditionally silenced [53].

Electronic microscope analysis shows a hierarchical system of chromatin fibers with different dimensions, made of DNA, histones and nonhistone proteins. The supramolecular organization of DNA has four different levels. The first level is represented by four core histone proteins (H2A, H2B, H3 and H4) which form an octamer wrapped around 1.75 times by 146 base of DNA, making together nucleosomes [54]. Nucleosomes are linked by a short fragment of free DNA (approximately 60 pairs of bases), closed tight by histone H1. The compactness of DNA at this level is 10:1 [54]. Nucleosomes seem to be dynamic structures, since they have to suffer structure modifications during transcription, replication or recombination of DNA. The second level of chromatin economy is represented by the chromatin fiber of 30 nm, creating a solenoid aspect. A fundamental unit in the interphase, this chromatin plays an important role by putting together regions of linear DNA, stimulating genic interaction. The solenoid has a heterogeneous structure, characterized by an alternation of spiral and not spiraled areas, creating a proper configuration for RNA polymerase action, during transcription. The third level of chromatin organization results from creation of lateral loops of 300 nm diameter, attached to a protein nonhistonic matrix. At the beginning of prophase, a matrix will be formed by a 20 times compaction a chromatid, the highest level of chromatin organization [55]. So, the basic DNA will suffer an overall 10000 times compaction, being able to fit a small place into a nucleus. This conformation offers sterically occlusion for nucleosomes, which will be there for protected against nucleases cleavage, while the linker DNA doesn't have this kind of protection [56].

Many cancers are associated with translocations which can be explained by mutual rearrangements due to misfit of two unrepaired double stranded breaks, determined by the close proximity of some genetic regions, thus suggesting the dynamic properties of chromatin [57, 58]. Translocation that characterizes tumorigenesis may depend on the physical distance between individual genetic elements. Chromatin is a dynamic structure, with its own mobility that influences either gene regulation (local diffusion of chromatin) or genomic stability (global chromatin immobility) [57]. In normal cells, as well as in tumor cells, there are similar nuclear layers, defined as center of nucleus-to-locus distance, with a random distribution of genetic loci inside it [59]. Polarization of some chromosomes, with their genes located in the interior of the nucleus and their centromeres located at the nuclear periphery, along with all the other data already presented, strongly support the existing relation between the chromatin pattern and tumor development, but still many aspects remain to be proved.

The debate concerning chromatin remodeling as a cause or a consequence of tumorigenesis is still on.

Many works indicate that DNA methylation and chromatin remodeling are in reciprocal causal relationship: DNA methylation may cause chromatin modifications and specific chromatin modification may induce DNA methylation [1]. Recent data suggest that chromatin remodeling is a combination between a CIS effect determined by the action of a proximal genetic sequence and a TRANS effect induced by sequence independent complexes, most likely by ATP dependent nucleosomes remodeling complexes [60, 61].

Alu sequences are a class of repetitive DNA characterized by a pattern of CG dinucleotides (CpG) repeating every 31-32 bases. They may modulate the nucleosome strength when the CG elements are methylated. Thus, epigenetic nucleosomes within Alu sequences may have methylation-dependent regulatory functions [62].

Emerging data are suggesting that since genome regulation might be influenced by nucleosome positioning and their compositional modifications, nucleosomes are regulating the initiation of transcription, therefore nucleosomes positioning is leading to cancer or developmental effects [17]. Nucleosomes adopt preferential positions near promoter regions and random positions inside genes [63]. Transcription needs exposed binding sites consisting in nucleosome free regions at the 5′ and 3′ ends of the genes, so any change in nucleosome positioning at this level might determine gene activation [64, 65].

Nucleosome positioning is also influenced by another protein complex that activates or represses transcription through biochemical processes, such as octamer transfer, nucleosome remodeling or nucleosome sliding: switch/sucrose nonfermentable (Swi/Snf) complex. It consists in approximately 10 subunits of 2 MDa, with many variants of combinations, first discovered in Saccharomyces cerevisiae [16, 66]. The multiple varieties of Swi/Snf complexes exist in many cell types [67]. Swi/ Snf performs a crucial function in gene regulation and chromosome organization by directly altering the contacts between nucleosomes and DNA [68], using the energy of ATP hydrolysis [69]. The *in vitro* studies revealed that two subunits of the complex, Brg1 or Brm, are able to remodel nucleosomes, with maximal results when subunits BAF155, BAF170 and Ini1 presents a 2:1 stoichiometry relative to Brg1 [70]. The activity of chromatin remodelers appears to be gene specific [71]. The subunits of Swi/ Snf complex seem to have a broad range of functions: BAF155 and BAF170 regulate the protein levels and ensure framing functions for other SWI/SNF subunits [72, 73]; BAF53 is an actin and β-actin related protein signaling, through phosphatidylinositol 4,5- bisphosphate, which binds to Brg1, stimulating the binding to the actin filaments [74-76]; Ini1 is involved in rare and aggressive pediatric cancers [77, 78] as well as in HIV 1 infection [79-81]. The role of SWI/SNF components in cancer stem cells and tumor suppression is still vaguely understood, but their transcriptional pathways are already described, including the cell cycle and p53 signaling [82], insulin signaling [83], and TGFb signaling [84], or signaling through several different nuclear hormone receptors [85]. The biological roles of Swi/Snf components and their involvement in human disease remain to be completed. It is also known that loss of Snf2h impairs embryonic development and differentiation [86] and contributes to tumor development [87]. These tumors are also characterized by polyploidy and chromosomal instability [88]. Since Swi/Snf complex plays also an important role in DNA double strand brake repair, alteration of its function may lead to genomic instability [89]. Critical subunits of Swi/Snf complex miss or are disrupted in approximately 17% of all human adenocarcinomas [90]. Another tumor suppressor gene is Ikaros, a molecule that plays a central role in lymphocyte development through its association with chromatin remodeling complexes [91]. Fusion protein BCR-ABL from preB lymphoblastic leukemia mediates an aberrant splicing of Ikaros, with consequences on cell differentiation [92].

Radiations have the ability to paradoxically induce or cure tumors. It seems that chromatin structure might be influenced by UV and gamma radiation. To study the changes in chromatin pattern under irradiation conditions, Fluorescence In Situ Hybridization (FISH), combined with high-resolution confocal microscopy has been used [93, 94]. FISH studies were performed in leukemia cells for tumor suppressor gene TP53, revealing that TP53 genes are getting closer to each other, as well with the nuclear center within 2 hours of exposure to gamma-radiation, returning during the following 2 hours to its pre-irradiation conditions [95, 96]. There is increasing evidence that CSCs have a higher intrinsic radioresistance than non-CSC tumor cells [97], explaining the difference of CSCs and non-CSC in their response to cancer therapy.

Such repressive complex for chromatin is "Nucleosome Remodeling and Histone Deacetylase" (NuRD) [98], suggested to play a role in acute promyelocytic leukemia (APL) [99]. Human APL is characterized by PML-RARa translocation, which represses gene transcription through several distinct epigenetic mechanisms: DNA methylation, chromatin compaction, heterochromatinization, histone deacetylation, histone modification. NuRD complex is strongly implicated in the epigenetic silencing, by PML-RARa. Earlier findings regarding carcinogenesis, such as the combination of both genetic and epigenetic factors, were confirmed. in this case, PML-RARa oncogenic fusion protein recruiting, induces DNA hypermethylation [100] and result in blocking of hematopoietic differentiation [101].

Covalent modification of histones is an important mechanism, involved in the epigenetic processes. Five types of histones are known to be involved in chromatin building: H1/H5, H2A, H2B, H3, and H4 [15, 102]. In their structure, histones have three distinct domains: a central globular conserved domain and two terminal domains; one short N-terminal tail and one longer C-terminal tail [54].

Generally, histone modifications affect gene transcription, DNA replication and DNA repair mechanisms. The post-translational modifications of the N-terminal tail domains include: methylation, acetylation, phosphorylation, citrullination, ADP-ribosylation, sumoylation and ubiquitination [18-20]. The most studied of these modifications are methylation and acetylation. Lysine residues acetylation in the histone H3 and H4 by histone acetyltransferase

(HAT) and lysine 4 methylation in the histone H3 (H3K4me) by histone methyltransferase (HMT), are generally correlated with active transcription of chromatin. In contrast, methylation of lysine 9 and lysine 27 (H3K9, H3K27me) in the histone 3 have been reported as markers in transcriptionally silenced-chromatin [21, 22].

During the last years, a major challenge in cancer biology is to elucidate how the histone modifications in stem cells, influence carcinogenesis.

Histones methylation is a post translational modification that occurs at the lysine residues and is considered a reversible process [103]. Transcriptional activation or repression, correlates with different degrees of methylation of histones. The binding of one to three methyl groups at each lysine amino acid in the histone structure, give rise to unmethylated, monomethylated, dimethylated and trimethylated degrees of methylation [104, 105]. The monomethylation state of histone has been reported to be associated with an open chromatin structure that lead to transcriptional activation. In contrast, the trimethylation state was shown to be associated with a condensed chromatin structure, which in turn inhibits transcription [106].

Some important exceptions from this rule have been reported by Strahl BD et al., they showed that H3K4 histone methylation state (mono-, di-, or tri-methylated level) is invariably associated with active chromatin, while H3K9 trimethylation can be connected to both transcriptionally active and inactive chromatin [107]. To explain this exception from the general rule, Vakoc et al., described a mechanism by which an association between meH3K9 with RNA polymerase II complexes induces chromatin modification and transcriptional activation [108]. However, it is not fully understood why these markers differs from the general rule.

The binding of the methyl group of each lysine 4, 36 or 79 in the histone 3 (H3K4, H3K36, H3K79) and H4 (k20, H2BK5) induces trnascriptional activation. In contrast, the binding of three methyl group of lysine 9, 27 in the histone 3 (H3K9, H33K27) AND h4k20 was show to be associated with inhibiton of transcription [109, 110]. The histone modifications are arising from the action of enzymes which are responsible for methylation/demethylation activity in the pattern of histone H3 and H4. The enzymes involved in histone modifications are histone acetyltransferases (HATs) and histone deacetylases (HDACs), histona methyltransferases (HMTs) and histone demethylases (HDMs). These enzymes add or remove acetyl or methyl groups, respectively [111, 112]. Several enzymes, like histone methyltransferase (HMTs), histone demethylases (HDMs) and histone deacetylases (HDACs), are connected with each other to create a strong link between chromatin state and transcription.

In addition to changes in histone acetylation, widespread changes in histone methylation patterns are described in cancer. Accordingly, in cancer, aberrant gene silencing was shown to be associated with changes in H3K9 and H3K27 methylation patterns [113].

A recent analysis in the context of histone modifications in cancer, illustrates different scenarios such as histone methylation and its consequences, describing the role of histone methyltransferases (HMTs) and histone demethylation (HDMS) by adding or removing a methyl group. It has been reported that the level of transcriptional activation is largely maintained by HMTs and HDMs which are involved in the histone methylation [103].

The histone lysine methyltransferase (HMT) that is responsible for the histone methylation, has a catalytically active site known as SET domain, which is formed by de 130 amino acid sequence. The major function of the SET domain is to modulate gene activity [114].

The binding of the methyl group at several lysine sites in histone H3 (H3K9, H3K27, H3K36, H3K79) and loss of acetylated H4 lysine 16 and H4 lysine 20 trimethylation have been reported to be associated with changes that occur during tumorigenesis[115]. The enzymes HDACs and HATs have been suggested to be responsible for these changes and are commonly found to be altered in various forms of cancer [116].

Various observations suggest the presence of a novel chromatin pattern in embryonic stem cell, which consists of lysine 27 and lysine 4 tri-methylation superposition, termed "bivalent domains" [117].

The bivalent domains have been analysed by the genome mapping of histone methylation profiles in embryonic stem cell and was reported to include both active and repressive chromatin marks. Developmentally, the "bivalent domains" is responsible for maintaining epigenomic plasticity, enabling embryonic stem cells to regulate gene expression [117]. Bivalency is lost during stem cell differentiation, allowing epigenetic plasticity and lineage commitment. Epigenetic plasticity in association with bivalent gene promoters is suggested to induce a transcriptionally repressive and permissive histone mark in embryonic stem cells [117, 118].

In cancer, bivalency has been suggested to stigmatize specific genes for DNA methylation, inducing aberrant reprogramming [119-121]. In analogy with embrionic stem cells, bivalent gene promoters were reported to be DNA-methylated in cancer cells, suggesting the provenience of cancer cells from embryonic stem cells [122]. In absence of DNA methylation, the repressive H3K27 trimethylation mark was also demonstrated to induce gene silencing in cancer cells.

Chromatin regulating complexes are commonly observed in cancer, and is hypothesized to involve multiple mechanisms, including DNA methylation and Polycomb repressive complexes (PRCs). Chromatin regulating complexes including two families of Polycomb repressive complexes (PRC1 and PRC1), mediate trimethylation on H3K27 in cancer cells [123, 124]. PRC2 complex has also been reported to intermediate H3K27 trimethylation in embryonic stem cell [125].

## 4. miRNA and DNA methylation in cancer stem cells

MicroRNAs (miRNAs) was first discovered in 1993 by Victor Ambros, Rosalind Lee and Rhonda Feinbaum. The recent definition of miRNA is: small non-coding RNA molecules (21-24 nucleotides long), implicated in posttranscriptional gene expression, regulation by two different mechanisms: splitting and subsequent degradation of targeted RNAm or inhibiting translation, both determining the stop or stimulation of cell reproduction [126-130].

However, the entire mechanism of miRNA is not yet fully understood [131, 132].

The study on Caenorhabditis elegans (C. elegans) has permitted the clonation of first miRNA, lin-4 and let-7 and their targets [133, 134]. This study discovered that the gene lin-14 was able to transcribe a precursor that matured to a 22 nucleotide mature RNA, which contained sequences partially complementary to multiple sequences in the 3′ UTR of the lin-14 mRNA, ensuring inhibition of translation of lin-14 mRNA. In addition, in 2000, along with the discovery that gene let-7 repressed the genes lin-41, lin-14, lin-28, lin-42 and daf12 mRNA during transition in developmental stages in C. Elegans, it was also established that non-coding RNA identified in 1993, was part of a wider phenomenon [133].

More than 700 miRNAs have been identified in humans and over 800 more are predicted to exist. These molecules have an important role in cellular physiological processes (e.g. cell cycle, cell proliferation, apoptosis, cell differentiation and development), by implication in gene regulation; miRNA has been found to control about 30% of all human genes.

In human embryonic stem cells and the differentiated embryonic bodies, over 100 miRNAs have been already described [101]. The self-renewal and pluripotency of embryonic stem cells are regulated by an array of protein-coding genes in a regulatory circuitry [135], which includes OCT4, SOX2, and KLF4 genes. Extensive studies have indicated the importance of OCT4 in self-renewal and pluripotency of embryonic stem cells [136, 137]. Multipotent cell lineages in early mouse development, have also been reported to be dependent on SOX2 function [138, 139] in the process of embryonic stem cells self-renewal and pluripotency. The miRNA genes are also connected to the transcriptional regulatory circuitry of embryonic stem cells [140] and are overexpressed in their differentiating processes.

The three key proteins of pluripotent cells, Oct4, Nanog and SOX2, and TCF3 were found in the promoters of miRNA specific stem cells, but also in promoters of miRNA, which controls cell proliferation (mir 92 si let7g) and differentiation (e.g., mir-9 or mir-124a for neutral line). OCT4 was reported to bind and repress miR-145 promoter in human embryonic stem cells. On the other hand, inhibition of Oct 4 increases the activity of these miRNAs that in turn inhibit the stem cell renewal.

miRNAs, occasionally causes DNA methylation of promoter sites and can regulate other epigenetic mechanisms. An altered miRNA gene methylation patterns in human cancers was reported to sustain in tumorigenesis. Half of these genes are associated with CpG islands and several studies indicated that miRNA gene methylation was often detectable, both in normal and malignant cells. Recent works have identified many types of miRNA, which allow cancer cells to multiply indefinitely by avoiding natural cellular aging mechanisms, thus suggesting a close relation between cancer development and miRNA expression [141].

There are several mechanisms which may lead to modification of mi RNA in cancer [142-145].

- *Chromosomal changes* - quantitative gene changes have been identified in approximately 283 miRNA, determined by either loosing heterozigotism by the action of a suppressive gene or by amplification of a chromosomal region of an oncogene either by chromosomal ruptures or translocations [146];
- *miRNA biosynthesis abnormalities*, mainly represented by gene amplification for proteins as Drosha (implicated in miRNA maturation process) or Ago2 (responsible for the interaction with target messengers);
- *Epigenetic changes*- recent data suggest the implication of DNA methylation in the disorder of miRNA expression. Gene analysis for miRNA established that these genes are usually associate with CpG islands and thus represent candidate targets of the DNA methylation machinery. A high level of miRNA genes methylation exists both in normal and malignant cells. Epigenetic changes of chromatin, for instance histone deacetylation, cause important alteration of miRNA expression as well [141];
- *miRNA as oncogenes or tumor suppressors* - miRNA always acts as negative regulator of gene expression. In cancer, miRNA were classifies as miRNA with oncogenic effect (oncomirs) and miRNA with suppressor effect (supressor mirs) [147-149].

Oncogenic activity of miRNA, initially determined for mir-17-92 and mir-155, was further sustained by the discovery of other potentially oncogenic miRNA [150]. Therefore it is logical that this classification of miRNA in oncogenes or tumor supressor genes may facilitate the identification of different tissues where they are expressed [151].

Embryonic stem cells gene expression of Oct4, Sox2, Klf4, and Nanog was observed in highly aggressive human tumors [152]. It has been reported that miR-200 known to mediate transcriptional repression, also play an important role in both cancer stem cells andembryonic stem cells [153, 154].

Several miRNAs have been reported to be overexpressed in human cancer. The mir-17-92 polycistron (cluster) is overexpressed in B-cell lymphoma [155, 156] and in testicular germ cell tumors miR-372 and miR-373 were identified as possible oncogenes [157].

Another theory supports the idea that some cancers such as Kaposi `s sarcoma, were induced by viral oncogenic miRNA [158]. It is clear that discovery of miRNA involvement in cancer stem cells function will be a crucial step in elucidating the process of oncogenesis [159].

## 5. Epigenetic targeting in cancer stem cells

Recently, several epigenetic drugs targeting epigenetic mechanisms have been tested *in vivo* and *in vitro*. The epigenetic mechanisms comprise modifications of histones and DNA methylation. Histone modifications includes several post translational modification of the: methylation, acetylation, phosphorylation, ubiquitination, sumoylation; commonly found in tumor cells. Thus, epigenetic modifications targeting is an important event in cancer therapy. Epigenetic targeting may be realized by two classes of substances with antitumor effect in malignancies: the hypomethylating agents and histone deacetylase inhibitors [160].

### 5.1. Targeting DNA methylation

DNA methylation is the most studied epigenetic marker. Abnormal DNA methylation of several regulatory genes is usually associated with cancer. The methylation process is reversible, therefore the reactivation of silenced genes can be realized using substances with hypomethylating activity [161].

The new development cancer therapies are based on molecules that can inhibit the classes of DNA methyltransferases (DNMT), histone deacetylases (HDACs), histone acetyltransferases (HATs) and new substances that target chromatin and nucleosome remodeling proteins. DNMT inhibitors (DNMTi) can be natural or synthetic compounds [148, 162].

As mentioned before, DNMTs are enzymes that catalyze the reaction between methyl groups and pyrimidine base cytosine. The methyl group donor is S-adenosyl-L-methionine (SAM), which is the active form of amino acid methionine.

The DNA hypomethylating agents are divided into two categories: nucleoside analogs drugs and non-nucleoside analogs drugs. The first description substances are 5-azacytidine (azacitidine, Vidaza™) and 5-aza-2′-deoxycytidine (decitabine, Dacogen™) that have the most powerful effect from nucleoside analogs drugs [1, 163-165].

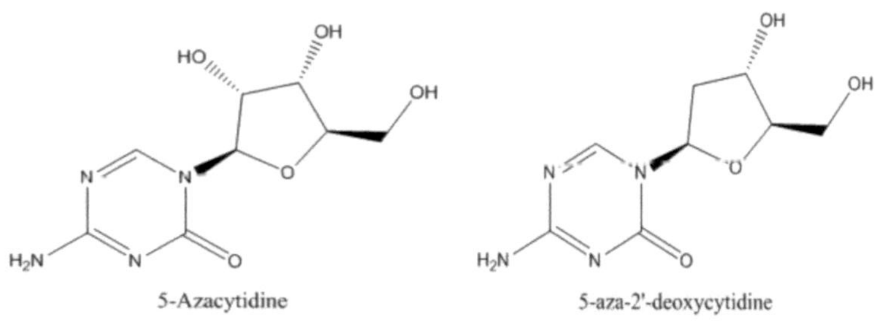


**Figure 2.** Nucleoside analog drugs. Their structure allows incorporation into the DNA and subsequent hypomethilation.

Other substances from this group are: 1-β-D-arabinosyl-5-azacytidine (fazarabine) [166], dihydro-5-azacytidine (DHAC), 5-fluoro-2′-deoxycytidine (FCDR) and zebularine [163]. Incorporation into the DNA structure of nucleoside analogs is facilitated by their similar chemical structure.

5-azacytidine is used as single-agent therapy or in combination with other therapies in treatment of myelodysplastic syndromes (MDS), acute myeloid leukemias (AML) and solid tumor. As associated substances are utilized valproic acid, cytarabine, entinostat, etanercept etc [137, 164].

5-aza-2′-deoxycytidine (DAC) has benefited as monotherapy in myelodysplastic syndromes, chronic myelomonocytic leukemia (CMML) and has been FDA approved on May 2006. The drug has been associated with: carboplatin useful in solid tumors treatment [167], valproic acid in acute myeloid leukemias and advanced leukemia [168, 169], imatinib mesylate in chronic myelogenous leukemia (CML) [170] and IL-2 in metastatic melanoma, renal carcinoma [171].

Zebularine (2-pyrimidone-1-β- D-riboside) is other nucleoside analog with hypomethylation activity [172] and also implicated in tumor gene expression [173].

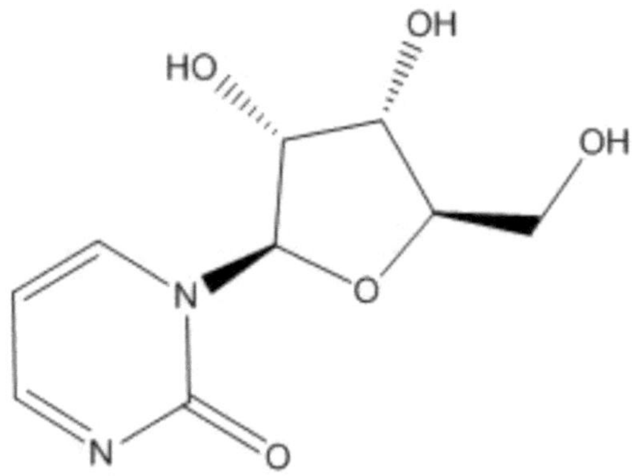


Zebularine

**Figure 3.** Structure of Zebularine. Zebularine is another nucleoside analog drug, with hypomethilation effect.

There are recent studies about another two molecules: NPEOC-DAC and SGI 110 (S110). NPEOC-DAC is the result of chemical reaction between azacytosine molecule and 2-(p-nitrophenyl) ethoxycarbonyl, with reported effect on DNA methyltransferases inhibition. Byun et al. demonstrated that NPEOC-DAC inhibited DNA methylation in two cell lines of liver cancer. The authors, also showed that SGI 110 (S110) has a pronounced effect on DNA methylation inhibition [174].

The non-nucleoside analogs category contains compounds with hypomethylation effect. This group contains hydralazine (the widely known as vasodilatator), procainamide (antiarhythmic), RG108 and SGI-1027.

Physiologically, acetylation of chromatin is realized by specific enzymes - histone deacetylases and acetyltransferases. A possible change in their normal function can promote tumors.

### 5.2. Targeting histone modification

At first glance, HDACs are enzymes that play a role in elimination of acetyl radical just from lysine molecules of histones, but their actions is not limited to histones, they can also act on non-histone proteins [175].

HDAC inhibitors are classified into four classes, based on their chemical structure: short-chain fatty acids, hydroxamic acids, cyclic peptides, benzamides (hybrid molecules) [176].

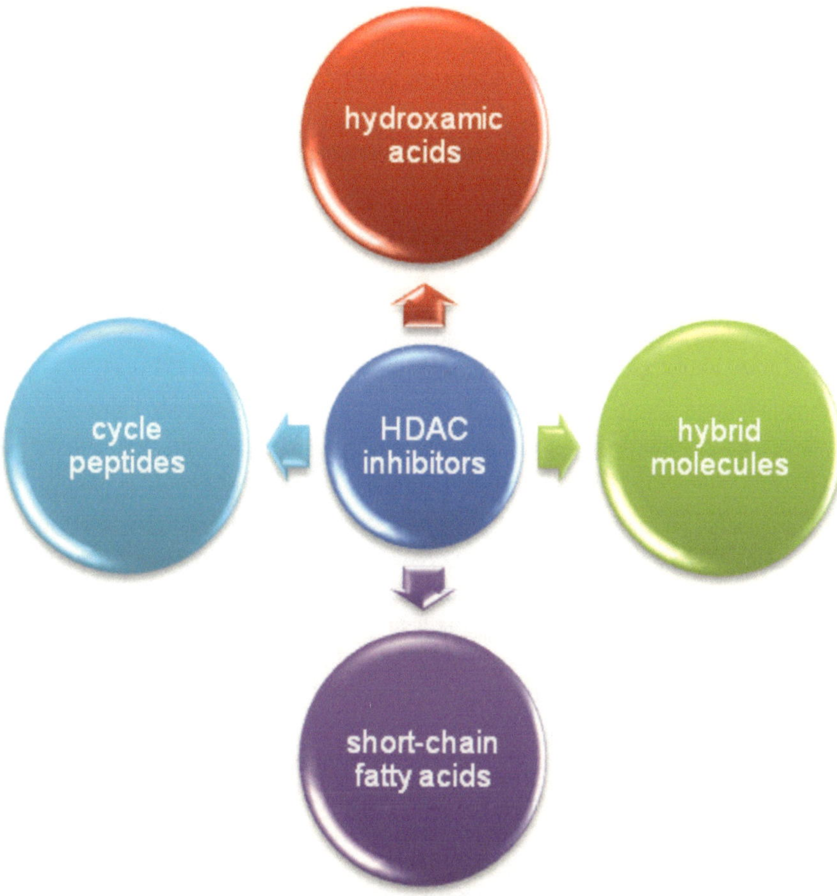


**Figure 4.** HDAC inhibitors. There are four classes of curently known HDAC inhibitors: short-chain fatty acids, hydroxamic acids, cyclic peptides, benzamides, with a great potential use as detection and prognosis markers.

Exemples of short-chain fatty acids are: sodium n-butyrate, sodium phenylacetate, phenylbutyrate, valproate, substances that in millimolar concentrations are involved in inhibition the growth of some carcinomas but their mechanism of action is not fully understood [163, 177-179].

One of the most studied agent from class of small fatty acids, is valproic acid (VPA), an antiepileptic drug reported to target histone deacetylase. Numerous research studies *in vitro* demonstrated that VPA was implicated in hyperacetylation of histones H3 and H4 and also *in vivo* tests confirmed the drug inhibiting action of HDACs. VPA antitumor activity was demanstrated by: cell growth inhibition, apoptosis inducing, antimetastatic and antiangiogenesis effect, etc. These benefits lead to FDA approving of VPA [14, 180].

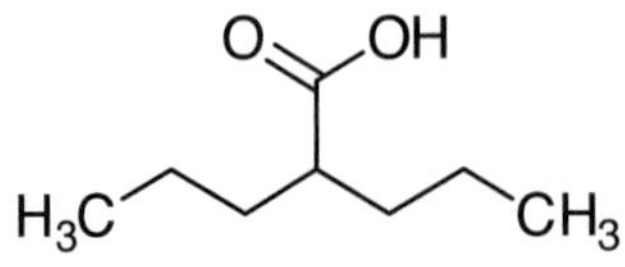


**Figure 5.** Structure of valproic acid. Valproic acid is a small fatty acid commonly used as an antiepileptic drug, but with recently emerged antitumor effects.

The class of hydroxamic acids include synthesized compounds such as: belinostat, panobinostat, vorinostat (SAHA) etc. Belinostat and panobinostat, have been used in clinical trials to treat solid tumors and blood malignancies [181-183]; MDL and CML [184-186], vorinostat (SAHA) that was approved by FDA for the treatment of chronic T-cell lymphoma (CTCL) and used in clinical trials for hematologic malignancies, mesothelioma, breast and ovarian cancer, etc [175].

A natural compound from cyclic peptides class is romidepsin, also known as Istodax (FK228), which was clinical tested in various lymphomas. The drug was shown to induce apoptosis in different tumor cell lines, due to blocking of HDACs [187].

Hybrid molecules (i.e. benzamides) includes two synthetic compounds: Entinostat (MS-275) and Mocetinostat (MGCD 0103). The mechanism by which Entinostat induced cytotoxic effect on tumor cells was suggested to be due to the upregulation of some tumor suppressor genes (p21]. Both Entinostat and Mocetinostat are currently approved by the FDA and are used in cancer treatment. Entinostat is used in the treatment of blood and lung tumor [181, 183] and Mocetinostatin in the treatment of chronic lymphocytic leukemia (CLL) [175].

HATs are a class of enzymes discovered twenty years ago, enzymes with demonstrated role in gene transcription [188]. HATs have been reported to be implicate in numerous types of diseases (i.e. viral infection, respiratory maladies, cancer etc). It has been suggested that the HATs enzymes may be used as biological markers for cancer prediction or recurrence [14]. Four families of HATs are known that share primary-structure homology: GNAT (Gcn5-related N-acetyltransferase), p300/CBP and MYST, Rtt109 [189]. The HAT enzymes have various chemical structure and their classification is still unclear.

Histone methylation process plays an important task in epigenetic regulation, which lead to synthesizing of new target drugs for cancer therapy [163].

Researchers describe a class of enzymes called histone methyltransferases. This class of enzymes includes lysine methyltransferases and arginine methyltransferases, both of them linked to many types of cancer.

There are 8 known lysine methyltransferases (KMT1-8) with suggested role in the epigenetic gene silencing in malignancies like: prostate, liver, colon, breast cancer [190, 191].

Few of the many types of arginine methyltransferases (PRMTs), are also closely linked to cancer [191].

Thus, the importance of DNMTs and HDACs, two classes of enzymes involved in epigenetic targeted therapy of malignant diseases, is obvious. The enzymes implicated in histone methylation and demethylation are mainly attractive as validated targets for cancer therapy.

http://dx.doi.org/10.5772/53263

## 6. Conclusions and perspectives

Epigenetic is a heritage mechanism involved in the process of stem cells differentiation to more specialized cells. According to the cancer stem cell model, dysregulation of epigenetic mechanisms (i.e. DNA methylation and histone modification) in pluripotent stem cells enable their transformation in cancer cells with high proliferation rates and poor prognosis.

DNA methylation is considered the most largely studied part of the epigenetic, but recent works associate the methylation with other epigenetic changes, such as histone modifications, chromatin remodeling and microRNA, suggesting a reciprocal relationship between them in cancer cells. The similarities between chromatin regulation process in stem cells and cancer cells have been mentioned in several studies.

It is therefore important to understand the epigenetic alterations that take place in cancer cells compared with normal cells and the importance of these modifications in carcinogenesis, according to the cancer stem cell theory. In addition, it is very useful to understand the potential of epigenetic marks in designing more effective treatment strategies that specifically target cancer stem cells.

## Acknowledgments

Grant support: 134/2011 UEFISCDI Romania

## Author details

Anica Dricu[1], Stefana Oana Purcaru[1], Alice Sandra Buteica[2], Daniela Elise Tache[1], Oana Daianu[1,3], Bogdan Stoleru[1], Amelia Mihaela Dobrescu[4], Tiberiu Daianu[5] and Ligia Gabriela Tataranu[3]

*Address all correspondence to: anica.dricu@live.co.uk anicadricu@webmail.umfcv.ro

1 Department of Biochemistry, University of Medicine and Pharmacy of Craiova, Romania

2 Department of Pharmacology, University of Medicine and Pharmacy of Craiova, Romania

3 Department of Neurosurgery, "Bagdasar-Arseni" Emergency Hospital, Bucharest, Romania

4 Department of Medical Genetics,University of Medicine and Pharmacy of Craiova, Romania

5 Department of Microbiology, University of Medicine and Pharmacy of Craiova, Romania

## References


[1] Jones PA, Baylin SB. The fundamental role of epigenetic events in cancer. Nat Rev Genet. 2002 Jun;3(6):415-28.

[2] Jones PA, Baylin SB. The epigenomics of cancer. Cell. (Research Support, N.I.H., Extramural Review). 2007 Feb 23;128(4):683-92.

[3] Bonnet D, Dick JE. Human acute myeloid leukemia is organized as a hierarchy that originates from a primitive hematopoietic cell. Nature Medicine. 1997 Jul;3(7):730-7.

[4] Nowell PC. The clonal evolution of tumor cell populations. Science. (Research Support, U.S. Gov't, P.H.S.). 1976 Oct 1;194(4260):23-8.

[5] Marquardt JU, Factor VM, Thorgeirsson SS. Epigenetic regulation of cancer stem cells in liver cancer: current concepts and clinical implications. J Hepatol. (Research Support, N.I.H., Intramural Review). 2010 Sep;53(3):568-77.

[6] Sell S. On the stem cell origin of cancer. Am J Pathol. (Research Support, N.I.H., Extramural Review). 2010 Jun;176(6):2584-494.

[7] Sell S, Pierce GB. Maturation arrest of stem cell differentiation is a common pathway for the cellular origin of teratocarcinomas and epithelial cancers. Lab Invest. 1994 Jan; 70(1):6-22.

[8] Mimeault M, Batra SK. Recent insights into the molecular mechanisms involved in aging and the malignant transformation of adult stem/progenitor cells and their therapeutic implications. Ageing Res Rev. 2009 Apr;8(2):94-112.

[9] Fillmore CM, Kuperwasser C. Human breast cancer cell lines contain stem-like cells that self-renew, give rise to phenotypically diverse progeny and survive chemotherapy. Breast Cancer Res. 2008;10(2):R25.

[10] Andrewes CH. Francis Peyton Rous 1879-1970. Biogr Mem Fellows R Soc. 1971;17:643-62.

[11] Hardy PA, Zacharias H. Reappraisal of the Hansemann-Boveri hypothesis on the origin of tumors. Cell Biol Int. 2005 Dec;29(12):983-92.

[12] Soto AM, Sonnenschein C. The tissue organization field theory of cancer: a testable replacement for the somatic mutation theory. Bioessays. 2011 May;33(5):332-40.

[13] Jaenisch R, Bird A. Epigenetic regulation of gene expression: how the genome integrates intrinsic and environmental signals. Nat Genet. 2003 Mar;33 Suppl:245-54.

[14] Feinberg AP, Ohlsson R, Henikoff S. The epigenetic progenitor origin of human cancer. Nat Rev Genet. 2006 Jan;7(1):21-33.

[15] Cedar H, Bergman Y. Linking DNA methylation and histone modification: patterns and paradigms. Nat Rev Genet. 2009 May;10(5):295-304.

[16] de la Serna IL, Ohkawa Y, Imbalzano AN. Chromatin remodelling in mammalian differentiation: lessons from ATP-dependent remodellers. Nat Rev Genet. 2006 Jun; 7(6):461-73.

[17] Jiang C, Pugh BF. Nucleosome positioning and gene regulation: advances through genomics. Nat Rev Genet. 2009 Mar;10(3):161-72.

[18] Sawan C, Vaissiere T, Murr R, Herceg Z. Epigenetic drivers and genetic passengers on the road to cancer. Mutat Res. 2008 Jul 3;642(1-2):1-13.

[19] Kouzarides T. Chromatin modifications and their function. Cell. 2007 Feb 23;128(4): 693-705.

[20] Hadnagy A, Beaulieu R, Balicki D. Histone tail modifications and noncanonical functions of histones: perspectives in cancer epigenetics. Mol Cancer Ther. 2008 Apr;7(4): 740-8.

[21] Sharma S, Kelly TK, Jones PA. Epigenetics in cancer. Carcinogenesis. 2010 Jan;31(1): 27-36.

[22] Marin-Husstege M, Muggironi M, Liu A, Casaccia-Bonnefil P. Histone deacetylase activity is necessary for oligodendrocyte lineage progression. J Neurosci. 2002 Dec 1;22(23):10333-45.

[23] Espada J, Esteller M. DNA methylation and the functional organization of the nuclear compartment. Semin Cell Dev Biol. 2010 Apr;21(2):238-46.

[24] Park YJ, Claus R, Weichenhan D, Plass C. Genome-wide epigenetic modifications in cancer. Prog Drug Res. 2011;67:25-49.

[25] Illingworth RS, Bird AP. CpG islands--'a rough guide'. FEBS Lett. 2009 Jun 5;583(11): 1713-20.

[26] Esteller M. Epigenetics in cancer. N Engl J Med. 2008 Mar 13;358(11):1148-59.

[27] Tsai HC, Baylin SB. Cancer epigenetics: linking basic biology to clinical medicine. Cell Res. 2011 Mar;21(3):502-17.

[28] Chang SC, Tucker T, Thorogood NP, Brown CJ. Mechanisms of X-chromosome inactivation. Front Biosci. 2006;11:852-66.

[29] Kacem S Fau - Feil R, Feil R. Chromatin mechanisms in genomic imprinting. 20100121 DCOM- 20100323(1432-1777 (Electronic)).

[30] Katto J Fau - Mahlknecht U, Mahlknecht U. Epigenetic regulation of cellular adhesion in cancer. 20110928 DCOM- 20111129(1460-2180 (Electronic)).

[31] Turek-Plewa J Fau - Jagodzinski PP, Jagodzinski PP. The role of mammalian DNA methyltransferases in the regulation of gene expression. 20051212 DCOM- 20060628(1425-8153 (Print)).

[32] Bestor TH. The DNA methyltransferases of mammals. Hum Mol Genet. 2000 Oct; 9(16):2395-402.

[33] Robertson KD. DNA methylation and chromatin - unraveling the tangled web. 20020802 DCOM- 20020822(0950-9232 (Print)).

[34] Schaefer M Fau - Lyko F, Lyko F. Solving the Dnmt2 enigma. 20100127 DCOM- 20100315(1432-0886 (Electronic)).

[35] Challen GA, Sun D, Jeong M, Luo M, Jelinek J, Berg JS, et al. Dnmt3a is essential for hematopoietic stem cell differentiation. Nat Genet. 2012 Jan;44(1):23-31.

[36] Van Emburgh BO, Robertson KD. Modulation of Dnmt3b function in vitro by interactions with Dnmt3L, Dnmt3a and Dnmt3b splice variants. Nucleic Acids Res. 2011 Jul;39(12):4984-5002.

[37] Riggs AD. X inactivation, differentiation, and DNA methylation. 19750822 DCOM- 19750822(0301-0171 (Print)).

[38] Holliday R Fau - Pugh JE, Pugh JE. DNA modification mechanisms and gene activity during development. 19750408 DCOM- 19750408(0036-8075 (Print)).

[39] Wicha Ms Fau - Liu S, Liu S Fau - Dontu G, Dontu G. Cancer stem cells: an old idea--a paradigm shift. 2006 20060220 DCOM- 20060413(0008-5472 (Print)).

[40] Costa Ff Fau - Le Blanc K, Le Blanc K Fau - Brodin B, Brodin B. Concise review: cancer/testis antigens, stem cells, and cancer. 2009 20070302 DCOM- 20070529(1066-5099 (Print)).

[41] Loriot A Fau - Reister S, Reister S Fau - Parvizi GK, Parvizi Gk Fau - Lysy PA, Lysy Pa Fau - De Smet C, De Smet C. DNA methylation-associated repression of cancer-germline genes in human embryonic and adult stem cells. 2009 20090423 DCOM- 20090623(1549-4918 (Electronic)).

[42] Kapoor A Fau - Agius F, Agius F Fau - Zhu J-K, Zhu JK. Preventing transcriptional gene silencing by active DNA demethylation. 2005 20051025 DCOM- 20051205(0014-5793 (Print)).

[43] Kress C Fau - Thomassin H, Thomassin H Fau - Grange T, Grange T. Local DNA demethylation in vertebrates: how could it be performed and targeted? 2001 20010420 DCOM- 20010517(0014-5793 (Print)).

[44] De Smet C, Loriot A. DNA hypomethylation in cancer: Epigenetic scars of a neoplastic journey. Epigenetics. 2010 Apr 10;5(3).

[45] Gama-Sosa Ma Fau - Slagel VA, Slagel Va Fau - Trewyn RW, Trewyn Rw Fau - Oxenhandler R, Oxenhandler R Fau - Kuo KC, Kuo Kc Fau - Gehrke CW, Gehrke Cw Fau - Ehrlich M, et al. The 5-methylcytosine content of DNA from human tumors. 1983 19831217 DCOM- 19831217(0305-1048 (Print)).

[46] Reya T, Morrison SJ, Clarke MF, Weissman IL. Stem cells, cancer, and cancer stem cells. Nature. 2001 Nov 1;414(6859):105-11.

[47] Taipale J Fau - Beachy PA, Beachy PA. The Hedgehog and Wnt signalling pathways in cancer. 2001 20010517 DCOM- 20010621(0028-0836 (Print)).

[48] Tang M Fau - Torres-Lanzas J, Torres-Lanzas J Fau - Lopez-Rios F, Lopez-Rios F Fau - Esteller M, Esteller M Fau - Sanchez-Cespedes M, Sanchez-Cespedes M. Wnt signaling promoter hypermethylation distinguishes lung primary adenocarcinomas from colorectal metastasis to the lung. 2006 20061026 DCOM- 20061212(0020-7136 (Print)).

[49] Gu Jw Fau - Rizzo P, Rizzo P Fau - Pannuti A, Pannuti A Fau - Golde T, Golde T Fau - Osborne B, Osborne B Fau - Miele L, Miele L. Notch signals in the endothelium and cancer "stem-like" cells: opportunities for cancer therapy. 2012 20120509(2045-824X (Electronic)).

[50] Dominguez M. Interplay between Notch signaling and epigenetic silencers in cancer. 2006 20060919 DCOM- 20061128(0008-5472 (Print)).

[51] Tamaru H. Confining euchromatin/heterochromatin territory: jumonji crosses the line. 2010 20100716 DCOM- 20100810(1549-5477 (Electronic)).

[52] Zhimulev If Fau - Belyaeva ES, Belyaeva ES. Intercalary heterochromatin and genetic silencing. 2003 20031027 DCOM- 20040318(0265-9247 (Print)).

[53] Dillon N. Heterochromatin structure and function. Biol Cell. 2004 Oct;96(8):631-7.

[54] Luger K, Mader AW, Richmond RK, Sargent DF, Richmond TJ. Crystal structure of the nucleosome core particle at 2.8 A resolution. Nature. 1997 Sep 18;389(6648): 251-60.

[55] Gilbert N, Allan J. Distinctive higher-order chromatin structure at mammalian centromeres. Proc Natl Acad Sci U S A. 2001 Oct 9;98(21):11949-54.

[56] Xi Y, Yao J, Chen R, Li W, He X. Nucleosome fragility reveals novel functional states of chromatin and poises genes for activation. Genome Res. 2011 May;21(5):718-24.

[57] Soutoglou E, Misteli T. Mobility and immobility of chromatin in transcription and genome stability. Curr Opin Genet Dev. 2007 Oct;17(5):435-42.

[58] Soutoglou E, Dorn JF, Sengupta K, Jasin M, Nussenzweig A, Ried T, et al. Positional stability of single double-strand breaks in mammalian cells. Nat Cell Biol. 2007 Jun; 9(6):675-82.

[59] Skalnikova M, Kozubek S, Lukasova E, Bartova E, Jirsova P, Cafourkova A, et al. Spatial arrangement of genes, centromeres and chromosomes in human blood cell nuclei and its changes during the cell cycle, differentiation and after irradiation. Chromosome Res. 2000;8(6):487-99.

[60] Weissman B, Knudsen KE. Hijacking the chromatin remodeling machinery: impact of SWI/SNF perturbations in cancer. Cancer Res. 2009 Nov 1;69(21):8223-30.

[61] Taby R, Issa JP. Cancer epigenetics. CA Cancer J Clin. 2010 Nov-Dec;60(6):376-92.

[62] Salih F, Salih B, Kogan S, Trifonov EN. Epigenetic nucleosomes: Alu sequences and CG as nucleosome positioning element. J Biomol Struct Dyn. 2008 Aug;26(1):9-16.

[63] Mavrich TN, Ioshikhes IP, Venters BJ, Jiang C, Tomsho LP, Qi J, et al. A barrier nucleosome model for statistical positioning of nucleosomes throughout the yeast genome. Genome Res. 2008 Jul;18(7):1073-83.

[64] Yuan GC, Liu YJ, Dion MF, Slack MD, Wu LF, Altschuler SJ, et al. Genome-scale identification of nucleosome positions in S. cerevisiae. Science. 2005 Jul 22;309(5734): 626-30.

[65] Schones DE, Cui K, Cuddapah S, Roh TY, Barski A, Wang Z, et al. Dynamic regulation of nucleosome positioning in the human genome. Cell. 2008 Mar 7;132(5):887-98.

[66] Clapier CR, Cairns BR. The biology of chromatin remodeling complexes. Annu Rev Biochem. 2009;78:273-304.

[67] Wu JI, Lessard J, Crabtree GR. Understanding the words of chromatin regulation. Cell. 2009 Jan 23;136(2):200-6.

[68] Euskirchen GM, Auerbach RK, Davidov E, Gianoulis TA, Zhong G, Rozowsky J, et al. Diverse roles and interactions of the SWI/SNF chromatin remodeling complex revealed using global approaches. PLoS Genet. 2011 Mar;7(3):e1002008.

[69] Gregory RI, Shiekhattar R. Chromatin modifiers and carcinogenesis. Trends Cell Biol. 2004 Dec;14(12):695-702.

[70] Phelan ML, Sif S, Narlikar GJ, Kingston RE. Reconstitution of a core chromatin remodeling complex from SWI/SNF subunits. Mol Cell. 1999 Feb;3(2):247-53.

[71] T P, K S. Chromatin remodeling in eukaryotes. Nature Education. 2008.

[72] Chen J, Archer TK. Regulating SWI/SNF subunit levels via protein-protein interactions and proteasomal degradation: BAF155 and BAF170 limit expression of BAF57. Mol Cell Biol. 2005 Oct;25(20):9016-27.

[73] Sohn DH, Lee KY, Lee C, Oh J, Chung H, Jeon SH, et al. SRG3 interacts directly with the major components of the SWI/SNF chromatin remodeling complex and protects them from proteasomal degradation. J Biol Chem. 2007 Apr 6;282(14):10614-24.

[74] Percipalle P, Visa N. Molecular functions of nuclear actin in transcription. J Cell Biol. 2006 Mar 27;172(7):967-71.

[75] Castano E, Philimonenko VV, Kahle M, Fukalova J, Kalendova A, Yildirim S, et al. Actin complexes in the cell nucleus: new stones in an old field. Histochem Cell Biol. 2010 Jun;133(6):607-26.

[76] Rando OJ, Zhao K, Janmey P, Crabtree GR. Phosphatidylinositol-dependent actin filament binding by the SWI/SNF-like BAF chromatin remodeling complex. Proc Natl Acad Sci U S A. 2002 Mar 5;99(5):2824-9.

[77] Versteege I, Sevenet N, Lange J, Rousseau-Merck MF, Ambros P, Handgretinger R, et al. Truncating mutations of hSNF5/INI1 in aggressive paediatric cancer. Nature. 1998 Jul 9;394(6689):203-6.

[78] Sevenet N, Lellouch-Tubiana A, Schofield D, Hoang-Xuan K, Gessler M, Birnbaum D, et al. Spectrum of hSNF5/INI1 somatic mutations in human cancer and genotype-phenotype correlations. Hum Mol Genet. 1999 Dec;8(13):2359-68.

[79] Van Maele B, Busschots K, Vandekerckhove L, Christ F, Debyser Z. Cellular co-factors of HIV-1 integration. Trends Biochem Sci. 2006 Feb;31(2):98-105.

[80] Turelli P, Doucas V, Craig E, Mangeat B, Klages N, Evans R, et al. Cytoplasmic recruitment of INI1 and PML on incoming HIV preintegration complexes: interference with early steps of viral replication. Mol Cell. 2001 Jun;7(6):1245-54.

[81] Das S, Cano J, Kalpana GV. Multimerization and DNA binding properties of INI1/hSNF5 and its functional significance. J Biol Chem. 2009 Jul 24;284(30):19903-14.

[82] Isakoff MS, Sansam CG, Tamayo P, Subramanian A, Evans JA, Fillmore CM, et al. Inactivation of the Snf5 tumor suppressor stimulates cell cycle progression and cooperates with p53 loss in oncogenic transformation. Proc Natl Acad Sci U S A. 2005 Dec 6;102(49):17745-50.

[83] Lee YS, Sohn DH, Han D, Lee HW, Seong RH, Kim JB. Chromatin remodeling complex interacts with ADD1/SREBP1c to mediate insulin-dependent regulation of gene expression. Mol Cell Biol. 2007 Jan;27(2):438-52.

[84] Xi Q, He W, Zhang XH, Le HV, Massague J. Genome-wide impact of the BRG1 SWI/SNF chromatin remodeler on the transforming growth factor beta transcriptional program. J Biol Chem. 2008 Jan 11;283(2):1146-55.

[85] Simone C. SWI/SNF: the crossroads where extracellular signaling pathways meet chromatin. J Cell Physiol. 2006 May;207(2):309-14.

[86] Stopka T, Skoultchi AI. The ISWI ATPase Snf2h is required for early mouse development. Proc Natl Acad Sci U S A. 2003 Nov 25;100(24):14097-102.

[87] Klochendler-Yeivin A, Fiette L, Barra J, Muchardt C, Babinet C, Yaniv M. The murine SNF5/INI1 chromatin remodeling factor is essential for embryonic development and tumor suppression. EMBO Rep. 2000 Dec;1(6):500-6.

[88] Vries RG, Bezrookove V, Zuijderduijn LM, Kia SK, Houweling A, Oruetxebarria I, et al. Cancer-associated mutations in chromatin remodeler hSNF5 promote chromosomal instability by compromising the mitotic checkpoint. Genes Dev. 2005 Mar 15;19(6):665-70.

[89] Chai B, Huang J, Cairns BR, Laurent BC. Distinct roles for the RSC and Swi/Snf ATP-dependent chromatin remodelers in DNA double-strand break repair. Genes Dev. 2005 Jul 15;19(14):1656-61.

[90] Rosson GB, Bartlett C, Reed W, Weissman BE. BRG1 loss in MiaPaCa2 cells induces an altered cellular morphology and disruption in the organization of the actin cytoskeleton. J Cell Physiol. 2005 Nov;205(2):286-94.

[91] Kathrein KL, Lorenz R, Innes AM, Griffiths E, Winandy S. Ikaros induces quiescence and T-cell differentiation in a leukemia cell line. Mol Cell Biol. 2005 Mar;25(5): 1645-54.

[92] Klein F, Feldhahn N, Herzog S, Sprangers M, Mooster JL, Jumaa H, et al. BCR-ABL1 induces aberrant splicing of IKAROS and lineage infidelity in pre-B lymphoblastic leukemia cells. Oncogene. 2006 Feb 16;25(7):1118-24.

[93] Pinkel D, Landegent J, Collins C, Fuscoe J, Segraves R, Lucas J, et al. Fluorescence in situ hybridization with human chromosome-specific libraries: detection of trisomy 21 and translocations of chromosome 4. Proc Natl Acad Sci U S A. 1988 Dec;85(23): 9138-42.

[94] Lichter P, Ledbetter SA, Ledbetter DH, Ward DC. Fluorescence in situ hybridization with Alu and L1 polymerase chain reaction probes for rapid characterization of human chromosomes in hybrid cell lines. Proc Natl Acad Sci U S A. 1990 Sep;87(17): 6634-8.

[95] Dolling JA, Boreham DR, Brown DL, Raaphorst GP, Mitchel RE. Rearrangement of human cell homologous chromosome domains in response to ionizing radiation. Int J Radiat Biol. 1997 Sep;72(3):303-11.

[96] Kozubek S, Bartova E, Kozubek M, Lukasova E, Cafourkova A, Koutna I, et al. Spatial distribution of selected genetic loci in nuclei of human leukemia cells after irradiation. Radiat Res. 2001 Feb;155(2):311-9.

[97] Krause M, Yaromina A, Eicheler W, Koch U, Baumann M. Cancer stem cells: targets and potential biomarkers for radiotherapy. Clin Cancer Res. 2011 Dec 1;17(23):7224-9.

[98] Lai AY, Wade PA. Cancer biology and NuRD: a multifaceted chromatin remodelling complex. Nat Rev Cancer. 2011 Aug;11(8):588-96.

[99] Morey L, Brenner C, Fazi F, Villa R, Gutierrez A, Buschbeck M, et al. MBD3, a component of the NuRD complex, facilitates chromatin alteration and deposition of epigenetic marks. Mol Cell Biol. 2008 Oct;28(19):5912-23.

[100] Di Croce L, Raker VA, Corsaro M, Fazi F, Fanelli M, Faretta M, et al. Methyltransferase recruitment and DNA hypermethylation of target promoters by an oncogenic transcription factor. Science. 2002 Feb 8;295(5557):1079-82.

[101] Morin RD, O'Connor MD, Griffith M, Kuchenbauer F, Delaney A, Prabhu AL, et al. Application of massively parallel sequencing to microRNA profiling and discovery in human embryonic stem cells. Genome Res. 2008 Apr;18(4):610-21.

[102] Bhasin M, Reinherz EL, Reche PA. Recognition and classification of histones using support vector machine. J Comput Biol. 2006 Jan-Feb;13(1):102-12.

[103] Chi P, Allis CD, Wang GG. Covalent histone modifications--miswritten, misinterpreted and mis-erased in human cancers. Nat Rev Cancer. 2010 Jul;10(7):457-69.

[104] Rice JC, Allis CD. Histone methylation versus histone acetylation: new insights into epigenetic regulation. Curr Opin Cell Biol. 2001 Jun;13(3):263-73.

[105] Brait M, Sidransky D. Cancer epigenetics: above and beyond. Toxicol Mech Methods. 2011 May;21(4):275-88.

[106] Baxter CS, Byvoet P. CMR studies of protein modification. Progressive decrease in charge density at the epsilon-amino function of lysine with increasing methyl substitution. Biochem Biophys Res Commun. 1975 May 19;64(2):514-8.

[107] Strahl BD, Ohba R, Cook RG, Allis CD. Methylation of histone H3 at lysine 4 is highly conserved and correlates with transcriptionally active nuclei in Tetrahymena. Proc Natl Acad Sci U S A. 1999 Dec 21;96(26):14967-72.

[108] Vakoc CR, Mandat SA, Olenchock BA, Blobel GA. Histone H3 lysine 9 methylation and HP1gamma are associated with transcription elongation through mammalian chromatin. Mol Cell. 2005 Aug 5;19(3):381-91.

[109] Barski A, Cuddapah S, Cui K, Roh TY, Schones DE, Wang Z, et al. High-resolution profiling of histone methylations in the human genome. Cell. 2007 May 18;129(4): 823-37.

[110] Steger DJ, Lefterova MI, Ying L, Stonestrom AJ, Schupp M, Zhuo D, et al. DOT1L/ KMT4 recruitment and H3K79 methylation are ubiquitously coupled with gene transcription in mammalian cells. Mol Cell Biol. 2008 Apr;28(8):2825-39.

[111] Haberland M, Montgomery RL, Olson EN. The many roles of histone deacetylases in development and physiology: implications for disease and therapy. Nat Rev Genet. 2009 Jan;10(1):32-42.

[112] Shi Y. Histone lysine demethylases: emerging roles in development, physiology and disease. Nat Rev Genet. 2007 Nov;8(11):829-33.

[113] Nguyen CT, Weisenberger DJ, Velicescu M, Gonzales FA, Lin JC, Liang G, et al. Histone H3-lysine 9 methylation is associated with aberrant gene silencing in cancer cells and is rapidly reversed by 5-aza-2'-deoxycytidine. Cancer Res. 2002 Nov 15;62(22):6456-61.

[114] Jenuwein T, Laible G, Dorn R, Reuter G. SET domain proteins modulate chromatin domains in eu- and heterochromatin. Cell Mol Life Sci. 1998 Jan;54(1):80-93.

[115] Fraga MF, Ballestar E, Villar-Garea A, Boix-Chornet M, Espada J, Schotta G, et al. Loss of acetylation at Lys16 and trimethylation at Lys20 of histone H4 is a common hallmark of human cancer. Nat Genet. 2005 Apr;37(4):391-400.

[116] Song J, Noh JH, Lee JH, Eun JW, Ahn YM, Kim SY, et al. Increased expression of histone deacetylase 2 is found in human gastric cancer. APMIS. 2005 Apr;113(4):264-8.

[117] Bernstein BE, Mikkelsen TS, Xie X, Kamal M, Huebert DJ, Cuff J, et al. A bivalent chromatin structure marks key developmental genes in embryonic stem cells. Cell. 2006 Apr 21;125(2):315-26.

[118] Weishaupt H, Sigvardsson M, Attema JL. Epigenetic chromatin states uniquely define the developmental plasticity of murine hematopoietic stem cells. Blood. 2010 Jan 14;115(2):247-56.

[119] Rodriguez J, Munoz M, Vives L, Frangou CG, Groudine M, Peinado MA. Bivalent domains enforce transcriptional memory of DNA methylated genes in cancer cells. Proc Natl Acad Sci U S A. 2008 Dec 16;105(50):19809-14.

[120] McGarvey KM, Van Neste L, Cope L, Ohm JE, Herman JG, Van Criekinge W, et al. Defining a chromatin pattern that characterizes DNA-hypermethylated genes in colon cancer cells. Cancer Res. 2008 Jul 15;68(14):5753-9.

[121] Mikkelsen TS, Ku M, Jaffe DB, Issac B, Lieberman E, Giannoukos G, et al. Genome-wide maps of chromatin state in pluripotent and lineage-committed cells. Nature. 2007 Aug 2;448(7153):553-60.

[122] Dreesen O, Brivanlou AH. Signaling pathways in cancer and embryonic stem cells. Stem Cell Rev. 2007 Jan;3(1):7-17.

[123] Widschwendter M, Fiegl H, Egle D, Mueller-Holzner E, Spizzo G, Marth C, et al. Epigenetic stem cell signature in cancer. Nat Genet. 2007 Feb;39(2):157-8.

[124] Schlesinger Y, Straussman R, Keshet I, Farkash S, Hecht M, Zimmerman J, et al. Polycomb-mediated methylation on Lys27 of histone H3 pre-marks genes for de novo methylation in cancer. Nat Genet. 2007 Feb;39(2):232-6.

[125] Ezhkova E, Pasolli HA, Parker JS, Stokes N, Su IH, Hannon G, et al. Ezh2 orchestrates gene expression for the stepwise differentiation of tissue-specific stem cells. Cell. 2009 Mar 20;136(6):1122-35.

[126] Olsen PH, Ambros V. The lin-4 regulatory RNA controls developmental timing in Caenorhabditis elegans by blocking LIN-14 protein synthesis after the initiation of translation. Dev Biol. 1999 Dec 15;216(2):671-80.

[127] Seggerson K, Tang L, Moss EG. Two genetic circuits repress the Caenorhabditis elegans heterochronic gene lin-28 after translation initiation. Dev Biol. 2002 Mar 15;243(2):215-25.

[128] Bartel DP. MicroRNAs: genomics, biogenesis, mechanism, and function. Cell. 2004 Jan 23;116(2):281-97.

[129] Humphreys DT, Westman BJ, Martin DI, Preiss T. MicroRNAs control translation initiation by inhibiting eukaryotic initiation factor 4E/cap and poly(A) tail function. Proc Natl Acad Sci U S A. 2005 Nov 22;102(47):16961-6.

[130] Pillai RS, Bhattacharyya SN, Artus CG, Zoller T, Cougot N, Basyuk E, et al. Inhibition of translational initiation by Let-7 MicroRNA in human cells. Science. 2005 Sep 2;309(5740):1573-6.

[131] Bagga S, Bracht J, Hunter S, Massirer K, Holtz J, Eachus R, et al. Regulation by let-7 and lin-4 miRNAs results in target mRNA degradation. Cell. 2005 Aug 26;122(4): 553-63.

[132] Lim LP, Lau NC, Garrett-Engele P, Grimson A, Schelter JM, Castle J, et al. Microarray analysis shows that some microRNAs downregulate large numbers of target mRNAs. Nature. 2005 Feb 17;433(7027):769-73.

[133] Lee RC, Feinbaum RL, Ambros V. The C. elegans heterochronic gene lin-4 encodes small RNAs with antisense complementarity to lin-14. Cell. 1993 Dec 3;75(5):843-54.

[134] Moss EG, Lee RC, Ambros V. The cold shock domain protein LIN-28 controls developmental timing in C. elegans and is regulated by the lin-4 RNA. Cell. 1997 Mar 7;88(5):637-46.

[135] Boyer LA, Lee TI, Cole MF, Johnstone SE, Levine SS, Zucker JP, et al. Core transcriptional regulatory circuitry in human embryonic stem cells. Cell. 2005 Sep 23;122(6): 947-56.

[136] Niwa H, Miyazaki J, Smith AG. Quantitative expression of Oct-3/4 defines differentiation, dedifferentiation or self-renewal of ES cells. Nat Genet. 2000 Apr;24(4):372-6.

[137] Zaehres H, Lensch MW, Daheron L, Stewart SA, Itskovitz-Eldor J, Daley GQ. High-efficiency RNA interference in human embryonic stem cells. Stem Cells. 2005 Mar; 23(3):299-305.

[138] Avilion AA, Nicolis SK, Pevny LH, Perez L, Vivian N, Lovell-Badge R. Multipotent cell lineages in early mouse development depend on SOX2 function. Genes Dev. 2003 Jan 1;17(1):126-40.

[139] Ivey KN, Muth A, Arnold J, King FW, Yeh RF, Fish JE, et al. MicroRNA regulation of cell lineages in mouse and human embryonic stem cells. Cell Stem Cell. 2008 Mar 6;2(3):219-29.

[140] Marson A, Levine SS, Cole MF, Frampton GM, Brambrink T, Johnstone S, et al. Connecting microRNA genes to the core transcriptional regulatory circuitry of embryonic stem cells. Cell. 2008 Aug 8;134(3):521-33.

[141] Weber B, Stresemann C, Brueckner B, Lyko F. Methylation of human microRNA genes in normal and neoplastic cells. Cell Cycle. 2007 May 2;6(9):1001-5.

[142] Visone R, Croce CM. MiRNAs and cancer. Am J Pathol. 2009 Apr;174(4):1131-8.

[143] Garzon R, Calin GA, Croce CM. MicroRNAs in Cancer. Annu Rev Med. 2009;60:167-79.

[144] Croce CM. Causes and consequences of microRNA dysregulation in cancer. Nat Rev Genet. 2009 Oct;10(10):704-14.

[145] Iorio MV, Croce CM. MicroRNAs in cancer: small molecules with a huge impact. J Clin Oncol. 2009 Dec 1;27(34):5848-56.

[146] Calin GA, Sevignani C, Dumitru CD, Hyslop T, Noch E, Yendamuri S, et al. Human microRNA genes are frequently located at fragile sites and genomic regions involved in cancers. Proc Natl Acad Sci U S A. 2004 Mar 2;101(9):2999-3004.

[147] Scott GK, Mattie MD, Berger CE, Benz SC, Benz CC. Rapid alteration of microRNA levels by histone deacetylase inhibition. Cancer Res. 2006 Feb 1;66(3):1277-81.

[148] Saito Y, Liang G, Egger G, Friedman JM, Chuang JC, Coetzee GA, et al. Specific activation of microRNA-127 with downregulation of the proto-oncogene BCL6 by chromatin-modifying drugs in human cancer cells. Cancer Cell. 2006 Jun;9(6):435-43.

[149] Calin GA, Dumitru CD, Shimizu M, Bichi R, Zupo S, Noch E, et al. Frequent deletions and down-regulation of micro- RNA genes miR15 and miR16 at 13q14 in chronic lymphocytic leukemia. Proc Natl Acad Sci U S A. 2002 Nov 26;99(24):15524-9.

[150] Iorio MV, Ferracin M, Liu CG, Veronese A, Spizzo R, Sabbioni S, et al. MicroRNA gene expression deregulation in human breast cancer. Cancer Res. 2005 Aug 15;65(16):7065-70.

[151] Esquela-Kerscher A, Slack FJ. Oncomirs - microRNAs with a role in cancer. Nat Rev Cancer. 2006 Apr;6(4):259-69.

[152] Ben-Porath I, Thomson MW, Carey VJ, Ge R, Bell GW, Regev A, et al. An embryonic stem cell-like gene expression signature in poorly differentiated aggressive human tumors. Nat Genet. 2008 May;40(5):499-507.

[153] Gotoh N. Control of stemness by fibroblast growth factor signaling in stem cells and cancer stem cells. Curr Stem Cell Res Ther. 2009 Jan;4(1):9-15.

[154] Shimono Y, Zabala M, Cho RW, Lobo N, Dalerba P, Qian D, et al. Downregulation of miRNA-200c links breast cancer stem cells with normal stem cells. Cell. 2009 Aug 7;138(3):592-603.

[155] He H, Jazdzewski K, Li W, Liyanarachchi S, Nagy R, Volinia S, et al. The role of microRNA genes in papillary thyroid carcinoma. Proc Natl Acad Sci U S A. 2005 Dec 27;102(52):19075-80.

[156] Dews M, Homayouni A, Yu D, Murphy D, Sevignani C, Wentzel E, et al. Augmentation of tumor angiogenesis by a Myc-activated microRNA cluster. Nat Genet. 2006 Sep;38(9):1060-5.

[157] Voorhoeve PM, le Sage C, Schrier M, Gillis AJ, Stoop H, Nagel R, et al. A genetic screen implicates miRNA-372 and miRNA-373 as oncogenes in testicular germ cell tumors. Cell. 2006 Mar 24;124(6):1169-81.

[158] Cai X, Lu S, Zhang Z, Gonzalez CM, Damania B, Cullen BR. Kaposi's sarcoma-associated herpesvirus expresses an array of viral microRNAs in latently infected cells. Proc Natl Acad Sci U S A. 2005 Apr 12;102(15):5570-5.

[159] Krutzfeldt J, Rajewsky N, Braich R, Rajeev KG, Tuschl T, Manoharan M, et al. Silencing of microRNAs in vivo with 'antagomirs'. Nature. 2005 Dec 1;438(7068):685-9.

[160] Donepudia S, Mattisonb RJ, E. J, Kihslingerb, A. L, Godleyb. Modulators of DNA methylation and histone acetylation Update on cancer therapeutics 2007:157-69.

[161] Datta J, Ghoshal K, Denny WA, Gamage SA, Brooke DG, Phiasivongsa P, et al. A new class of quinoline-based DNA hypomethylating agents reactivates tumor suppressor genes by blocking DNA methyltransferase 1 activity and inducing its degradation. Cancer Res. (Research Support, N.I.H., Extramural). 2009 May 15;69(10): 4277-85.

[162] Snykers S, Henkens T, De Rop E, Vinken M, Fraczek J, De Kock J, et al. Role of epigenetics in liver-specific gene transcription, hepatocyte differentiation and stem cell reprogrammation. J Hepatol. 2009 Jul;51(1):187-211.

[163] Mai A, Altucci L. Epi-drugs to fight cancer: from chemistry to cancer treatment, the road ahead. Int J Biochem Cell Biol. 2009 Jan;41(1):199-213.

[164] Yang X, Lay F, Han H, Jones PA. Targeting DNA methylation for epigenetic therapy. Trends Pharmacol Sci. 2010 Nov;31(11):536-46.

[165] Jones PA, Taylor SM. Cellular differentiation, cytidine analogs and DNA methylation. Cell. 1980 May;20(1):85-93.

[166] Ghoshal K, Bai S. DNA methyltransferases as targets for cancer therapy. Drugs Today (Barc). 2007 Jun;43(6):395-422.

[167] Appleton K, Mackay HJ, Judson I, Plumb JA, McCormick C, Strathdee G, et al. Phase I and pharmacodynamic trial of the DNA methyltransferase inhibitor decitabine and carboplatin in solid tumors. J Clin Oncol. 2007 Oct 10;25(29):4603-9.

[168] Garcia-Manero G, Kantarjian HM, Sanchez-Gonzalez B, Yang H, Rosner G, Verstovsek S, et al. Phase 1/2 study of the combination of 5-aza-2'-deoxycytidine with valproic acid in patients with leukemia. Blood. 2006 Nov 15;108(10):3271-9.

[169] Blum W, Klisovic RB, Hackanson B, Liu Z, Liu S, Devine H, et al. Phase I study of decitabine alone or in combination with valproic acid in acute myeloid leukemia. J Clin Oncol. 2007 Sep 1;25(25):3884-91.

[170] Oki Y, Kantarjian HM, Gharibyan V, Jones D, O'Brien S, Verstovsek S, et al. Phase II study of low-dose decitabine in combination with imatinib mesylate in patients with accelerated or myeloid blastic phase of chronic myelogenous leukemia. Cancer. 2007 Mar 1;109(5):899-906.

[171] Gollob JA, Sciambi CJ, Peterson BL, Richmond T, Thoreson M, Moran K, et al. Phase I trial of sequential low-dose 5-aza-2'-deoxycytidine plus high-dose intravenous bolus

interleukin-2 in patients with melanoma or renal cell carcinoma. Clin Cancer Res. 2006 Aug 1;12(15):4619-27.

[172] Billam M, Sobolewski MD, Davidson NE. Effects of a novel DNA methyltransferase inhibitor zebularine on human breast cancer cells. Breast Cancer Res Treat. 2010 Apr; 120(3):581-92.

[173] Flotho C, Claus R, Batz C, Schneider M, Sandrock I, Ihde S, et al. The DNA methyltransferase inhibitors azacitidine, decitabine and zebularine exert differential effects on cancer gene expression in acute myeloid leukemia cells. Leukemia. 2009 Jun;23(6): 1019-28.

[174] Byun HM, Choi SH, Laird PW, Trinh B, Siddiqui MA, Marquez VE, et al. 2'-Deoxy-N4-(2-(4-nitrophenyl)ethoxycarbonyl)-5-azacytidine: a novel inhibitor of DNA methyltransferase that requires activation by human carboxylesterase 1. Cancer Lett. 2008 Aug 8;266(2):238-48.

[175] Seidel C, Florean C, Schnekenburger M, Dicato M, Diederich M. Chromatin-modifying agents in anti-cancer therapy. Biochimie. 2012 May 22.

[176] Lafon-Hughes L, Di Tomaso MV, Mendez-Acuna L, Martinez-Lopez W. Chromatin-remodelling mechanisms in cancer. Mutat Res. 2008 Mar-Apr;658(3):191-214.

[177] Terao Y, Nishida J, Horiuchi S, Rong F, Ueoka Y, Matsuda T, et al. Sodium butyrate induces growth arrest and senescence-like phenotypes in gynecologic cancer cells. Int J Cancer. 2001 Oct 15;94(2):257-67.

[178] Gilbert J, Baker SD, Bowling MK, Grochow L, Figg WD, Zabelina Y, et al. A phase I dose escalation and bioavailability study of oral sodium phenylbutyrate in patients with refractory solid tumor malignancies. Clin Cancer Res. 2001 Aug;7(8):2292-300.

[179] Carducci MA, Gilbert J, Bowling MK, Noe D, Eisenberger MA, Sinibaldi V, et al. A Phase I clinical and pharmacological evaluation of sodium phenylbutyrate on an 120-h infusion schedule. Clin Cancer Res. 2001 Oct;7(10):3047-55.

[180] Duenas-Gonzalez A, Candelaria M, Perez-Plascencia C, Perez-Cardenas E, de la Cruz-Hernandez E, Herrera LA. Valproic acid as epigenetic cancer drug: preclinical, clinical and transcriptional effects on solid tumors. Cancer Treat Rev. 2008 May;34(3): 206-22.

[181] Costa FF. Epigenomics in cancer management. Cancer Manag Res. 2010;2:255-65.

[182] Gimsing P, Hansen M, Knudsen LM, Knoblauch P, Christensen IJ, Ooi CE, et al. A phase I clinical trial of the histone deacetylase inhibitor belinostat in patients with advanced hematological neoplasia. Eur J Haematol. 2008 Sep;81(3):170-6.

[183] Tan J, Cang S, Ma Y, Petrillo RL, Liu D. Novel histone deacetylase inhibitors in clinical trials as anti-cancer agents. J Hematol Oncol. 2010;3:5.

[184] Gupta M, Ansell SM, Novak AJ, Kumar S, Kaufmann SH, Witzig TE. Inhibition of histone deacetylase overcomes rapamycin-mediated resistance in diffuse large B-cell

lymphoma by inhibiting Akt signaling through mTORC2. Blood. 2009 Oct 1;114(14): 2926-35.

[185] Chen S, Ye J, Kijima I, Evans D. The HDAC inhibitor LBH589 (panobinostat) is an inhibitory modulator of aromatase gene expression. Proc Natl Acad Sci U S A. 2010 Jun 15;107(24):11032-7.

[186] Kauh J, Fan S, Xia M, Yue P, Yang L, Khuri FR, et al. c-FLIP degradation mediates sensitization of pancreatic cancer cells to TRAIL-induced apoptosis by the histone deacetylase inhibitor LBH589. PLoS One. 2010;5(4):e10376.

[187] Grant C, Rahman F, Piekarz R, Peer C, Frye R, Robey RW, et al. Romidepsin: a new therapy for cutaneous T-cell lymphoma and a potential therapy for solid tumors. Expert Rev Anticancer Ther. 2010 Jul;10(7):997-1008.

[188] Kleff S, Andrulis ED, Anderson CW, Sternglanz R. Identification of a gene encoding a yeast histone H4 acetyltransferase. J Biol Chem. 1995 Oct 20;270(42):24674-7.

[189] Dekker FJ, Haisma HJ. Histone acetyl transferases as emerging drug targets. Drug Discov Today. 2009 Oct;14(19-20):942-8.

[190] Allis CD, Berger SL, Cote J, Dent S, Jenuwien T, Kouzarides T, et al. New nomenclature for chromatin-modifying enzymes. Cell. 2007 Nov 16;131(4):633-6.

[191] Spannhoff A, Sippl W, Jung M. Cancer treatment of the future: inhibitors of histone methyltransferases. Int J Biochem Cell Biol. 2009 Jan;41(1):4-11.

Chapter 8

# DNA Methylation in the Pathogenesis of Head and Neck Cancer

Zvonko Magić, Gordana Supić,
Mirjana Branković-Magić and Nebojša Jović

Additional information is available at the end of the chapter

http://dx.doi.org/10.5772/51169

## 1. Introduction

Head and neck cancer is the sixth most common cancer worldwide and one of the most aggressive malignancies in human population. The most common histologic type among the head and neck tumors are the squamous cell carcinomas (*SCC*). Despite the significant efforts committed during the last decades in its early detection, prevention and treatment, head and neck cancer prognosis remains very poor with the rising incidence in developed countries and younger population. Carcinogenesis of Head and Neck Squamous Cell Carcinoma (*HNSCC*) is a multistep process, which arises through an accumulation of genetic and epigenetic alterations. Although the impact of genetic changes in oral carcinogenesis is well-known, over the last decade it has been demonstrated that epigenetic changes, especially aberrant DNA methylation, play a significant role in *HNSCC*.

### 1.1. Head and neck cancer – Etiology and risk factors

Head and Neck Squamous Cell Carcinoma is the sixth most common cancer in males and tenth in females worldwide [1]. Despite the fact that significant results have been achieved during the last decades in its early detection, prevention and treatment, the survival rate has remained less than 40%, and *HNSCC* remains one of the most aggressive malignancies. Furthermore, the incidence of this carcinoma is rising in developed countries and younger population, particularly young women [2, 3]. Early stages of the disease are associated with minimal symptoms, thus small percentage of *HNSCC* has been diagnosed at an early clinical stage. Advanced stages respond poorly to current cancer therapies, with high incidence of local and regional relapse and lymph node metastasis [2, 4, 5].

Head and neck cancers include malignancies arising from different anatomical sites within the upper aero-digestive tract. Head and neck cancers are characterized by heterogeneous histology. The majority carcinomas that arise from squamous cell epithelia are head and neck squamous cell carcinomas (*HNSCC*), while other cancer types that can occur in the head and neck include thyroid cancer, malignant salivary gland tumors, lymphomas and sarcomas. *HNSCC* include cancers of the oral cavity, larynx, pharynx (oropharynx, hypopharynx, nasopharynx), and esophagus, [4, 5], Figure 1.

### 1.2. Risk factors for HNSCC

Both environmental and genetic factors play an important role in the etiology of head and neck cancers but the causal relationship between environmental factors, lifestyle and tumor development is not yet fully elucidated. The mucosa of the upper aerodigestive tract is exposed to number of carcinogens attributed to cause genetic and epigenetic changes that ultimately lead to head and neck cancer development. *HNSCC* incidence is influenced by age, genetic factors, geographic region and different lifestyle factors, including alcohol, smoking, betel quid use, oral hygiene, and Human Papilloma Virus (HPV) infection [5]. Emerging evidences are indicating that environmental factors, such as smoking, alcohol and diet could directly or indirectly affect epigenetic mechanisms of gene expression regulation and DNA methylation in *HNSCC*.

### 1.3. Tobacco and alcohol use in HNSCC

Smoking and alcohol consumption are the major risk factors for head and neck cancers [6, 7]. In addition, the combination of both alcohol and tobacco use synergically increases the risk for *HNSCC*development more than 10 times [8]. Cigarette smoking is the major cause of lung cancer and is associated with head and neck, esophagus, bladder, breast and kidney cancer [9]. Increased risk with smoking may be due to the direct effect of tobacco carcinogens or due to genetic polymorphisms in enzymes that activate or detoxify carcinogens.

Several carcinogens present in cigarette smoke are inactivated by a family of enzymes cytochrome P-450 (CYP), which convert carcinogens into reactivated intermediates. These intermediates form DNA adducts that need to be detoxified by a number of enzymes, including glutathione S-transferase [GST) [10]. Single nucleotide polymorphisms (SNPs) in these genes could be an alternative mechanism that modulates the effects of cigarette smoke. Even though alcohol and smoking are known risk factors, only a fraction of smokers and alcohol consumers develop *HNSCC,* suggesting that genetic susceptibility and interactions between genetic, epigenetic and environmental factors could play an important role in the etiology of *HNSCC* [11, 12].

Alcohol consumption has been associated with an increased risk of the head and neck, esophagus, liver, colorectal, and breast cancer [13]. Possible mechanisms by which alcohol exerts its harmful effect includes the genotoxic effect of ethanol metabolite acetaldehyde, production of reactive oxygen- and nitrogen species, changes in folate metabolism, generation of DNA adducts and inhibition of DNA repair. Also, alcohol could exert its damaging effect directly, either acting as a solvent of carcinogens from tobacco smoke or damaging the oral mucosa, that enhances the penetration of carcinogens from tobacco smoke [7]. Genetic polymorphisms of ethanol-metabolizing enzymes, including alcohol dehydrogenases (ADH) (which metabolizes alcohol into acetaldehyde), with a different ability to generate carcinogen acetaldehyde, may determine individual susceptibility to head and neck cancer. Acetaldehyde can form adducts with DNA, interfering with DNA synthesis and repair [7, 13]. "Fast-metabolizing" ADHs genotype was associated with the increase of *OSCC* and *HNSCC* risk [14, 15, 16]. By the contrast, in other studies "fast-metabolizing" ADHs genotype was found to be associated with decreased risk of *HNSCC* [11, 17, 18]. Therefore, the mechanism by which smoking and alcohol causes increased risk for *HNSCC* and the role of alcohol and tobacco-related polymorphisms have not been fully elucidated.

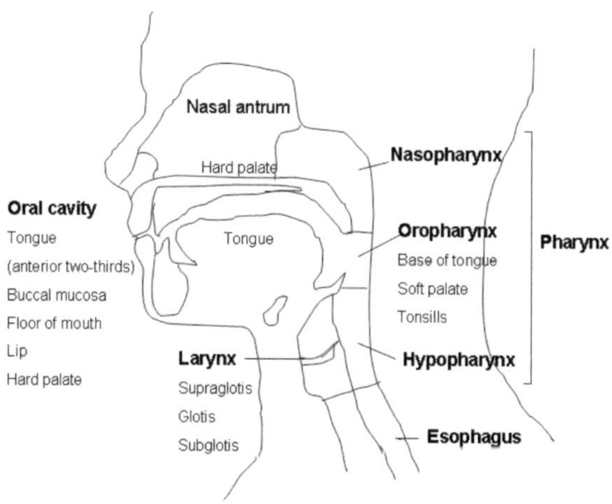


**Figure 1.** Diverse anatomical localization of Head and Neck Squamous Cell Carcinomas. Although head and neck cancers are characterized by heterogeneous histology, the majority carcinomas arise from squamous cell epithelia of the oral cavity (tongue, buccal mucosa, floor of the mouth), oropharynx (soft palate, base of tongue, tonsils), hypopharynx, nasopharynx, larynx (supraglotis, glottis, subglotis) and esophagus.

### 1.4. HPV infection in HNSCC

In addition to alcohol and tobacco exposure, human papilloma virus (HPV) infection has also a significant part in the etiology of head and neck cancer. HPV cancers predominantly arise from tongue and palatine tonsils within the oropharynx [5, 19]. Acting in synergy with tobacco use and heavy alcohol consumption, HPV infection with high-risk types is considered as an etiological factor in the development of *HSCC* and *OSCC* [5]. Reported incidence of high-risk HPVs in oral carcinoma patients varied from 0% to 100% [20], depending on the methods used for HPV detection, tumor-host characteristics of the examined group of patients, varying numbers of included tissue samples, but it is also affected with different distribution of oncogenic HPVs in different world regions. The DNA of oncogenic HPVs is present in 20% of all *HNSSCs* and in nearly 60% of tonsillar cancers [5, 8]. There is increasing evidence that HPV-associated *HNSCC* carcinomas are distinct clinical and pathological tumor entity from alcohol and smoking-associated *HNSCCs* with regards to risk factors, tumor biology and progression [5]. Infection with oncogenic HPV types, predominantly HPV16 and HPV18 is associated with increased risk of *HNSSC* [5, 19].

HPV infection causes deregulation of cell cycle and apoptosis by inactivation of *Rb* and *p53* tumor suppressor gene protein products, involved in the maintenance of genome stability. E6 protein of high risk HPVs affects the *p53* protein function by ubiquitin-dependent degradation. Although *p53* tumor suppressor gene is the most often mutated gene in human oncology, in tumors with HPV etiology is not clear in which extent the mechanism of *p53* mutation is included in *p53* inactivation. It can be assumed that *p53* mutations occur most frequently in HPV negative than in the HPV positive head and neck cancers, but it is questionable if the presence of *p53* mutation in HPV infected tumors additionally influences prognosis of the patients. Numerous studies with conflicting results deal with the influence of oncogenic HPV types and prognosis of *HSCC*. The majority of them reported that *HSCC* patients with HPV infection have better prognosis than the patients who are HPV negative [5, 21, 22]. On the contrary, our previous results concerning *OSCC* patients in stage III of the disease showed worse overall and disease-free survival for patients infected with high-risk HPV types (HPV 16, 18 and 31) [23], indicating the presence of more aggressive disease in these patients. Our study comparing disease-free interval (DFI) and overall survival (OS) between patients with HPV infection only and the patients with HPV infection and *p53* mutation showed significantly shorter disease-free interval as well as overall survival in patients with both HPV infection and *p53* mutation. Presence of *p53* mutations in HPV infected tumors confer a higher risk of recurrence in this disease. In addition, since all patients were treated with postoperative radiotherapy, shorter DFI indicate that the response to radiotherapy may be influenced by *p53* status [24]. However, it has been recently reported that it is unlikely that HPV infection plays significant role in mobile tongue carcinogenesis in young *OSCC* patients [25].

The role of HPV infection in the etiology, as well as in prognosis of head and neck cancers varies and it depends on head and neck cancer subtypes and different anatomic site of tumors. From that point of view, it is clear that HPV typing, together with other molecular markers may help in defining a particular group of tumors in regard to prognosis and response to anti cancer therapies.

### 1.5. Diet and HNSCC

Recent studies provide growing evidence that some dietary components, might affect the process of carcinogenesis. There is a growing body of evidence that bioactive food components, such as isothiocyanates from cruciferous vegetables (cauliflower, cabbage, and broccoli), diallyl sulfide (an organosulphur compound from garlic), green tea flavonoids, folate, and selenium, effect on cancer might be mediated through epigenetic mechanisms. Several recent studies indicate that dietary habits and fruit and vegetable intake could be associated with cancer risk [26, 27]. Increased fruit and vegetable consumption was recently associated with reduced occurrence of *HNSCC* [28]. However, the findings of association of diet and cancer risk are still confounding.

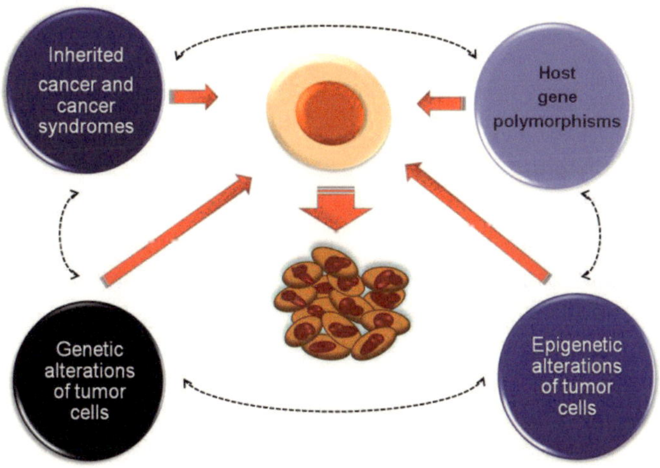


**Figure 2.** Schematic presentation of synergistic effect of different genetic alterations in transformation of normal to malignant cell. Gene mutations can be inherited (BRCA1, BRCA2, RET, VHL, APC) and associated with a predisposition to certain cancer or cancer syndromes. Also, mutations can be acquired leading to the strong predisposition to malignant transformation of cells (K-*ras*, p53, HER2, *bcr-abl, bcl-2*, Rb). The human genome is characterized with enormous number of genetic polymorphisms that sometimes results with impaired function of the gene product, especially when cells are exposed to environmental or host risk factors. Hypermethylation of gene promoter sequences causes gene silencing that is of great importance for tumor suppressor genes. All these genetic alterations can impair function of other genes and further contribute to increased risk of malignant transformation.

## 2. Molecular changes In *HNSCC*

Second half of 20$^{th}$ century and beginning of 21$^{st}$ century are marked with almost revolutionary breakthrough in our understanding of human gene structure and functions. The rapid development of biotechniques led to the sequencing of complete human genome and later of genome and transcriptome of many human tumors [29, 30]. Even before these achievements, it was well accepted that malignant tumors, on the molecular level, are disease of genes. This knowledge led to enormous number of worldwide research projects and publications concerning association of gene alterations in tumor cells with cancerogenesis and early diagnosis, tumor progression, tumor staging and response to therapy. In spite of many practical/

clinical results of these studies [Her-2/neu, *BRCA-1* and *BRCA-2* in Breast Cancer; *K-ras* and *EGFR* in Colon Cancer; *bcr-abl* in Chronic Myeloid Leukemia; *B-RAF* and *c-KIT* in Melanoma; detection of dominant clone of B- and T-lymphocytes in tracking minimal residual disease in lymphomas and leukemia's [29-33], still much more questions concerning significance of gene alterations for tumor development and treatment remains unanswered. In the last 10-15 years significant efforts are done to fulfill these gaps in our understanding of molecular pathogenesis of cancer by studying epigenetic changes of tumor tissues.

These alterations are of special interest because epigenetic changes are tumor/tissue specific, although inheritable epigenetic alterations are under strong influence of environmental risk factors and patient behavior and they are potentially reversible. Intensive research of epigenetic alterations in human tumors and their association with environmental risk factors and patient behavior put an attention to another group of gene alterations, i.e. on inherited gene polymorphisms. These researches tried to elucidate connection of certain gene polymorphisms with environmental and host risk factors and epigenetic alterations in different human tumors and in *HNSCC* [12, 16, 34-36], Figure 2.

Carcinogenesis of *HNSCC* is a multistep process, which arises through an accumulation of genetic and epigenetic alterations. These genetic alterations result in inactivation of multiple tumor suppressor genes and activation of proto-oncogenes by deletions, point mutations, promoter methylation, and gene amplification [3], Table 1.

| Genetic changes | Locus / gene | Cancer type | Frequency | Ref. |
|---|---|---|---|---|
| LOH | 9p21-22/ **p16INK4a/p14ARF** | *HNSCC*<br>*OSCC* | 70–80% | 37, 38,39, 40 |
| | 3p/ **RASSF1A, FHIT, RARB2** | *OSCC*<br>*HNSCC* | 30–70% | 37, 39, 40, 47 |
| | 17p13/**p53** | *HNSCC* | 76% | 39 |
| | 11q | *OSCC* | 20-33% | 37 |
| | 13q14/**Rb** | *HNSCC* | 68% | 39 |
| | 8p | *OSCC* | 53-83% | 37 |
| Mutation | 9p21-22/ **p16** | *OSCC* | 70% | 41 |
| | 5q21-22/**APC** | *OSCC* | 50% | 37 |
| | 17p13/**p53** | *HNSCC* | 40-79% | 49 |
| | 11p15/**H-ras** | *OSCC* | 35-55% | 37 |
| Amplification | 11q13/(**PRAD-1/Cyclin D1/hst-1/int-2**) | *HNSCC* | 30–50% | 46, 47 |
| | 7p12/**EGFR** | *OSCC* | 30% | 53, 54 |

**Table 1.** Frequent genetic abnormalities in head and neck cancer.

Genetic instability in regions leads to loss of chromosomal region that contains tumor suppressor genes. A high incidence of Loss of heterozygosity (LOH) observed at 9p, 8p, 3p, 9q, and 11q regions were associated with tumor stage, and poor histological differentiation in *HNSCC* [37]. Loss of heterozygosity (LOH) of 9p21 appears is an early and frequent event in head and neck carcinogenesis [37, 38-40]. The CDKN2A gene locus found in 9p21 region encodes two different transcripts, *p16* and *p14*ARF, which are responsible for G1 cell cycle regulation and MDM2 mediated degradation of *p53*. *P16* and *p14* are often inactivated in *HNSCC* through homozygous deletion, by promoter methylation, and by point mutations [41-44].

Loss of chromosome region 3p is a common early genetic event in *HNSCC* [2, 40, 45]. Genetic alterations at 3p that are common in *HNSCC* and *OSCC* contains tumor suppressor genes Fragile histidine triad (*FHIT*) gene mapped at *3p14*, Ras association family (*RASSF1A*) gene, mapped at 3p21, and Retinoic acid receptor B2 gene (*RARB2*), mapped to chromosome region 3p24 [37, 40]. Amplification of 11q13 leads to overexpression of cyclin D1 [46], detected in 30–60% of *HNSCC* and 40% of cases of oral squamous dysplasia [47].

There has been much research on the tumor suppressor gene *p53* and its role in *HNSCC* and *OSCC* carcinogenesis. The *p53* protein blocks cell division at the G1 to S boundary, stimulates DNA repair after DNA damage, and induces apoptosis. *P53* has been shown to be functionally inactivated in oral and head and neck tumors [48]. LOH of 17p13, which contains *p53* and point mutations of the *p53* are seen in more than 50% of *HNSCC* cases [39, 49]. Cigarette smoking has been associated with the mutation of *p53* in head and neck cancers [14]. Investigations about the prognostic value of *p53* status in head and neck cancer subtypes hardly can get a clear result due to the presence of large heterogeneity in regard to patients characteristics, and methods for *p53* detection. Meta-analysis of Tandon et al [50] pointed out that evidence about the prognostic value of *p53* in head and neck cancer squamous cell carcinomas has been inconclusive. However, determination of *p53* status of *HNSCC* may be of particular interests due to its possible role in prediction of the response to cisplatin based chemotherapy. Cisplatin chemotherapy is widely used chemotherapeutical approach in the treatment of head and neck cancers and data that patients with *p53* mutations respond better to cisplatin chemotherapy need further confirmation [51]. Chemotherapy responses in *HNSCC* patients is also influenced by polymorphism at codon 72 of *p53* gene. In patients with wild type *p53*, arginine at codon 72 is associated with better response to chemotherapy. On the contrary, if *p53* is mutated, proline at position 72 is better option [52]. Better understanding of cellular processes and their actors such as *p53* network and their relation to clinical settings will help in appropriate biomarker characterization. Epidermal growth factor receptor (*EGFR*) is overexpressed in 90% of *HNSCC* [53], often due to amplification [54]. Thus, frequent molecular abnormalities in head and neck squamous cell carcinoma include alterations in tumor suppressor genes *p16*INK4A, *p53*, *p14*ARF, *FHIT*, *RASSF1A*, *Rb*, cyclin D1, and activation of oncogenes, such as members of the *ras* gene family, *c-myc*, and *EGFR* [2-4], Table 1.

A large number of previous studies have also suggested the correlation between polymorphisms of genes involved in cell cycle control, angiogenesis and metabolism of alcohol and carcinogens and susceptibility to head and neck cancer [10, 16, 34-36].

Although the impact of genetic changes in oral carcinogenesis is well-known, over the last decade it has been demonstrated that epigenetic changes, especially aberrant DNA methylation, play a significant role in *HNSCC* [55]. Epigenetic modifications are heritable changes in gene expression that are not coded in the DNA sequence [56]. These changes are mitoticaly (clonally) heritable and potentially reversible, which provides large possibilities of epigenetic therapy. Additionally, epigenetic changes could be modulated by the nutrition, environmental and genetic factors and/or gene-by-environment interactions. Main mechanisms of epigenetic control in mammals include DNA methylation, histone modifications and RNA interference (RNA silencing).

## 3. DNA methylation

DNA methylation of cytosine in a CpG dinucleotide is the key epigenetic modification in mammals. The covalent addition of a methyl group to the 5-carbon (C5) position of cytosine that are located 5' to a guanosine base in a CpG dinucleotide are catalyzed by a family of enzymes DNA methyltransferases (*DNMTs*). CpG dinucleotides are asymmetrically distributed in the genome. Throughout the genome rare solitary CpGs are heavily methylated. In contrast, CpG clustered in small stretches of DNA (0.5-4kb regions), with greater than 50% GC content, are termed 'CpG islands'. Of approximately 50% the genes in the genome CpG islands are associated with promoter regions. In normal cells, most CpG sites outside of CpG islands are methylated, whereas CpG islands in gene promoters are usually unmethylated, independently of the gene transcription status [56]. During the process of cancerogenesis paradoxical changes in DNA methylation patterns occurs, with simultaneous global hypomethylation and regional hypermethylation changes. Global DNA hypomethylation may activate, 'unlock' repetitive elements that could affect genome stability or could lead to transcriptional activation of latent viruses or oncogenes. Simultaneously, regional hypermethylation leads to transcriptional silencing of tumor suppressor genes. Cytosine methylation of CpG islands in the promoters of tumor suppressor genes causes their inactivation, transcriptional silencing and consequently malignant transformation. Investigations showed that the number of cancer-related genes that are inactivated by epigenetic modifications equals or even exceeds the number of genes inactivated by mutation. Furthermore, genetic and epigenetic changes have almost identical biological effect and pattern of gene expression [56]. Pattern of tumor suppressor genes hypermethylation shows tumor-type specificity.

While *DNMT3A* and *DNMT3B* are mostly involved in *de novo* methylation, *DNMT1* is involved in the maintenance of DNA methylation after replication [56]. Several studies have shown *DNMT* overexpression (mainly *DNMT1* and *DNMT3B*) in cancer, including *HNSCC* [57]. The analysis of *DNMT* knockout cells revealed that individual enzymes also interact between each other, and interact with other chromatin modifying enzymes, histone deacetylases (*HDAC*) and methyl-CpG binding proteins (MBPs). Methylation of cytosine within CpG islands is associated with binding of MBPs, which recruit *HDAC* to methylated DNA in regions of transcriptional silencing. Histone deacetylation, catalyzed by *HDACs*, leads to the chromatin condensation and suppression of DNA transcription. Thus, DNA methylation and histone modifications are not isolated events, but highly coordinated [56].

### 3.1. DNA methylation in *HNSCC*

Frequent hypermethylation of tumor-related genes were observed in cancer tissue of *OSCC* and *HNSCC*, in the normal adjacent mucous in the *OSCC* [58], dysplastic tissue [59], and leukoplakia [60]. Promoter hypermethylation can also be detected in buccal swabs samples of tobacco and alcohol users [58], Thus, DNA methylation has been considered as an early event in head and neck carcinogenesis.

The list of genes that are found to be inactivated by DNA methylation events in *HNSCC* is growing rapidly and includes genes involved in the cell cycle control (*p14,* p15, *p16* and p53), DNA damage repair (*MGMT, hMLH1,* and ATM), apoptosis (*DAPK, RASSF1A,* and RARβ), *Wnt* signalling (*APC, RUNX3, WIF1, E-cad* and *DCC*) *SFRP* family genes, *TCF21*, etc. [42, 44, 55, 58-62], Table 2.

| FUNCTION | *Gene* | Gene name | Locus | Gene Action | *HNSCC methylation* | Ref. |
|---|---|---|---|---|---|---|
| **Cell Cycle Control** | ***p16*** | Cyclin-dependent kinase inhibitor 2A (CDKN2A) | 9p21 | Regulation of the *Rb* pathway | 10-70% | 42, 96 |
| | ***p15*** | Cyclin-dependent kinase inhibitor 2B | 9p21 | TGF beta-mediated cell cycle arrest | 23-80% | 151 |
| **Apoptosis** | ***p14*** | Alternative open reading frame (ARF) of INK4a locus | 9p21 | Pro-apoptosis | 18-46% | 75-77, 96 |
| | ***DAPK1*** | Death-associated protein kinase 1 | 19q34 | p53-dependent apoptosis | 18-77% | 42, 44, 61, 68, 72, 78 |
| ***Wnt signaling pathway*** | ***APC*** | Adenomatous polyposis coli | 5q21-22 | *Wnt* signaling and adhesion | 20-68% | 44, 92-95 |
| | ***CDH1*** | *E-cad*herin | 16q22 | Cell–cell adhesion | 2-66% | 44, 72, 81-88 |
| | ***SFRP*** | Soluble frizzled receptor protein genes family | 10q24 | Antagonists of the Wnt pathway | 30-94% | 97-99 |

| FUNCTION | Gene | Gene name | Locus | Gene Action | HNSCC methylation | Ref. |
|---|---|---|---|---|---|---|
| | ***WIF1*** | Wnt inhibitory factor 1 | 12q14 | Secreted Wnt antagonist | 25-90% | 62, 97, 102 |
| | ***RUNX3*** | Runt-related transcription factor 3 | 1p36 | *Wnt* signaling inhibitor, TGF-β-induced tumor suppression | 18-36% | 62, 99-101 |
| **DNA damage repair** | ***hMLH1*** | human mutL homolog 1 | 3p21 | DNA mismatch repair | 8-76% | 96, 106, 107 |
| | ***MGMT*** | O$^6$-mehylguanine DNA methyltransferase | 10q26 | DNA repair for alkylated guanine | 10-57% | 59, 44, 72, 103-105 |
| **Tumor suppressor** | ***FHIT*** | Fragile Histidine Triad | *3p14* | Control of cell cycle | 33-84% | 96, 110 |
| | ***RASSF1A*** | Ras association (RalGDS/AF-6) domain family member 1A | 3p21 | RAS pathway regulation and tumor suppression | 10-76% | 45, 72, 78, 79, 96 |
| | ***DCC*** | Deleted in Colorectal Cancer | 18q21 | Cell–cell adhesion | 17-75% | 108, 109 |
| | ***RARβ*** | Retinoic acid receptor beta | 3p24 | Regulatory protein and apoptosis | 53-88% | 59, 78 |

**Table 2.** Genes commonly methylated in *HNSCC*.

### 3.2. DNA methylation association with progression and prognosis in *HNSCC*

A number of tumor suppressor genes hypermethylation has been associated with worse outcome in various cancer types. Hypermethylation of the *p16* and *WIF1* genes [63] and *RASSF1A* and *RUNX3* methylation status [64] were found to be independent prognostic factors non-small cell lung cancers. *DAPK* promoter hypermethylation has been associated with tumor aggressiveness and poor prognosis in lung cancer [65]. *E-cad*herin promoter hypermethylation was found to be the prognostic factor of worse prognosis in diffuse gastric cancer [66], and in non-small cell lung carcinoma [67]. Epigenetic inactivation of several genes by DNA methylation has been found to associate with *HNSCC* progression [44, 58, 61, 68].

*p16$^{INK4a}$* is cyclin-dependent kinase inhibitor which regulates the *Rb* pathway, leading to inhibition of cell cycle progression. An alternate spliced product of the same INK4a locus is another tumor suppressor gene *p14ARF* (Alternative open reading frame). Loss of *p16* in head and neck and oral tumors has been frequently reported [69, 70]. *p16* methylation was correlated with malignant transformation of oral epithelial dysplasia and is a potential biomarker for prediction of prognosis of mild or moderate oral epithelial dysplasia, with the overall sensitivity and specificity of >60% [71]. Previously, *p16* methylation status has been correlated with tumor stage, lymph node metastasis and tumor size in *HNSCC* [72], and poorly differentiated *HNSCC* [73]. *p16* hypermethylation has been associated with poor prognosis in *HNSCC* [55, 74] and *OSCC* [75]. Interestingly, *p16INK4A* and *p14ARF* genes, transcribed from the same locus INK4A by alternate splicing, could have a diametrically opposite clinical effect in oral cancer patients when methylated. Promoter methylation of *p16* was associated with increased disease recurrences and worse prognosis, whereas *p14* methylation was strongly associated with lower disease recurrence and was found to be a good prognostic predictor for oral carcinoma [75]. However, other studies associated *p14* methylation with tumor stage and lymph node involvement of *OSCC* [76] and poor prognosis [77]. These findings indicate that DNA methylation status of *INK4A/ARF* locus could be used as a prognostic biomarker for assessing the aggressiveness of disease in oral and head and neck carcinoma patients.

*Death associated protein-kinase (DAPK)*, plays a critical role in apoptosis regulation in tumor development, and commonly is hypermethylated in *HNSCC* [42] and *OSCC* [68]. *DAPK* promoter methylation showed the positive correlation with lymph node involvement [42, 72, 78] and advanced disease stage in *HNSCC* [42, 72]. The presence of *DAPK* promoter hypermethylation detected in surgical margins was associated with the decreased overall survival and was shown to be an independent prognostic factor for overall survival in *OSCC* patients [61].

*RASSF1A* Ras association (RalGDS/AF-6) domain family member 1A, involved in RAS pathway regulation and tumor suppression, is frequently inactivated by promoter hypermethylation in *HNSCC* [45, 72]. *RASSF1A* methylation correlates with head and neck tumor stage [72], poor disease-free survival of *OSCC* [79] and lymph node metastasis in nasophageal carcinomas [78].

*E-cadherin* (*E-cad*) has a dual role in a mammalian cell, as a $Ca^{+2}$-dependent cell adhesion molecule, and as a part of the complex signaling Wnt pathway interacting with β- and α-catenine [80]. Hypermethylation of *E-cad* is a common event in *HNSCC* [44, 72, 81, 82]. Reduced *E-cad* expression as a consequence of promoter hypermethylation leads to the development of the invasive phenotype in the *OSCC* [83], and is associated with lymph node metastasis in the *OSCC* [84] and *HNSCC* [85]. Hypermethylation of *E-cad* has previously been associated with tumor stage of *HNSCC* [72] and nasopharyngeal carcinomas [86] and lymph node metastasis of oral [82] and nasopharyngeal carcinomas [87]. Down-regulation of CDH1 due to hypermethylation contributed to the progression of esophageal cancer [88], led to poor differentiation and the development of the invasive phenotype in the *OSCC* [83], and salivary gland carcinomas [89]. Furthermore, *E-cad* hypermethylation was associated with poor survival in *the OSCC* [84] and *HNSCC* [85]. Recently published investigations showed that *E-cad* gene hypermethylation was associated with the decreased survival in *HNSCC* patients [90]. In addition, advanced *OSCC* patients with *E-cad* promoter methylation had significantly worse 3- and 5-year survival rates [44], and *E-cad* hypermethylation was found to be an independent prognostic factor in oral tongue carcinoma [81]. However, *HNSCC* patients with *E-cad* promoter methylation had lower rates of local recurrences and better disease-specific survival and outcome [91], which indicates that the role of *E-cad* gene methylation in head and neck carcinomas has not been fully elucidated.

*APC* gene plays an integral role in *the Wnt* signaling pathway in binding and degrading of β-catenine. Hypermethylation of *the APC* gene promoter is frequent in *HNSCC* [92-94], and *OSCC* [44]. *APC* methylation status has previously been associated with worse prognosis of esophageal carcinoma [95]. However, in another study on esophageal cancer, hypermethylation of the *APC* gene was related to a lower number of metastatic lymph nodes and better recurrence rates [96].

*SFRP* (soluble frizzled receptor protein) family genes are involved in the inhibition of *Wnt* signaling. Promoters of SFRP-2, SFRP-4, SFRP-5 genes showed methylation in *OSCC*, whereas SFRP-1 was demethylated in oral cancer [97]. SFRP-1 has been associated with tumor grade in *OSCC* [98]. Hypermethylation of SFRP-1 was associated with an increased risk of esophageal cancer recurrence [99].

*RUNX3* Runt-related transcription factor 3 gene plays a role in the transforming growth factor-beta (TGF-β) -induced tumor suppression pathway. *RUNX3* may have an oncogenic role in *HNSCC* and its expression may predict malignant behavior [100]. In contrast to *HNSCC*, in *OSCC* the *RUNX3* gene is downregulated due to promoter hypermethylation [101] and associated with lymph node involvement and tumor stage in tongue carcinomas [62]. Hypermethylation of *RUNX3* detected in the plasma of esophageal cancer patients was significantly associated with an increased risk of cancer recurrence [99].

*WIF1* Wnt inhibitory factor 1, gene involved in the inhibition of *Wnt* signaling, is commonly methylated in the *HNSCC* [102] and *OSCC* [62, 97]. Its methylation status was correlated with lymph node metastasis in nasopharyngeal carcinoma [102].

*MGMT* O(6)-methylguanine-DNAmethyltransferase a DNA repair gene that removes mutagenic $O^6$-guanine adducts from DNA, is inactivated by hypermethylation in *HNSCC* [59] and *OSCC* [44]. *MGMT* promoter hypermethylation was associated with tumor stage of *HNSCC* [72] and with lymph node involvement in laryngeal carcinomas [103]. In addition, the methylation of *MGMT* was associated with poor survival and reduced disease-free survival in *OSCC* [104] and increased recurrences rate and poor prognosis of *HNSCC* [105].

*hMLH1* mutL homolog 1 is involved in the DNA repair process. The *hMLH1* promoter methylation occurred in high frequency of the majority of the early stage *OSCC* and in about half of the late stage carcinomas [106], indicating its potential role in the tumor progression. Promoter methylation of *hMLH1* gene is also a common event in *HNSCC*, and was correlated with poor survival in *HNSCC* [107].

*RARß* Retinoic acid receptor beta is commonly methylated in *HNSCC* [59] and associated with highly differentiated tumors, advanced tumor stage and the presence of lymph node metastasis of nasopharyngeal carcinomas [78].

*TIMP3* Tissue inhibitor of metalloproteinases 3 gene is involved in the inhibition of angiogenesis and tumor growth. Promoter methylation of TIMP3 predicts better outcome in *HNSCC* treated by radiotherapy [91].

*DCC* Deleted in colorectal cancer, tumor suppressor gene highly methylated in *HNSCC* [108] was correlated with mandibular invasion and poor survival in oral cancer [109].

*FHIT* Fragile Histidine Triad gene is associated highly methylated in *HNSCC* [96], and associated with poor prognosis in early stage esophageal squamous cell carcinoma [110].

*MINT1* and *MINT 31,* are the members of Methylated in tumor gene family, which methylation was previously associated with invasiveness and poor survival in the *OSCC* [109].

A number of recent data suggests that promoter hypermethylation of specific genes does not occur independently or randomly, but concurrently, which indicate that during the tumor progression progressive accumulation of epigenetic alterations could occur. High degree of methylation of multiple genes CpG island regions, associated with microsatellite instability and *hMLH1* gene hypermethylation, has been defined as a CpG island methylator phenotype (CIMP) in colorectal cancer, and is characterized by a poor outcome [111]. It has been suggested that a form of the CpG island methylator phenotype (CIMP) exists in other solid tumors, including *HNSCC* [112]. As opposed of CIMP positive colorectal cancers In oral cancer CIMP is characterized by less aggressive tumor biology [113],. The panel of tumor-related genes used to classify multiple methylation and CIMP differs substantially between studies [12, 112, 113], which could likely affect the results of association with clinical parameters and prognosis. Future extensive investigations are needed to establish a reliable set of reference cancer-related genes whose methylation status should be examined in the specific types of tumors. Further investigations are needed to better characterize the etiology of this methylation phenotype as well as to determine if this phenotype has important prognostic or clinical use.

### 3.3. DNA methylation in early detection of *HNSCC*

The detection of aberrant DNA hypermethylation emerged as a potential biomarker strategy for early detection of various carcinomas. Since DNA methylation is an early event in tumorigenesis of *HNSCC,* identification of methylation markers could provide great promise for early detection and treatment in *HNSCC* [68]. As opposed to advanced *HNSCC* diagnosis, early *HNSCC* detection increases survival to 80%. Therefore, early detection markers may potentially serve as a predictive tool for diagnosis and recurrence of *HNSCC.* However, even though such markers provide great promise for early detection, epigenetic biomarkers have not yet been clinically implemented [114, 115].

Routine oral visual screening could significantly reduce oral cavity mortality [116]. However, oral cavity screening will not identify cancers deep in the pharynx or larynx which requires special instrumentation and examination. In addition, screening of *HNSCC* should involve noninvasive detection of *OSCC* and *HNSCC,* such as detection in saliva and oral rinses, or minimally invasive detection, such as blood and serum analysis. Saliva presents an ideal means for *HNSCC* biomarker detection because of its proximity to the primary tumor site, availability of exfoliated cancer cells, and ease of sampling [117, 118].

Soluble CD44 promoter gene hypermethylation detected in saliva samples has been indicated as an early detection marker in *HNSCC* screening [119]. Recently, *NID2* and *HOXA9* promoter hypermethylation have been identified as biomarkers for prevention and early detection in oral carcinoma tissues and saliva [120]. Hypermethylation of multiple tumor-related genes (*RAR-β, DAPK, CDH1, p16* and *RASSF1A*) analyzed in combination could serve as a biomarker for early diagnosis of esophageal squamous cell carcinoma [57]. Moreover, these multiple tumor-related gene hypermethylation were associated with the increase of *DNMT3b* expression in early stages of esophageal cancer [57].

The development methylation-specific polymerase chain reaction (PCR) techniques has resulted in the identification of methylated genes specific to *HNSCC* detected in tumor samples [68], including *DAPK* [42], and *RASSF1A* [72].

Saliva and oral rinses could be ideal diagnostic and predictive biofluids for head and neck cancer since they samples cells from the entire lesion and the entire oral cavity. The detection of hypermethylated marker genes from oral rinse and saliva samples has a great potential for the noninvasive detection of *OSCC* and *HNSCC* [118, 68, 121, 122, 123, 124]. DNA hypermethylation of *p16, MGMT,* and *DAPK* in saliva showed aberrant methylation in 56% of samples from *HNSCC* patients, and only in one of the 30 control subjects [68]. The aberrant methylation of a combination of marker genes *E-cadherin,* transmembrane protein with epidermal growth factor-like and 2 follistatin-like domains 2 (*TMEFF2*), and *MGMT,* present in oral rinses was used to detect *OSCC* with >90% sensitivity and specificity [124].

Using the approach of gene selection according to previous studies on promoter methylation in *HNSCC* Carvalho et al. analyzed both saliva and serum in 211 *HNSCC* patients and 527 normal controls, and showed high specificity of promoter hypermethylation in *HNSCC* patients compared with normal subjects (>90%); however, the sensitivity of this panel was 31.4% [118]. In another study with different approaches, genome-wide methylation array analysis of 807 cancer-associated genes, was conducted on the matched preoperative saliva, postoperative saliva, and oral cancer tissue, and compared to saliva of normal subjects. Multiple potential diagnostic gene panels that consisted of 4 to 7 genes ranged in their sensitivity from 62% to 77% and in their specificity from 83% to 100% [123], significantly higher than previous studies of aberrant methylation detected in saliva in head and neck cancer patients [121, 122, 118]. Using this approach, new genes could be discovered that can be used as a reliable biomarker for the early detection of oral and head and neck cancer.

The *KIF1A* (Kinesin family member 1A) gene, that encodes a microtubule-dependent molecular motor protein involved in organelle transport and cell division, has recently been associated with aberrant DNA methylation in *HNSCC* [125]. *EDNRB* (Endothelin receptor type B) is a G protein coupled receptor, which activates a phosphatidylinositol calcium second messenger system, has previously been associated with nasopharyngeal carcinomas [126] and *HNSCC* [125]. Promoter hypermethylation of *KIF1A* and *EDNRB* is a frequent event in primary *HNSCC,* and these genes are preferentially methylated in salivary rinses from *HNSCC* patients. *KIF1A* (97.8% specificity and 36.6% sensitivity) and *EDNRB* (93.2% specificity and 67.6% sensitivity) are highly sensitive markers that could potentially be used as biomarkers for *HNSCC* detection. In addition, combining the markers improves sensitivity while maintains good specificity (93.1% specificity and 77.4% sensitivity) [125].

### 3.4. Predictive significance of DNA methylation

Epigenetic alterations such as DNA methylation could be a marker of response to radio and/or chemotherapy in the treatment of cancer. DNA methylation could play an important role in the regulation of gene expression for genes involved in cell cycle and apoptosis, thus affecting the chemosensitivity of cancers. Treatment of cancer cells with demethylating agent could lead to re-expression of gene involved in the activation of the apoptotic process and restore the sensitivity to the chemotherapy. Targeting the epigenetic mechanisms of apoptosis related genes inactivation may increase the efficacy of chemotherapy in various cancer types. Studies in vitro and in model systems certainly suggest that treatment with epigenetic agents can reverse drug resistance.

The best known example of DNA promoter hypermethylation and response to chemotherapy is *MGMT* promoter methylation in glioma patients treated with alkylating agents [127]. The expression of DNA repair gene *MGMT,* which removes alkyl groups added to guanine in DNA, is controlled by its promoter methylation. A cell that expresses a low amount of *MGMT* is known to be more sensitive to the antiproliferative effects of alkylating agents. It has been shown that hypermethylation of *MGMT* is the predictor of good response to temozolomide therapy in gliomas [128], to carmustine therapy in gliomas [127], and to cyclophosphamide therapy in diffuse B cell lymphoma [129]. Acquired hypermethylation of DNA mismatch repair gene *hMLH1* (detectable in peripheral blood) during carboplatinum/taxane therapy of ovarian cancer predicts poorer outcome [130]. In addition, *WRN* gene promoter hypermethylation was associated with hypersensitivity to topoisomerase inhibitor irinotecan in primary colon cancer [131].

It has been shown that DNA methylation could have the predictive significance in *OSCC* and *HNSCC.* Hypermethylation of *MGMT* was the predictor of good response to temozolomide therapy in oral squamous cell carcinoma [105]. GPx3 promoter hypermethylation was associated with tumorigenesis and chemotherapy response in *HNSCC* [132]. A correlation between methylation of mitotic checkpoint gene CHFR (checkpoint with ring finger) and sensitivity to microtubule inhibitors (docetaxel or paclitaxel) was observed in *OSCC* cells [133]. Downregulation of *SMG-1* (suppressor with morphogenetic effect on genitalia) due to promoter hypermethylation in HPV-Positive *HNSCC* resulted in increased radiation sensitivity and correlated with improved survival, whereas *SMG-1* overexpression protected HPV-positive tumor cells from irradiation [134]. DNA methylation could be a regulatory mechanism for chemosensitivity to 5-fluorouracil and cisplatin by zebularine, a novel DNA methyltransferase inhibitor, in oral squamous cell carcinomas [135]. It has been shown that zebularine suppresses the apoptotic potential of 5-fluorouracil via cAMP/PKA/CREB pathway in human oral carcinoma cells [136].

Radiotherapy is the standard adjuvant treatment for *OSCC* and the Ras/PI3K/AKT pathway plays an important role in *OSCC* radioresistance. A combination of *RASSF1A, RASSF2A,* and *HIN-1* methylation was found to be significantly associated with poor disease-free survival in patients treated with radiotherapy after surgery but not in patients treated with surgery alone [79].

*TGF-β* signaling has been found to be disrupted in *HNSCC* progression [137], thus this pathway has been targeted for therapy [138]. Downregulation of disabled homolog 2 (*DAB2*) gene expression via promoter DNA methylation frequently occurs in *HNSCC* and acts as an independent predictor of metastasis and poor prognosis [139]. Epigenetic downregulation of *DAB2* switches *TGF-β* from a tumor suppressor to a tumor promoter, suggest a way to stratify patients with advanced SCC who may benefit from anti-TGF-β therapies [139].

Although methylation of certain genes appears to influence the sensitivity to chemotherapeutic drugs, the majority of studies were performed on cell line models, or a small number of subjects. In addition, combination therapies of epigenetic agents and standard chemotherapy/radiotherapy have to be carefully investigated due to potential harmful effects in the clinical application of *DNMT* inhibitors. Epigenetic profile in predicting the chemosensitivity of individual cancers would contribute to personalized therapy [140]. Studies of pharmacoepigenomics will require large-scale analyses and genome-wide methylation analyses using microarrays and next-generation sequencers, necessary to confirm the usage of epigenetic changes in predicting responses to chemotherapeutic drugs.

### 3.5. Epigenetic therapy of *HNSCC*

Unlike mutations, epigenetic changes are reversible, which provides large possibilities of epigenetic therapy [141]. Demethylating agents that inhibit DNA methyltransferases *DNMTs*, could have a utility to effectively activate expression of previously epigenetically silenced genes. 5-azanucleosides, nucleoside analogs that inhibit *DNMTs*, with consequent hypomethylation of DNA, have long been known to have DNA demethylating activities, but are too toxic for clinical use [141]. However, recent studies have shown that therapeutic efficacy could be achieved at low drug doses [142 -4]. 5-Azacytidine, a cytosine analog treatment has been tested in multiple cancer cell lines and are shown to reexpress methylated genes in myelodysplastic syndromes (MDS) [142, 143]. Low doses were used in a large trial in patients with MDS, and showed an increase in the time of conversion of MDS to leukemia, and increased overall survival [144].

5-Azacytidine application resulted in partial demethylation of the *MGMT* and *RASSF1A* tumor suppressor genes and reduced proliferation of the tumor cells suggesting further investigation of 5-azacytidine for *HNSCC* treatment [145]. Methylation status and expression of *HIC1*, a potential tumor suppressor gene, was restored after demethylation treatment of *HNSCC* cell lines with 5-azacytidine [146].

Epigenetic therapy in monotherapy could reactivate tumor suppressor genes or in combination therapy may enhance the anti-proliferative effect of standard chemotherapy, such as cisplatin, 5-fluorouracil, etc. The low dose of a novel DNA methyltransferase inhibitor, zebularine may sensitize oral cancer cells to cisplatin, an important characteristic of solid cancer treatment. DNA methylation could be a regulatory mechanism for dihydropyrimidine dehydrogenase (*DPD),* known to be a principal factor in 5-fluorouracil (5-FU) resistance and that DPD activated by zebularine in *OSCC* could be an inhibiting factor in the response to apoptosis induced by 5-FU [135].

The epidermal growth factor receptor (*EGFR*) has been extensively investigated and validated as a therapeutic target in lung, colorectal, pancreatic, and head and neck cancers. However, patients with wild type *EGFR* obtain little sustained benefit from anti-*EGFR* monotherapy Broad restoration of tumor suppressor function by demethylation could enhance the anti-proliferative and pro-apoptotic effect of *EGFR* blockade in solid malignancy. Re-expression of *p15, p21,* or *p27,* cell cycle inhibitors downstream of *EGFR,* or *PTEN,* a PI3K/Akt inhibitory protein, may have particular synergy with anti-*EGFR* therapy. Recent phase I study evaluated the combination of anti-*EGFR* erlotinib and 5-azacytidine in solid carcinomas showed the beneficial clinical effect in lung and head and neck cancers [147]. Efficacy of erlotinib could be enhanced by concurrent hypomethylating therapy with 5-azacytidine, secondary to re-expression of tumor suppressors interacting with the *EGFR* signaling cascade. In recent study of resistance to anti-*EGFR* therapy agents, promoter methylation of commonly methylated genes was investigated in two parental non-small cell lung cancer (*NSCLC*) and *HNSCC* cell lines and their resistant derivatives to either erlotinib or cetuximab [148]. It was found that *DAPK* gene promoter was hypermethylated in drug-resistant derivatives generated from both parental cell lines. Restoration of *DAPK* into the resistant *NSCLC* cells by stable transfection re-sensitized the cells to both erlotinib and cetuximab [148], thus indicating that *DAPK* promoter methylation could be a potential biomarker of drug response.

These results demonstrate that DNA methylation could play an important role in both chemotherapy and radiotherapy resistance, and that gene silencing through promoter methylation is one of the key mechanisms of developed resistance to anti-*EGFR* therapeutic agents. Epigenetic therapy could be a novel treatment to overcome chemo- and/or radiotherapy resistance and to improve the benefits of current therapies.

### 3.6. DNA methylation in *HNSCC* and etiological factors

Epidemiological studies have reported the association of DNA methylation status in *HNSCC* with exposure to environmental factors, including tobacco smoke, alcohol intake, genotoxic betel quid consumption, HPV infection, diet and environmental pollutants.

Recent studies have shown a correlation between tobacco and/or alcohol use and hypermethylation of tumor related genes. DNA global hypomethylation was associated with alcohol consumption [149]. *p16* methylation has been correlated with alcohol use and smoking [72]. Promoter methylation of *p16* was previously correlated with alcohol intake [150], while *RASSF1A* methylation was associated with tobacco use in *HNSCC* [72]. Smoking and drinking was associated with *p15* promoter methylation in the upper aerodigestive tract of healthy individuals and *HNSCC* patients [151]. Promoter methylation of *SFRP1* occurred more often in both heavy and light drinkers compared to nondrinkers in head and neck squamous cell carcinoma [152]. Significant association of tumor-associated genes hypermethylation with alcohol use was observed in *HNSCC* [153].

Recent studies are indicating that increased fruit and vegetable consumption are associated with reduced head and neck cancer risk [28]. There is a growing body of evidence that bioactive food components, such as isothiocyanates from cruciferous vegetables (cauliflower, cabbage, and broccoli), diallyl sulfide, an organosulphur compound from garlic, isoflavone, phytosterole, folate, selenium, vitamin E, flavonoids might reduce cancer risk through epigenetic mechanisms. The chemoprevention of cancer by natural compounds could be a promising approach with less side effects and toxicity. Main polyphenols with the properties of *DNMT* inhibition are tea polyphenols, soy isoflavones, organosulphur compounds from garlic, and isothiocyanates from cruciferous vegetables. Dietary folate intake was associated with *p16* promoter methylation in head and neck squamous cell carcinoma [154]. Epigallocatechin-3-gallate (*EGCG*), the major polyphenol in green tea, is believed to be a key active ingredient with anti-cancer properties. *EGCG* is methylated by catechol-O-methyltransferase and inhibits DNA methyltransferase (*DNMT*), thus reversing the hypermethylation and inducing the re-expression of the silenced genes [141].

*EGCG* has been reported to reverse hypermethylation and reactivate several tumor suppressor genes in human esophageal squamous cell carcinoma cell lines [155]. The reversion-inducing cysteine-rich protein with Kazal motifs (*RECK*), a novel matrix metalloproteinases (*MMP*) inhibitor, is involved in the inhibition of tumor angiogenesis, invasion, and metastasis. *EGCG* treatment enhanced *RECK* expression by reversal of hypermethylation of *RECK* promoter and inhibiting *MMP* activities and invasion in *OSCC* cell lines [156]. Genistein, soy dietary isoflavone, reversed DNA hypermethylation and reactivated *RARβ*, *p16*, and *MGMT* in esophageal cancer cells [157]. However, the findings of association of diet and epigenetic modifications in the head and cancer and other carcinomas are still confounding.

## 4. Conclusions

Head and neck squamous cell carcinoma (*HNSCC*) is one of the most common and highly aggressive malignancies worldwide, despite the significant efforts committed in the last decades in its detection, prevention and treatment. Therefore, early detection and better disease prediction via genetic and epigenetic biomarkers is crucial. However, very few reliable markers are currently known. Recent studies provide strong evidence that DNA methylation could have an important role in head and neck cancer. The detection of promoter methylation status may be a useful molecular marker for early detection of *HNSCC* from tissue, saliva, and serum samples and in real time analysis of margins during surgery. In addition, the creation of methylation gene panels could be useful for *HNSCC* screening in the timely inclusion of treatment and thorough surveillance during follow-up period. Unlike genetic changes, epigenetic modifications are heritable and potentially reversible, thus providing the potential for therapy. Frequent DNA methylation detected in *HNSCC* and association with tumor progression and survival indicates that DNA methylation plays an important role in head and neck carcinogenesis and may be a useful diagnostic marker and a potential therapeutic target for *HNSCC*.

## Author details

Zvonko Magić[1,2*], Gordana Supić[1,2], Mirjana Branković-Magić[3] and Nebojša Jović[4,2]

*Address all correspondence to: zvonkomag@yahoo.co.uk

1 Institute for Medical Research, Military Medical Academy, Belgrade, Serbia

2 Faculty of Medicine, Military Medical Academy, University of Defense, Belgrade, Serbia

3 Institute for Oncology and Radiology of Serbia, Belgrade, Serbia

4 Clinic for Maxillofacial Surgery, Military Medical Academy, Belgrade, Serbia

## References

[1] Jemal, A., Siegel, R., Ward, E., Murray, T., Xu, J., & Thun, M. J. (2007). Cancer statistics. *CA Cancer J Clin.*, 57(1).

[2] Perez-Ordonez, B., Beauchemin, M., & Jordan, R. (2006). Molecular biology of squamous cell carcinoma of the head and neck. *J. Clin Pathol*, 57, 445-453.

[3] Williams, H.K. (2000). Molecular pathogenesis of oral squamous carcinoma. *Mol Pathol.*, 53(4), 165-72.

[4] Forastiere, A., Koch, W., Trotti, A., & Sidransky, D. (2001). Head and neck cancer. *N Engl J Med.*, 345(26), 1890-900.

[5] Ragin, C. C., & Taioli, E. (2007). Survival of squamous cell carcinoma of the head and neck in relation to human papillomavirus infection: review and meta-analysis. *Int J Cancer.*, 121, 1813-1820.

[6] Pelucchi, C., Talamini, R., Negri, E., et al. (2003). Folate intake and risk of oral and pharyngeal cancer. *Ann Oncol.*, 14, 1677-1681.

[7] Pöschl, G., & Seitz, H. K. (2004). Alcohol and cancer. *Alcohol Alcohol.*, 39(3), 155-65.

[8] Gillison, M. L., Koch, W. M., Capone, R. B., Spafford, M., Westra, W. H., Wu, L., et al. (2000). Evidence for a causal association between human papillomavirus and a subset of head and neck cancers. *J Natl Cancer Inst.*, 92, 709-720.

[9] Doll, R. (1998). Uncovering the risks of smoking: historical perspective. *Stat. Meth. Med Res.*, 7, 87-11.

[10] Zhang, Z. J., Hao, K., Shi, R., Zhao, G., Jiang, G. X., Song, Y., Xu, X., & Ma, J. (2011). Glutathione S-transferase M1 (GSTM1) and glutathione S-transferase T1 (GSTT1) null polymorphisms, smoking, and their interaction in oral cancer: a HuGE review and meta-analysis. *Am J Epidemiol.*, 173(8), 847-57.

[11] Solomon, P., Selvam, G., & Shanmugam, G. (2008). Polymorphism in ADH and MTHFR genes in oral squamous cell carcinoma of Indians. *Oral Diseases.*, 14, 633-639.

[12] Supic, G., Jovic, N., Kozomara, R., Zeljic, K., & Magic, Z. (2011). Interaction between the MTHFR C677T polymorphism and alcohol--impact on oral cancer risk and multiple DNA methylation of tumor-related genes. *J Dent Res.*, 90, 65-70.

[13] Seitz, H. K., & Stickel, F. (2007). Molecular mechanisms of alcohol-mediated carcinogenesis. *Nat Rev Cancer*, 7(8), 599-612.

[14] Brennan, A., Boyle, J. O., & Koch, W. M. (1995). Association between cigarette smoking and mutation of the 53 gene in squamous cell carcinoma of the head and neck. *N Engl J Med.*, 332, 712-17.

[15] Visapaa, J. P., Gotte, K., Benesova, M., et al. (2004). Increased cancer risk in heavy drinkers with the alcohol dehydrogenase 1C*1 allele, possibly due to salivary acetaldehyde. *Gut.*, 53, 871-6.

[16] Brocic, M., Supic, G., Zeljic, K., Jovic, N., Kozomara, R., Zagorac, S., Zlatkovic, M., & Magic, Z. (2011). Genetic polymorphisms of ADH1C and CYP2E1 and risk of oral squamous cell carcinoma. *Otolaryngol Head Neck Surg.*, 145(4), 586-93.

[17] Schwartz, S., Doody, D., Fitzgibbons, E., Ricks, S., Porter, P., & Chen, C. (2001). Oral squamous cell cancer risk in relation to alcohol consumption and alcohol dehydrogenase-3 genotypes. *Cancer Epidemiol Biomarkers Prev.*, 10, 1137-44.

[18] Peters, E., Mc Clean, M., Liu, M., Eisen, E., Mueller, N., & Kelsey, K. T. (2005). The ADH1C polymorphism modifies the risk of squamous cell carcinoma of the head and neck associated with alcohol and tobacco use. *Cancer Epidemiol Biomarkers Prev.*, 14, 476-82.

[19] Klussmann, J. P., Weissenborn, S., & Fuchs, P. G. (2001). Human papillomavirus infection as a risk factor for squamous-cell carcinoma of the head and neck. *N Engl J Med.*, 345, 376-81.

[20] Termine, N., Panzarella, V., Falaschini, S., Russo, A., Matranga, D., Lo, Muzio. I., & Campisi, G. (2008). HPV in oral squamous cell carcinoma vs Head and Neck squamous cell carcinoma biopsies: a meta-analysis (1998-2007). *Ann Oncol.*, 19, 1681-1690.

[21] Dahlgren, L., Dahlstrand, H. M., Linquist, D., Hogmo, A., Bjornestal, L., Lindholm, J., Lundberg, B., Dalianis, T., & Munck-Wikland, E. (2004). Human papillomavirus is more common in base of tongue than in mobile tongue and is a favorable prognostic factor in base of tongue cancer patients. *Int J Cancer.*, 112, 1015-1019.

[22] Mellin, H., Friesland, S., Lewensohn, R., Dalianis, T., & Munck Wikland, E. (2000). Human papillomavirus (HPV) DNA in tonsillar cancer: clinical correlates, risk of relapse, and survival. *Int J Cancer.*, 89, 300-304.

[23] Kozomara, R., Jovic, N., Magic, Z., Brankovic-Magic, M., & Minic, V. (2005). Mutations and human papillomavirus infection in oral squamous cell carcinomas: correlation with overall survival. J Cranio-Maxillofacial Surg. ., 33, 342-348.

[24] Kozomara, R. J., Brankovic-Magic, M. V., Jovic, N. R., Stosic, S. M., & Magic, Z. M. (2007). Prognostic significance of TP53 mutations in oral squamous cell carcinoma with human papilloma infection. *Int J Biol Markers.*, 22, 252-257.

[25] Kabeya, M., Furuta, R., Kawabata, K., Takahashi, S., & Ishikawa, Y. (2012). Prevalence of human papillomavirus in mobile tongue cancer with particular reference to young patients. *Cancer Sci.*, 103, 161-168.

[26] Bekkering, T., Beynon, R., Davey, Smith. G., Davies, A., Harbord, R., Sterne, J., Thomas, S., & Wood, L. (2006). A systematic review of RCTs investigating the effect of dietal and physical activity interventions on cancer survival, updated report. *World Cancer Research Fund.*, http://www.dietandcancerreport.org/, (accessed 15 January 2012).

[27] Djuric, Z. (2011). The Mediterranean diet: Effects on proteins that mediate fatty acid metabolism in the colon. *Nutr Rev.*, 69(12), 730-744.

[28] Freedman, N., Park, Y., Subar, A., Hollenbeck, A., Leitzmann, M., Schatzkin, A., et al. (2008). Fruit and vegetable intake and head and neck cancer risk in a large United States prospective cohort study. *Int J Cancer.*, 122, 2330-6.

[29] Magić, Z. (1999). Apoptosis and cancer. Ed. In: Antypas G, editor. 2nd Balkan Congress of Oncology. *Kushadasi October 1998, Turkey. Bologna: Monduzzi Ed.*, 343-348.

[30] Magic, Z., Radulovic, S., & Brankovic Magic, M. (2007). cDNA microarrays: identification of gene signatures and their application in clinical practice. *J BUON. 12(Suppl 1)*, S39-S44.

[31] Kandolf-Sekulović, L., Cikota, B., Jović, M., Skiljević, D., Stojadinović, O., Medenica, Lj., & Magić, Z. (2009). The role of apoptosis and cell-proliferation regulating genes in mycosis fungoides. *J Dermatol Sci.*, 55, 53-56.

[32] Cikota, B., Tukić, Lj., Tarabar, O., & Magić, Z. (2007). p53 and ras gene mutations and quantification of residual disease in patients with B-cell non-hodgkin's lymphoma. *J Exp Clin Cancer Res*, 26(4), 515-522.

[33] Branković-Magić, M., Janković, R., Dobričić, J., Borojević, N., Magić, Z., & Radulović, S. (2008). TP53 mutations in breast cancer: association with ductal histology and early relapse of disease. *Int J Biol Markers.*, 23, 147-153.

[34] Hiyama, T., Yoshihara, M., Tanaka, S., & Chayama, K. (2008). Genetic polymorphisms and head and neck cancer risk (Review). *Int J Oncol.*, 32, 945-73.

[35] Zeljic, K., Supic, G., Stamenkovic, Radak. M., Jovic, N., Kozomara, R., & Magic, Z. (2012). Vitamin D receptor, CYP27B1 and CYP24A1 genes polymorphisms association with oral cancer risk and survival. *J Oral Pathol Med.*, doi: j.16000714x.

[36] Supic, G., Jovic, N., Zeljic, K., Kozomara, R., & Magic, Z. (2012). Association of VEGF-A Genetic Polymorphisms with Cancer Risk and Survival in Advanced-Stage Oral Squamous Cell Carcinoma Patients. *Oral Onc.*, http://dx.doi.org/10.1016/j.oraloncology.2012.05.023.

[37] El -Nagger, A. K., Hurr, K., Batsakis, J. G., et al. (1995). Sequential loss of heterozygosity at microsatellite motifs in preinvasive and invasive head and neck squamous carcinoma. *Cancer Res.*, 55, 2656-9.

[38] Califano, J., van der , R. P., Westra, W., Nawroz, H., Clayman, G., Piantadosi, S., Corio, R., Lee, D., Greenberg, B., Koch, W., & Sidransky, D. (1996). Genetic progression model for head and neck cancer: implications for field cancerization. *Cancer Res.*, 56, 2488-2492.

[39] Hu, N., Wang, C., Hu, Y., Yang, H., Kong, L., Lu, N., et al. (2006). Genome-wide loss of heterozygosity and copy number alteration in esophageal squamous cell carcinoma using the Affymetrix GeneChip Mapping 10 K array. *BMC Genomics*, 7(299).

[40] Partridge, M., Emilion, G., Pateromichelakis, S., et al. (1999). Location of candidate tumour suppressor gene loci at chromosomes 38p and 9p for oral squamous carcinomas. *Int J Cancer*, 84, 318-25.

[41] Sartor, M., Steingrimsdottir, H., Elamin, F., Gaken, J., Warnakulasuriya, S., Patridge, M., et al. (1999). Role of 16 MTS1, cyclin D1 and RB in primary oral cancer and oral cancer cell lines. *Br. J Cancer*, 80, 79-86.

[42] Sanchez-Cespedes, M., Esteller, M., Wu, L., Nawroz-Danish, H., Yoo, G. H., Koch, W. M., Jen, J., Herman, J. G., & Sidransky, D. (2000). Gene promoter hypermethylation in tumors and serum of head and neck cancer patients. *Cancer Res.*, 60, 892-895.

[43] Ha, P. K., & Califano, J. A. (2006). Promoter methylation and inactivation of tumour-suppressor genes in oral squamous-cell carcinoma. *Lancet Oncol.*, 7, 77-82.

[44] Supic, G., Kozomara, R., Brankovic-Magic, M., Jovic, N., & Magic, Z. (2009). Gene hypermethylation in tumor tissue of advanced oral squamous cell carcinoma patients. *Oral Oncol.*, 45, 1051-7.

[45] Hogg, R. P., Honorio, S., Martinez, A., et al. (2002). Frequent 3p allele loss and epigenetic inactivation of the RASSF1A tumour suppressor gene from region 321 in head and neck squamous cell carcinoma. *Eur J Cancer*, 38, 1585-92.

[46] Ambatipudi, S., Gerstung, M., Gowda, R., Pai, P., Borges, A. M., et al. (2011). Genomic Profiling of Advanced-Stage Oral Cancers Reveals Chromosome 11q Alterations as Markers of Poor Clinical Outcome. *PLoS ONE*, 6(2), e17250.

[47] Kim, M. M., & Califano, J. A. (2004). Molecular pathology of head-and neck cancer. *Int J Cancer*, 112, 545-553.

[48] Langdon, J. D., & Partidge, M. (1992). Expression of the tumour suppressor gene 53 in oral cancer. *Br J Oral Maxillofac Surg.*, 30, 214-20.

[49] Brachman, D. G., Graves, D., Vokes, E., Beckett, M., Haraf, D., Montag, A., et al. (1992). Occurrence of 53 gene deletions and human papilloma virus infection in human head and neck cancer. *Cancer Res.*, 52, 4832, 4836.

[50] Tandon, S., Tudur-Smith, C., Riley, R. D., Boyd, M. T., & Jones, T. M. (2010). A systematic review of 53 as a prognostic factor of survival in squamous cell carcinoma of the four main anatomical subsites of the head and neck. *Cancer Epidemiol Biomarkers Prev.*, 19, 574-587.

[51] Perrone, F., Bossi, P., Cortelazzi, B., et al. (2010). TP53 mutations and pathologic complete response to neoadjuvant cisplatin and fluorouracil chemotherapy in resected oral cavity squamous cell carcinoma. *J Clin Oncol.*, 28, 761-766.

[52] Mroz, E. A., & Rocco, J. W. (2010). Functional 53 status as a biomarker for chemotherapy response in oral-cavity cancer. *J Clin Oncol.*, 28, 715-717.

[53] Grandis, J. R., & Tweardy, D. J. (1993). Elevated levels of transforming growth factor alpha and epidermal growth factor receptor messenger R.N.A. are early markers of carcinogenesis in head and neck cancer. *Cancer Res.*, 53, 3579-3584.

[54] Scully, C. (1993). Oncogenes, tumor suppressors and viruses in oral squamous carcinoma. *J Oral Pathol Med.*, 22, 337-347.

[55] Shaw, R. (2006). The epigenetics of oral cancer. *Int J Oral Maxillofac Surg.*, 35, 101-108.

[56] Herman, J. G., & Baylin, S. B. (2003). Gene silencing in cancer in association with promoter hypermethylation. *N Eng. J Med.*, 349, 2042-2054.

[57] Li, B., Wang, B., Niu, L. J., Jiang, L., & Qiu, C. C. (2011). Hypermethylation of multiple tumor-related genes associated with D.N.M.T.3b up-regulation served as a biomarker for early diagnosis of esophageal squamous cell carcinoma. *Epigenetics*, 6(3), 307-16.

[58] Kulkarni, V., & Saranath, D. (2004). Concurrent hypermethylation of multiple regulatory genes in chewing tobacco associated oral squamous cell carcinomas and adjacent normal tissues. *Oral Oncol.*, 40, 145-153.

[59] Maruya, S., et al. (2004). Differential methylation status of tumor-associated genes in head and neck squamous carcinoma: incidence and potential implications. *Clin Cancer Res.*, 10, 3825-3830.

[60] Lopez, M., Aguirre, J. M., Cuevas, N., Anzola, M., Videgain, J., Aguirregaviria, J., & Martinez, D. P. (2003). Gene promoter hypermethylation in oral rinses of leukoplakia patients-a diagnostic and/or prognostic tool? *Eur J. Cancer*, 39, 2306-2309.

[61] Supic, G., Kozomara, R., Jovic, N., Zeljic, K., & Magic, Z. (2011). Prognostic significance of tumor-related genes hypermethylation detected in cancer-free surgical margins of oral squamous cell carcinomas. *Oral Oncol.*, 47(8), 702-8.

[62] Supic, G., Kozomara, R., Jovic, N., Zeljic, K., & Magic, Z. (2011). Hypermethylation of RUNX3 but not WIF1 gene and its association with stage and nodal status of tongue cancers. *Oral Dis.*, 17(8), 794-800.

[63] Yoshino, M., Suzuki, M., Tian, L., Moriya, Y., Hoshino, H., Okamoto, T., Yoshida, S., Shibuya, K., & Yoshino, I. (2009). Promoter hypermethylation of the 16 and Wif-1 genes as an independent prognostic marker in stage IA non-small cell lung cancers. *Int J Oncol.*, 35(5), 1201-9.

[64] Yanagawa, N., Tamura, G., Oizumi, H., Kanauchi, N., Endoh, M., Sadahiro, M., & Motoyama, T. (2007). Promoter hypermethylation of RASSF1A and RUNX3 genes as an independent prognostic prediction marker in surgically resected non-small cell lung cancers. *Lung Cancer.*, 58(1), 131-8.

[65] Inbal, B., Cohen, O., Polak-Charcon, S., Kopolovic, J., Vadai, E., Eisenbach, L., & Kimchi, A. (1997). DAP kinase links the control of apoptosis to metastasis. *Nature*, 390, 180-184.

[66] Graziano, F., Arduini, F., Ruzzo, A., Bearzi, I., Humar, B., More, H., et al. (2004). Prognostic analysis of E-cadherin gene promoter hypermethylation in patients with surgically resected, node-positive, diffuse gastric cancer. *Clin Cancer Res.*, 10, 2784-2789.

[67] Nakata, S., Sugio, K., Uramoto, H., Oyama, T., Hanagiri, T., Morita, M., & Yasumoto, K. (2006). The methylation status and protein expression of CDH1, p16 (INK4A), and fragile histidine triad in nonsmall cell lung carcinoma: epigenetic silencing, clinical features, and prognostic significance. *Cancer*, 106, 2190-2199.

[68] Rosas, S. L., Koch, W., Costa, Carvalho. M. G., Wu, L., Califano, J., Westra, W., Jen, J., & Sidransky, D. (2001). Promoter hypermethylation patterns of p16 O-6-methylguanine-DNA-methyltransferase, and death-associated protein kinase in tumors and saliva of head and neck cancer patients. *Cancer Res.*, 61, 939-942.

[69] Auerkari, E.I. (2006). Methylation of tumor suppressor genes p16 (INK4a), p27(Kip1) and E-cadherin in carcinogenesis. *Oral Oncol.*, 42, 5-13.

[70] Reed, A. L., Califano, J., Cairns, P., et al. (1996). High frequency of 16 (CDKN2/MTS-1/INK4A) inactivation in head and neck squamous cell carcinoma. *Cancer Res.*, 56, 3630-3.

[71] Cao, J., Zhou, J., Gao, Y., Gu, L., Meng, H., Liu, H., & Deng, D. (2009). Methylation of 16 CpG Island Associated with Malignant Progression of Oral Epithelial Dysplasia: A Prospective Cohort Study. *Clin Cancer Res.*, 15(16), 5178-83.

[72] Hasegawa, M. (2002). Nelson, H.H., Peters, E., Ringstrom, E., Posner, M., and Kelsey, K.T. Patterns of gene promoter methylation in squamous cell cancer of the head and neck. *Oncogene*, 21, 4231-4236.

[73] Steinmann, K., Sandner, A., Schagdarsurengin, U., & Dammann, R. H. (2009). Frequent promoter hypermethylation of tumor-related genes in head and neck squamous cell carcinoma. *Oncol Rep.*, 22(6), 1519-26.

[74] Koscielny, S., Dahse, R., Ernst, G., & von, Eggeling. F. (2007). The prognostic relevance of 16 inactivation in head and neck cancer. *ORL J Otorhinolaryngol Relat Spec.*, 69(1), 30-6.

[75] Sailasree, R., Abhilash, A., Sathyan, K., Nalinakumari, K., Thomas, S., & Kannan, S. (2008). Differential Roles of p16 INK4Aand p14ARF Genes in Prognosis of Oral Carcinoma. *Cancer Epidemiol Biomarkers Prev.*, 17(2), 414-20.

[76] Ishida, E., Nakamura, M., Shimada, K., Higuchi, T., Takatsu, K., Yane, K., & Konishi, N. (2007). DNA hypermethylation status of multiple genes in papillary thyroid carcinomas. *Pathobiology*, 74(6), 344-52.

[77] Dominguez, G., Silva, J., Garcia, J. M., et al. (2003). Prevalence of aberrant methylation of p14 ARFover p16INK4a in some human primary tumors. *Mutat Res.*, 530, 9-17.

[78] Fendri, A., Masmoudi, A., Khabir, A., Sellami-Boudawara, T., Daoud, J., Frikha, M., Ghorbel, A., Gargouri, A., & Mokdad-Gargouri, R. (2009). Inactivation of RASSF1A, RARbeta2 and DAP-kinase by promoter methylation correlates with lymph node metastasis in nasopharyngeal carcinoma. *Cancer Biol Ther.*, 8(5), 444-51.

[79] Huang, K. H., Huang, S. F., Chen, I. H., Liao, C. T., Wang, H. M., & Hsieh, L. L. (2009). Methylation of RASSF1A, RASSF2A, and HIN-1 is associated with poor outcome after radiotherapy, but not surgery, in oral squamous cell carcinoma. *Clin Cancer Res.*, 15(12), 4174-80.

[80] Kudo, Y., Kitajima, S., Ogawa, I., Hiraoka, M., Sargolzaei, S., Keikhaee, M. R., et al. (2004). Invasion and metastasis of oral cancer cells require methylation of E-cadherin and/or degradation of membranous beta-catenin. *Clin Cancer Res.*, 10, 5455-5463.

[81] Chang, H. W., Chow, V., Lam, K. Y., Wei, W. I., & Yuen, A. (2002). Loss of E-cadherin expression resulting from promoter hypermethylation in oral tongue carcinoma and its prognostic significance. *Cancer*, 94, 386-392.

[82] De Moraes, R. V., Oliveira, D. T., Landman, G., de Carvalho, F., Caballero, O., Nonogaki, S., et al. (2008). E-cadherin Abnormalities Resulting From CpG Methylation Promoter In Metastatic And Nonmetastatic Oral Cancer. *Head Neck*, 30, 85-92.

[83] Saito, Y., Takazawa, H., Uzawa, K., Tanzawa, H., & Sato, K. (1998). Reduced expression of Ecadherin in oral squamous cell carcinoma: relationship with DNA methylation of 5'CpG island. *Int J Oncol.*, 12, 293-298.

[84] Foschini, M. P., et al. (2008). E-cadherin Loss and DNP73l expression in oral squamous cell carcinomas showing aggressive behavior. *Head Neck.*, 30, 1475-1482.

[85] Kurtz, K. A., Hoffman, H. T., Zimmerman, M. B., & Robinson, R. A. (2006). Decreased E-cadherin but not beta-catenin expression is associated with vascular inva-

sion and decreased survival in head and neck squamous carcinomas. *Otolaryngol Head Neck Surg.*, 134, 142-146.

[86] Niemhom, S., Kitazawa, S., Kitazawa, R., Maeda, S., & Leopairat, J. (2008). Hypermethylation of epithelial-cadherin gene promoter is associated with Epstein-Barr virus in nasopharyngeal carcinoma. *Cancer Detect Prev.*, 32(2), 127-34.

[87] Ayadi, W., Karray-Hakim, H., Khabir, A., Feki, L., Charfi, S., Boudawara, T., Ghorbel, A., Daoud, J., Frikha, M., Busson, P., & Hammami, A. (2008). Aberrant methylation of p16 DLEC1, BLU and E-cadherin gene promoters in nasopharyngeal carcinoma biopsies from Tunisian patients. *Anticancer Res.*, 28(4B), 2161-7.

[88] Ling, Z. Q., Li, P., Ge, M. H., Zhao, X., Hu, F. J., Fang, X. H., Dong, Z. M., & Mao, W. M. (2011). Hypermethylation-modulated down-regulation of CDH1 expression contributes to the progression of esophageal cancer. *Int J Mol Med.*, 27(5), 625-35.

[89] Zhang, C. Y., Mao, L., Li, L., Tian, Z., Zhou, X. J., Zhang, Z. Y., & Li, J. (2007). Promoter methylation as a common mechanism for inactivating E-cadherin in human salivary gland adenoid cystic carcinoma. *Cancer*, 110(1), 87-95.

[90] Marsit, C. J., Posner, M. R., Mc Clean, M. D., & Kelsey, K. T. (2008). Hypermethylation of E-cadherin Is an Independent Predictor of Improved Survival in Head and Neck Squamous Cell Carcinoma. *Cancer*, 113, 1566-71.

[91] De Schutter, H., Geeraerts, H., Verbeken, E., & Nuyts, S. (2009). Promoter methylation of TIMP3 and CDH1 predicts better outcome in head and neck squamous cell carcinoma treated by radiotherapy only. *Oncol Rep.*, 21, 507-513.

[92] Esteller, M., et al. (2000). Analysis of Adenomatous Polyposis Coli Promoter Hypermethylation in Human. *Cancer Canc Res.*, 60, 4366-4371.

[93] Chen, K. (2007). Sawhney, R., Khan, M., Benninger, M.S., Hou, Z., Sethi, S., et al. Methylation of multiple genes as diagnostic and therapeutic markers in primary head and neck squamous cell carcinoma. *Arch Otolaryngol Head Neck Surg.*, 133, 1131-1138.

[94] Brock, M. V., Gou, M., Akiyama, Y., Muller, A., Wu, T. T., Montgomery, E., Deasel, M., Germonpré, P., Rubinson, L., Heitmiller, R. F., Yang, S. C., Forastiere, A. A., Baylin, S. B., & Herman, J. G. (2003). Prognostic importance of promoter hypermethylation of multiple genes in esophageal adenocarcinoma. *Clin Cancer Res.*, 9(8), 2912-9.

[95] Zare, M., Jazii, F., Alivand, M., Nasseri, N., Malekzadeh, R., & Yazdanbod, M. (2009). Qualitative analysis of Adenomatous Polyposis Coli promoter: Hypermethylation, engagement and effects on survival of patients with esophageal cancer in a high risk region of the world, a potential molecular marker. *BMC Cancer.*, 9, 24-35.

[96] Kim, Y. T., Park, J. Y., Jeon, Y. K., Park, S. J., Song, J. Y., Kang, C. H., Sung, S. W., & Kim, J. H. (2009). Aberrant promoter CpG island hypermethylation of the adenomatosis polyposis coli gene can serve as a good prognostic factor by affecting lymph

node metastasis in squamous cell carcinoma of the esophagus. *Dis Esophagus.*, 22(2), 143-50.

[97] Pannone, G., Bufo, P., Santoro, A., Franco, R., Aquino, G., Longo, F., Botti, G., Serpico, R., Cafarelli, B., Abbruzzese, A., Caraglia, M., Papagerakis, S., & Lo Muzio, L. (2010). WNT pathway in oral cancer: epigenetic inactivation of WNT-inhibitors. *Oncol Rep.*, 24(4), 1035-41.

[98] Sogabe, Y., Suzuki, H., Toyota, M., Ogi, K., Imai, T., Nojima, M., Sasaki, Y., Hiratsuka, H., & Tokino, T. (2008). Epigenetic inactivation of SFRP genes in oral squamous cell carcinoma. *Int J Oncol.*, 32(6), 1253-61.

[99] Liu, J. B., Qiang, F. L., Dong, J., Cai, J., Zhou, S. H., Shi, M. X., Chen, K. P., & Hu, Z. B. (2011). Plasma DNA methylation of Wnt antagonists predicts recurrence of esophageal squamous cell carcinoma. *World J Gastroenterol.*, 28; 17(44), 4917-21.

[100] Tsunematsu, T., Kudo, Y., Iizuka, S., Ogawa, I., Fujita, T., Kurihara, H., et al. (2009). RUNX3 has an oncogenic role in head and neck cancer. *PLoS ONE.*, 4, 1-12.

[101] Gao, F., Huang, C., Lin, M., et al. (2009). Frequent inactivation of RUNX3 by promoter hypermethylation and protein mislocalization in oral squamous cell carcinomas. *J Cancer Res Clin Oncol.*, 135, 739-747.

[102] Fendri, A., Khabir, A., Hadri-Guiga, B., Sellami-Boudawara, T., Daoud, J., Frikha, M., Ghorbel, A., Gargouri, A., & Mokdad-Gargouri, R. (2010). Epigenetic alteration of the Wnt inhibitory factor-1 promoter is common and occurs in advanced stage of Tunisian nasopharyngeal carcinoma. *Cancer Invest.*, 28(9), 896-903.

[103] Paluszczak, J., Misiak, P., Wierzbicka, M., Woźniak, A., & Baer-Dubowska, W. (2011). Frequent hypermethylation of DAPK, RARbeta, MGMT, RASSF1A and FHIT in laryngeal squamous cell carcinomas and adjacent normal mucosa. *Oral Oncol.*, 47(2), 104-7.

[104] Taioli, E., Ragin, C., Wang, X. H., Chen, J., Langevin, S. M., Brown, A. R., Gollin, S. M., Garte, S., & Sobol, R. W. (2009). Recurrence in oral and pharyngeal cancer is associated with quantitative MGMT promoter methylation. *BMC Cancer*, 9, 354.

[105] Zuo, C., Ai, L., Ratliff, P., Suen, J. Y., Hanna, E., Brent, T. P., & Fan, C. Y. (2004). O6-methylguanine-DNA methyltransferase gene: epigenetic silencing and prognostic value in head and neck squamous cell carcinoma. *Cancer Epidemiol Biomarkers Prev.*, 13(6), 967-75.

[106] González-Ramírez, I., Ramírez-Amador, V., Irigoyen-Camacho, M. E., Sánchez-Pérez, Y., Anaya-Saavedra, G., Granados-García, M., García-Vázquez, F., & García-Cuellar, C. M. (2011). hMLH1 promoter methylation is an early event in oral cancer. *Oral Oncol.*, 47(1), 22-6.

[107] Zuo, C., Zhang, H., Spencer, H. J., Vural, E., Suen, J. Y., Schichman, S. A., Smoller, B. R., Kokoska, M. S., & Fan, C. Y. (2009). Increased microsatellite instability and epige-

netic inactivation of the hMLH1 gene in head and neck squamous cell carcinoma. *Otolaryngol Head Neck Surg.*, 141(4), 484-90.

[108] Carvalho, A. L., Chuang, A., Jiang, W. W., Lee, J., Begum, S., Poeta, L., et al. (2006). Deleted in colorectal cancer is a putative conditional tumor-suppressor gene inactivated by promoter hypermethylation in head and neck squamous cell carcinoma. *Cancer Res.*, 66(19), 9401-7.

[109] Ogi, K., Toyota, M., Ohe-Toyota, M., Tanaka, N., Noguchi, M., Sonoda, T., Kohama, G., & Tokino, T. (2002). Aberrant methylation of multiple genes and clinicopathological features in oral squamous cell carcinoma. *Clin Cancer Res.*, 8, 3164-3171.

[110] Lee, E. J., Lee, B. B., Kim, J. W., Shim, Y. M., Hoseok, I., Han, J., Cho, E. Y., Park, J., & Kim, D. H. (2006). Aberrant methylation of Fragile Histidine Triad gene is associated with poor prognosis in early stage esophageal squamous cell carcinoma. *Eur J Cancer.*, 42(7), 972-80.

[111] Issa, J.P. (2004). CpG island methylator phenotype in cancer. *Nat Rev Cancer.*, 4(12), 988-93.

[112] Marsit, C. J., Houseman, E. A., Christensen, B. C., et al. (2006). Examination of a CpG island methylator phenotype and implications of methylation profiles in solid tumors. *Cancer Res.*, 66, 10621-9.

[113] Shaw, R. J., Hall, G. L., Lowe, D., Bowers, N. L., Liloglou, T., Field, J. K., Woolgar, J. A., & Risk, J. M. (2007). CpG island methylation phenotype (CIMP) in oral cancer: associated with a marked inflammatory response and less aggressive tumour biology. *Oral Oncol.*, 43(9), 878-86.

[114] Freedman, L. (2007). Quantitative science methods for biomarker validation in chemoprevention trials. *Cancer Biomark*, 3, 135-40.

[115] Papadimitrakopoulou, V. A., & Hong, W. K. (2000). Biomolecular markers as intermediate end points in chemoprevention trials of upper aerodigestive tract cancer. *Int J Cancer.*, 88, 852-5.

[116] Sankaranarayanan, R., Ramadas, K., Thomas, G., Muwonge, R., Thara, S., Mathew, B., et al. (2005). Effect of screening on oral cancer mortality in Kerala, India: a cluster-randomised controlled trial. *Lancet*, 365, 1927-33.

[117] Califano, J. A., Ahrendt, S., Meininger, G., Westra, W. H., Koch, W. M., & Sidransky, D. (1996). Detection of telomerase activity in oral rinses from head and neck squamous cell cancer patients. *Cancer Res.*, 56, 5720-5722.

[118] Carvalho, A. L., Jeronimo, C., Kim, M. M., Henrique, R., Zhang, Z., Hoque, M. O., Chang, S., Brait, M., Nayak, C. S., Jiang, W. W., Claybourne, Q., Tokumaru, Y., et al. (2008). Evaluation of promoter hypermethylation detection in body fluids as a screening/diagnosis tool for head and neck squamous cell carcinoma. *Clin Cancer Res.*, 14, 97-107.

[119] Franzmann, E. J., Reategui, E. P., Pedroso, F., et al. (2007). Soluble CD44 is a potential marker for the early detection of head and neck cancer. *Cancer Epidemiol Biomarkers Prev.*, 16, 1348-55.

[120] Guerrero-Preston, R., Soudry, E., Acero, J., Orera, M., Moreno-López, L., Macía-Colón, G., et al. (2011). NID2 and HOXA9 promoter hypermethylation as biomarkers for prevention and early detection in oral cavity squamous cell carcinoma tissues and saliva. *Cancer Prev Res (Phila)*, 4(7), 1061-72.

[121] Righini, C. A., de Fraipont, F., Timsit, J. F., et al. (2007). Tumor-specific methylation in saliva: a promising biomarker for early detection of head and neck cancer recurrence. *Clin Cancer Res.*, 13, 1179-85.

[122] Viet, C., Jordan, R. C. K., & Schmidt, B. L. (2007). DNA promoter hypermethylation in saliva for the early diagnosis of oral cancer. *J Calif Dent Assoc.*, 34, 844.

[123] Viet, C., & Schmidt, B. (2008). Methylation Array Analysis of Preoperative and Postoperative Saliva DNA in Oral Cancer Patients. *Cancer Epidemiol Biomarkers Pre.*, 17(12), 3603-11.

[124] Nagata, S., Hamada, T., Yamada, N., Yokoyama, S., Kitamoto, S., Kanmura, Y., et al. (2012). Aberrant DNA methylation of tumor-related genes in oral rinse a noninvasive method for detection of Oral Squamous Cell Carcinoma. *Cancer*, DOI: cncr.27417.

[125] Demokan, S., Chang, X., Chuang, A., Mydlarz, W., Kaur, J., Huang, P., et al. (2010). KIF1A and EDNRB are differentially methylated in primary HNSCC and salivary rinses. *Int. J. Cancer*, 127, 2351-2359.

[126] Lo, K. W., Tsang, Y. S., Kwong, J., To, K. F., Teo, P. M., & Huang, D. P. (2002). Promoter hypermethylation of the EDNRB gene in nasopharyngeal carcinoma. *Int J Cancer*, 98, 651-5.

[127] Esteller, M., Garcia-Foncillas, J., Andion, E., Goodman, S. N., Hidalgo, O. F., Vanaclocha, V., Baylin, S. B., & Herman, J. G. (2000). Inactivation of the DNA-repair gene MGMT and the clinical response of gliomas to alkylating agents. *N Engl J Med.*, 343(19), 1350-4.

[128] Hegi, M. E., Diserens, A. C., Gorlia, T., Hamou, M. F., de Tribolet, N., Weller, M., Kros, J. M., Hainfellner, J. A., Mason, W., Mariani, L., Bromberg, J. E., Hau, P., Mirimanoff, R. O., Cairncross, J. G., Janzer, R. C., & Stupp, R. (2005). MGMT gene silencing and benefit from temozolomide in glioblastoma. *N Engl J Med.*, 352(10), 997-1003.

[129] Esteller, M., Gaidano, G., Goodman, S. N., Zagonel, V., Capello, D., Botto, B., Rossi, D., Gloghini, A., Vitolo, U., Carbone, A., Baylin, S. B., & Herman, J. G. (2002). Hypermethylation of the DNA repair gene O(6)-methylguanine DNA methyltransferase and survival of patients with diffuse large B-cell lymphoma. *J Natl Cancer Inst.*, 94(1), 26-32.

[130] Gifford, G., Paul, J., Vasey, P. A., Kaye, S. B., & Brown, R. (2004). The acquisition of hMLH1 methylation in plasma DNA after chemotherapy predicts poor survival for ovarian cancer patients. *Clin Cancer Res.*, 10(13), 4420-6.

[131] Agrelo, R., Cheng, W. H., Setien, F., Ropero, S., Espada, J., Fraga, M. F., Herranz, M., Paz, M. F., Sanchez-Cespedes, M., Artiga, M. J., Guerrero, D., Castells, A., von, Kobbe. C., Bohr, V. A., & Esteller, M. (2006). Epigenetic inactivation of the premature aging Werner syndrome gene in human cancer. *Proc Natl Acad Sci USA.*, 103(23), 8822-7.

[132] Chen, B., Rao, X., House, M. G., Nephew, K. P., Cullen, K. J., & Guo, Z. (2011). GPx3 promoter hypermethylation is a frequent event in human cancer and is associated with tumorigenesis and chemotherapy response. *Cancer Lett.*, 309(1), 37-45.

[133] Ogi, K., Toyota, M., Mita, H., Satoh, A., Kashima, L., Sasaki, Y., et al. (2005). Small interfering RNA-induced CHFR silencing sensitizes oral squamous cell cancer cells to microtubule inhibitors. *Cancer Biol Ther.*, 4(7), 773-80.

[134] Gubanova, E., Brown, B., Ivanov, S. V., Helleday, T., Mills, G. B., Yarbrough, W. G., et al. (2012). Downregulation of SMG-1 in HPV-Positive Head and Neck Squamous Cell Carcinoma Due to Promoter Hypermethylation Correlates with Improved Survival. *Clin Cancer Res.*, 18(5), 1257-1267.

[135] Suzuki, M., Shinohara, F., Endo, M., Sugazaki, M., Echigo, S., & Rikiishi, H. (2009). Zebularine suppresses the apoptotic potential of 5-fluorouracil via cAMP/PKA/CREB pathway against human oral squamous cell carcinoma cells. *Cancer Chemother Pharmacol*, 64(2), 223-32.

[136] Suzuki, M., Shinohara, F., Nishimura, K., Echigo, S., & Rikiishi, H. (2007). Epigenetic regulation of chemosensitivity to 5-fluorouracil and cisplatin by zebularine in oral squamous cell carcinoma. *Int J Oncol*, 31(6), 1449-56.

[137] Logullo, A. F., Nonogaki, S., Miguel, R. E., Kowalski, L. P., Nishimoto, I. N., Pasini, F. S., Federico, M. H., Brentani, R. R., & Brentani, M. M. (2003). Transforming growth factor beta1 (TGFbeta1) expression in head and neck squamous cell carcinoma patients as related to prognosis. *J Oral Pathol Med.*, 32(3), 139-45.

[138] Tavassoli, M., Soltaninia, J., Rudnicka, J., et al. (2002). Tamoxifen inhibits the growth of head and neck cancer cells and sensitizes these cells to cisplatin induced-apoptosis: role of TGF-beta1. *Carcinogenesis.*, 23, 1569-75.

[139] Hannigan, A., Smith, P., Kalna, G., Lo, Nigro. C., Orange, C., O.'Brien, D. I., et al. (2010). Epigenetic downregulation of human disabled homolog 2 switches TGF-beta from a tumor suppressor to a tumor promoter. *J Clin Invest.*, 120(8), 2842-57.

[140] Toyota, M., Suzuki, H., Yamashita, T., Hirata, K., Imai, K., Tokino, T., & Shinomura, Y. (2009). Cancer epigenomics: implications of DNA methylation in personalized cancer therapy. *Cancer Sci.*, 100(5), 787-91.

[141] Magic, Z., Supic, G., & Brankovic-Magic, M. (2009). Towards targeted epigenetic therapy of cancer. *Journal of Buon.*, 14, S79-S88.

[142] Silverman, L. R., & Mufti, G. J. (2005). Methylation inhibitor therapy in the treatment of myelodysplastic syndrome. *Nature Clin Pract Oncol.*, 2, S12-S23.

[143] Issa, J. P., & Kantarjian, H. (2005). Azacitidine. *Nature Rev Drug Discov.* [5], S6-S7.

[144] Fenaux, P., et al. (2009). Efficacy of azacitidine compared with that of conventional care regimens in the treatment of higher-risk myelodysplastic syndromes: a randomised, open-label, phase III study. *Lancet Oncol.*, 10, 223-232.

[145] Koutsimpelas, D., Pongsapich, W., Heinrich, U., Mann, S., Mann, W. J., & Brieger, J. (2012). Promoter methylation of MGMT, MLH1 and RASSF1A tumor suppressor genes in head and neck squamous cell carcinoma: pharmacological genome demethylation reduces proliferation of head and neck squamous carcinoma cells. *Oncol Rep.*, 27(4), 1135-41.

[146] Brieger, J., Pongsapich, W., Mann, S. A., Hedrich, J., Fruth, K., Pogozelski, B., & Mann, W. J. (2010). Demethylation treatment restores hic1 expression and impairs aggressiveness of head and neck squamous cell carcinoma. *Oral Oncol.*, 46(9), 678-83.

[147] Bauman, J., Verschraegen, C., Belinsky, S., Muller, C., Rutledge, T., Fekrazad, M., Ravindranathan, M., Lee, S. J., & Jones, D. (2012). A phase I study of 5-azacytidine and erlotinib in advanced solid tumor malignancies. *Cancer Chemother Pharmacol.*, 69(2), 547-54.

[148] Ogawa, T., Liggett, T. E., Melnikov, A. A., Monitto, C. L., Kusuke, D., Shiga, K., et al. (2012). Methylation of death-associated protein kinase is associated with cetuximab and erlotinib resistance. *Cell Cycle.*, 11(8), 1656-63.

[149] Smith, I. M., Mydlarz, W. K., Mithani, S. K., et al. (2007). DNA global hypomethylation in squamous cell head and neck cancer associated with smoking, alcohol consumption and stage. *Int J Cancer.*, 121(8), 1724-8.

[150] Puri, S. K., Si, L., Fan, C. Y., & Hanna, E. (2005). Aberrant promoter hypermethylation of multiple genes in head and neck squamous cell carcinoma. *Am J Otolaryngol.*, 26(1), 12-7.

[151] Chang, H. W., Ling, G. S., Wei, W. I., & Yuen, A. P. (2004). Smoking and drinking can induce p15 methylation in the upper aerodigestive tract of healthy individuals and patients with head and neck squamous cell carcinoma. *Cancer*, 101(1), 125-32.

[152] Marsit, C., Mc Clean, M., Furniss, C., & Kelsey, K. (2006). Epigenetic inactivation of the SFRP genes is associated with drinking, smoking and HPV in head and neck squamous cell carcinoma. *Int. J. Cancer*, 119, 1761-1766.

[153] Bennett, K. L., Lee, W., Lamarre, E., Zhang, X., Seth, R., Scharpf, J., Hunt, J., & Eng, C. (2010). HPV status-independent association of alcohol and tobacco exposure or prior radiation therapy with promoter methylation of FUSSEL18, EBF3, IRX1, and SEPT9,

but not SLC5A8, in head and neck squamous cell carcinomas. *Genes Chromosomes Cancer*, 49, 319-26.

[154] Kraunz, K. S., Hsiung, D., Mc Clean, M. D., Liu, M., Osanyingbemi, J., Nelson, H. H., & Kelsey, K. T. (2006). Dietary folate is associated with p16 (INK4A) methylation in head and neck squamous cell carcinoma. *Int J Cancer.*, 119(7), 1553-7.

[155] Fang, M. Z., Wang, Y. W., Ai, N., Hou, Z., Sun, Y., Lu, H., Welsh, W., & Yang, C. S. (2003). Tea polyphenol (_)-epigallocatechin-3-gallate inhibits DNA methyltransferase and reactivates methylation-silenced genes in cancer cell lines. *Cancer Res.*, 63, 7563-7570.

[156] Kato, K., Long, N. K., Makita, H., Toida, M., Yamashita, T., Hatakeyama, D., Hara, A., Mori, H., & Shibata, T. (2008). Effects of green tea polyphenol on methylation status of RECK gene and cancer cell invasion in oral squamous cell carcinoma cells. *Br J Cancer*, 99(4), 647-54.

[157] Fang, M. Z., Chen, D., Sun, Y., Jin, Z., Christman, J. K., & Yang, C. S. (2005). Reversal of hypermethylation and reactivation of 16INK4aRARbeta, and MGMT genes by genistein and other isoflavones from soy. *Clin Cancer Res.*, 11(19 Pt 1), 7033-41.

Section 5

# Bacteria, Viruses and Metals Methylation: Risk and Benefit for Human Health

Chapter 9

# Host-Mimicking Strategies in DNA Methylation for Improved Bacterial Transformation

Hirokazu Suzuki

Additional information is available at the end of the chapter

http://dx.doi.org/10.5772/51691

## 1. Introduction

In 1928, Griffith [1] reported that soluble substances from virulent pneumococcal cells transformed non-virulent pneumococcus to virulent forms. This substance has now been demonstrated to be DNA [2-4]. This is considered to be the first report on genetic transformation of bacteria by exogenous DNA. Subsequently, natural competence of *Bacillus subtilis* was reported in 1958 by Young and Spizizen [5]. They also demonstrated genetic transformation of natural competent *B. subtilis* cells using exogenous DNA. It was in 1970 that genetic transformation of *Escherichia coli* using chemically competent cells was reported [6]. Thus, genetic transformation of common bacterial models was established at an early stage in the development of bacteriology. The alternative view is that bacterial models such as *B. subtilis* and *E. coli* have become the mainstay of this field because of high transformation ability. Genetic transformation techniques remain important for studying numerous bacteria and for the advancement of bacteriology, biochemistry, applied microbiology, and microbial biotechnology. Moreover, recent developments in the search for new bacteria and genome sequencing have provided numerous effective bacteria that are useful for biological studies and industrial applications. With these developments, there is a greater demand for establishing genetic transformation methods for more bacteria.

DNA introduction is an essential process for transforming target bacterium by exogenous DNA. Various methods for introducing DNA into bacteria have been developed to date, including chemotransformation, electroporation, sonopolation, tribos, and conjugational transfer [7]. In spite of these developments, it is often difficult to establish transformation methods for target bacterium. A possible reason is the difficulty faced while exploring suitable conditions for introducing DNA, which requires not only theoretical understanding but also a trial and error approach. Circumventing bacterial RM systems is a major challenge.

These systems defend bacteria against transformation by exogenous DNA, such as bacteriophages, and effectively hamper genetic transformation by exogenous plasmids. RM systems selectively digest exogenous DNA by differentiating them from host-endogenous DNA on the basis of host-specific DNA methylation [8]. Therefore, DNA that imitates the methylation patterns of the host bacterium (host-mimicking DNA) is incorporated into the bacterium without restriction. Thus, RM systems can be overcome by theoretical host-mimicking strategies (Figure 1), rather than exploring conditions for introducing DNA. This chapter explains host-mimicking strategies and provides tips for establishing transformation methods for new bacteria.

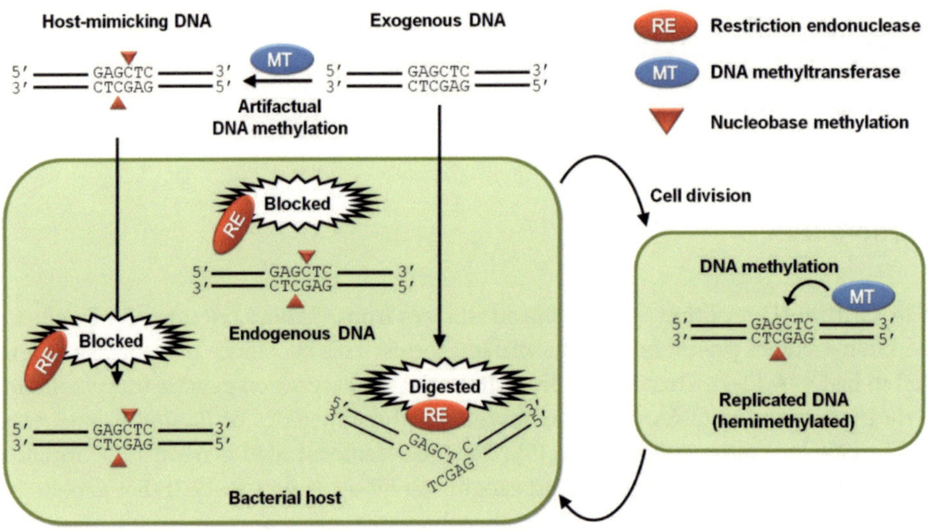


**Figure 1.** Host-mimicking strategies for circumventing restriction–modification (RM) systems in bacteria.RM systems serve to defend bacteria against invasion by exogenous DNA, and thereby hamper genetic transformation by exogenous plasmids. In typical RM systems, restriction endonuclease (RE) digests exogenous DNA but not endogenous DNA that has been methylated by cognate DNA methyltransferase (MT). Host-mimicking DNA that imitates the methylation patterns of the bacterial host is recognized as endogenous DNA by the host because RM systems depend on host-specific DNA methylation to distinguish between exogenous and endogenous DNA.

## 2. RM systems

In 1962, Arber and Dussoix [9] found that bacteriophage λ carried specificity for *E. coli* strains in which they were produced. For examples, bacteriophage λ from *E. coli* K-12 was efficiently transfected into K-12 and C strains, but not strains B and K(P1) (efficiencies were $<10^{-4}$ fold). Meanwhile, bacteriophage λ produced by *E. coli* C efficiently transformed strain C, but not strains K-12, B, and K(P1) (efficiencies were $<4\times10^{-4}$ fold). Thus, bacteriophage λ vectors readily infected *E. coli* strains that produced them but the infection to other strains was "restricted". This occurrence, termed restriction, is explained by *E. coli* RM systems that act as host defense against exogenous DNA.

RM systems selectively digest exogenous DNA and greatly influence the efficiency of genetic transformation by exogenous DNA. Numerous RM systems have been found in bacteria and archaea, and are classified into four main types (type I–IV) [10]. Their general properties are summarized in Table 1. The REBASE database (rebase.neb.com) [11] has accumulated large amounts of information about RM systems, including types, gene sequences, recognition sites, and origin organisms. Among the four types of RM systems, type II consists of RE and MT. In this type, RE cuts exogenous DNA at specific sites but not endogenous DNA that has been methylated by MT (Figure 1). Type I and III systems also cut exogenous DNA by similar mechanisms, but comprise protein complexes of some subunits. Type IV is known as a modification-specific restriction system to cut DNA with heterologous modifications. Intriguingly, RM systems behave as selfish elements like viruses and transposons [12], implying that RM systems have been irreversibly distributed in bacteria. The following sections describe more details of RM systems.

## 2.1. DNA modifications involved in DNA restriction

Several DNA modifications have been elucidated and in almost all cases the modifications that are involved in restriction are nucleobase methylations. The main forms of methylated nucleobases are $N^6$-methyladenine ($^{6m}$A; Figure 2), 5-methylcytosine ($^{5m}$C), and $N^4$-methylcytosine ($^{4m}$C). These modifications are performed for double-stranded DNA using methyltransferases or other methyltransfer machinery. In addition, some bacteriophage DNA contain 5-hydroxymethylcytosine ($^{5hm}$C) instead of cytosine. This modification is incorporated during phage DNA replication using 5-hydroxymethyldeoxycytidine triphosphate as the substrate [13]. The hydroxyl group is further glucosylated to produce β-glucosyl-5-hydroxymethylcytosine ($^{ghm}$C) in a phage-specific pattern by glucosyltransferase [14]. This modification has various biological functions, including circumvention of restriction barriers of RM systems in phage hosts [13, 14]. The modified cytosine $^{5hm}$C is also found in mammalians [15-17]. Unlike phages, it is produced by oxidation of $^{5m}$C in double-stranded DNA [18]. In bacteria, there are no known type I–III RM systems involving $^{5hm}$C or $^{ghm}$C. However, several type IV systems that restrict DNA containing $^{5hm}$C and/or $^{ghm}$C have been reported [19-21].

| RM system | Restriction | | Methylation | |
|---|---|---|---|---|
| | Machinery | Cleavage site | Machinery | Nucleobase |
| Type I | $R_2M_2S$ | Variable | $M_2S$ | $^{6m}$A |
| Type II | RE | Fixed | MT | $^{6m}$A, $^{5m}$C, $^{4m}$C |
| Type III | $R_2M_2$ | Variable | $M_2$ | $^{6m}$A |
| Type IV | RE | Variable | | |

**Table 1.** General properties of four types of RM systems.Type I comprises R, M, and S subunits. Methylation is performed by subunits M and S. Type III comprises R and M subunits. The M subunit alone catalyzes methylation. Type II comprises two independent proteins, RE and MT. Type IV comprises only RE and restricts DNA with heterologous modifications. Methylation produces $^{6m}$A, $^{5m}$C, or $^{4m}$C.

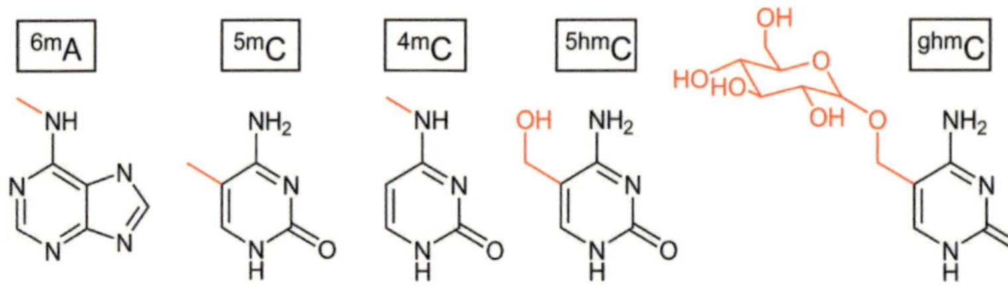


**Figure 2.** Chemical structures of modified nucleobases (modification moieties are indicated in red).

In addition to the methyl-based modifications described above, sulfur modification (phosphorothioation) of DNA backbones has been observed [22, 23]. Notably, it is suggested that this modification is involved in DNA restriction in *Salmonella enterica* [24]. The gene cluster for this RM system consists of eight genes, of which four are involved in phosphorothioation, while seven genes are essential for restricting unphosphorothioated DNA. Similar gene clusters, along with DNA containing phosphorothiol bonds, are found in many bacteria, implying that phosphorothioation is a widespread DNA modification [24, 25]. A type IV system that restricts phosphorothioated DNA has been also reported [26].

### 2.2. Type I RM systems

The *E. coli* strain K-12 harbors one type I RM system (EcoKI) encoded by the genes *hsdR* (R subunit), *hsdM* (M subunit), and *hsdS* (S subunit). This system constructs a multi-subunit complex that comprises two R subunits, two M subunits, and one S subunit ($R_2M_2S$), and scans double-stranded DNA after replication [27, 28]. When the complex recognizes DNA that is unmethylated at recognition sites, it acts as an ATP dependent endonuclease to digest DNA. The sequences of recognition sites are asymmetric but not palindromic. Examples include 5′-AACN$_6$GTGC-3′ and 5′-GCACN$_6$GTT-3′ for EcoKI, 5′-TGAN$_8$TGCT-3′ and 5′-AGCAN$_8$TCA-3′ for EcoBI, and 5′-TTAN$_7$GTCY-3′ and 5′-RGACN$_7$TAA-3′ for EcoDI (methylated adenine is underlined; R: A/G, Y: C/T, N: A/C/G/T) [29, 30].

The cleavage positions are distal from recognition sites and are variable. It is believed that the complex of type I RM system, while binding to recognition sites, translocates (or pulls) the DNA along in an ATP dependent fashion, and cleaves DNA when the translocation is impended by collision and/or by stalling with another translocating complex [27, 31, 32]. Electron microscopy analysis has been used to detect ATP-dependent formation of loop DNA during DNA cleavage by a type I RM complex [32]. The R subunit is responsible for ATP hydrolysis, translocation, and endonuclease activity, but not DNA binding. The binding depends on subunits M and S, which are therefore essential for both endonuclease and methyltransferase activities.

The complex of type I RM system acts similar to methyltransferase when it recognizes DNA that is hemimethylated (methylated on one strand) at recognition sites [27]. The methylation is performed by M and S subunits using *S*-adenosyl-L-methionine as the methyl donor [8]. The M subunit has the binding site for *S*-adenosyl-L-methionine, while the S subunit is essential for determining recognition sites. The R subunit is unnecessary for methyltransferase

http://dx.doi.org/10.5772/51691

activity. In all cases reported so far, methylation by type I RM systems occurs in adenine to produce $^{6m}$A.

### 2.3. Type II RM systems

Type II RM systems are extremely diverse and are currently classified into 11 subfamilies [8]. Generally, these comprise two enzymes, RE and MT. Cleavages of exogenous DNA at unmethylated recognition sites is carried out by RE, which spares endogenous DNA that has been methylated by the cognate MT. Most REs require $Mg^{2+}$ ions as a cofactor for cleavage. Although RE may form monomers, dimers, or tetramers, it functions without forming complexes with the cognate MT. The recognition of cleavage sites is highly precise and recognition sequences are often palindromic. Such sites include 5′-GAATTC-3′ for EcoRI and 5′-GGATCC-3′ for BamHI, which are cleaved symmetrically within the sites. Because of these useful properties, more than 3,500 REs have been characterized, and many are widely utilized in recombinant DNA technology [8]. The enzyme MT catalyzes methylation at recognition sites using *S*-adenosyl-L-methionine as the substrate and generally acts as a monomer. The nucleobases produced are $^{6m}$A, $^{5m}$C, or $^{4m}$C. For example, EcoRI and BamHI methyltransferases produce 5′-GA$^{6m}$ATTC-3′ and 5′-GGAT$^{4m}$CC-3′, respectively.

### 2.4. Type III RM systems

Type III RM systems operate with multi-subunit machinery comprising two R subunits and two M subunits ($R_2M_2$) [33]. Subunit M contains recognition domain for binding to specific sites and also a methyltransferase domain. It can thereby bind at recognition sites independently, and methylate DNA using *S*-adenosyl-L-methionine as a substrate. The nucleobase produced is $^{6m}$A in all cases reported so far. Unlike type I and II RM systems, full modification is actually hemimethylation (methylation on one strand). The recognition sequences are asymmetric, such as 5′-CAGCAG-3′ for EcoP15I (methylated adenine is underlined).

Subunit R has an ATP dependent DNA helicase and endonuclease domains that are responsible for DNA cleavage. This subunit is unable to bind to DNA and therefore requires subunit M to cleave DNA. Two unmethylated sites that are inversely oriented (head-to-head orientation) serve as the target for DNA cleavage. Cleavage occurs at 25–27 bp downstream of one of the recognition sites, which is chosen randomly from the two sites. Even DNA with 3.5 kb between the two sites is cleaved. The cleavage requires ATP similar to type I RM systems. However, the amount of ATP consumed is only ~1% of that required for cleavage by type I RM systems. This fact makes it difficult to transpose the translocation model that is proposed in type I RM systems to type III RM systems. Thus, some alternative models have now been proposed [33].

### 2.5. Type IV restriction systems

Several enzymes specifically restrict modified DNA [10, 19-21, 26, 34-36]. These systems offer very efficient to defense from bacteriophages with highly-modified DNA. Among these, the enzymes for which cleavage sites are very specific and precise are classified into the M subfamily of type II RM systems [21]. Examples include DpnI (recognition sequence: 5′-G$^{6m}$ATC-3′), GlaI (5′-G$^{5m}$CG$^{5m}$C-3′), BisI (5′-G$^{5m}$CNGC-3′; N: A/G/C/T), and MspJI (5′-$^{5m}$CNNR-3′; R: G/A). The enzymes with non-specific and variable cleavage sites are classified as type IV restriction systems. The *E. coli* strain K-12 harbors three type IV systems encoded by *mcrA, mcrB-mcrC,* and *mrr*. The enzyme McrA recognizes 5′-Y$^{5m}$CGR-3′ site (Y: C/T; R: G/A) [37], whereas McrBC recognizes pairs of 5′-R$^{m}$C-3′ ($^{m}$C: $^{5m}$C or $^{4m}$C) separated by 40–3000 bp, and cleaves DNA ~30 bp distal from one of the sites [36]. The Mrr system recognizes DNA containing $^{6m}$A, $^{5m}$C, or $^{4m}$C, but its recognition sites have not been well defined [36]. The enzyme SauUSI of *Staphylococcus aureus* recognizes 5′-S$^{5m}$CNGS-3′ and 5′-S$^{5hm}$CNGS-3′ (S: C/G; N: A/G/C/T) and cleaves at position 2–18 bp downstream of the recognition site [21]. The enzyme GmrSD restriction system of *E. coli* CT596 cuts DNA containing $^{ghm}$C [20]. Thus, all species of modified nucleobases are potentially restricted by type IV restriction systems.

| Microbe | Host-mimicking DNA | | Reference |
|---|---|---|---|
| | Production | Introduction | |
| *Bacillus anthracis* | *In vivo* (MF) | Electroporation | [50] |
| *Bacillus cereus* | *In vitro* (EX) | Electroporation | [51] |
| *Bacillus weihenstephanensis* | *In vitro* (EX) | Electroporation | [51] |
| *Bifidobacterium adolescentis* | *In vivo* (GM) | Electroporation | [52] |
| *Bifidobacterium longum* | *In vitro* (MT/SD) | Electroporation | [53] |
| *Borrelia burgdorferi* | *In vitro* (MT) | Electroporation | [54] |
| *Clostridium acetobutylicum* | *In vivo* (HG) | Electroporation | [55] |
| *Clostridium difficile* | *In vivo* (HG/SD) | Conjugation | [56] |
| *Clostridium thermocellum* | *In vivo* (IG) | Electroporation | [57] |
| *Geobacillus kaustophilus* | *In vivo* (GM/IG) | Conjugation | [41] |
| *Helicobacter pylori* | *In vitro* (EX) | Competency | [58] |
| *Salmonella typhimurium* | *In vivo* (DS) | Competency | [59] |
| *Staphylococcus aureus* | *In vivo* (DS) | Electroporation | [60] |
| *Streptomyces avermitilis* | *In vivo* (MF) | Protoplast | [61] |
| *Streptomyces bambergiensis* | *In vivo* (MF) | Conjugation | [62] |
| *Streptomyces coelicolor* | *In vivo* (MF) | Protoplast | [35] |
| *Streptomyces griseus* IFO 13350 | *In vivo* (GM/HG) | Protoplast | [40] |
| | *In vivo* (DS) | Protoplast | [63] |
| *Streptomyces griseus* NRRL B-2682 | *In vitro* (MT) | Protoplast | [64] |
| *Streptomyces natalensis* | *In vivo* (MF) | Conjugation | [65] |
| *Sulfolobus acidocaldarius* | *In vivo* (HG) | Electroporation | [38] |
| *Thermoanaerobacter* sp. X514 | *In vivo* (IG) | Sonoporation | [66] |

**Table 2.** Microbial transformation using host-mimicking DNA.DS: *in vivo* methylation in a strain that is related to the target bacterium and is deficient in restriction and proficient in methylation; EX: *in vitro* methylation using a crude extract of the target bacterium; GM: *in vivo* methylation using methyltransferase genes in the target bacterial genome; HG: *in vivo* methylation using heterologous genes; IG: *in vivo* methylation using *E. coli* intrinsic genes; MF: methyl-free DNA; MT: *in vitro* methylation using commercially available methyltransferases; and SD: transformation using DNA with specifically abolished recognition sites.

## 3. Host-mimicking strategies

Circumvention of RM systems is critical for establishing transformation methods for target bacteria (Table 2). This is true not only for bacteria but also archaea [38]. This section describes some strategies for circumventing RM systems and focuses on host-mimicking. Because all types of RM systems digest exogenous DNA after distinguishing it from endogenous DNA on the basis of host-specific methylation patterns, DNA modification that mimic these patterns evade digestion. A general flowchart for producing host-mimicking DNA is shown in Figure 3. The details are described in the following sections.

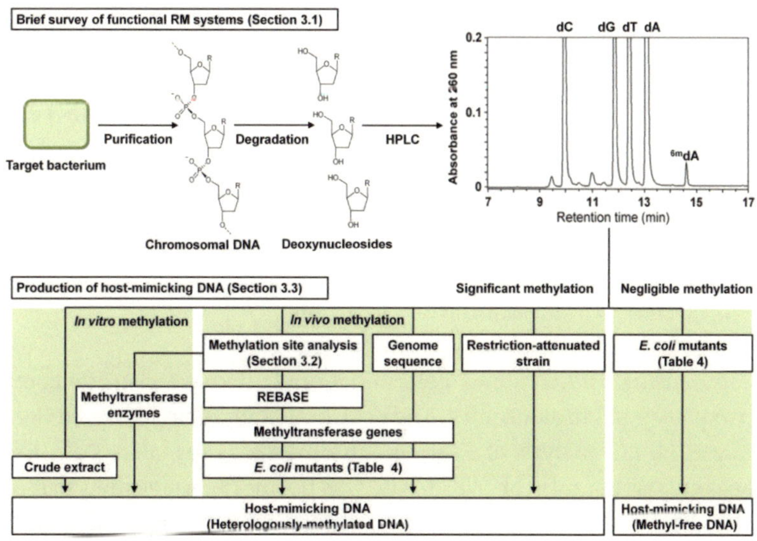


**Figure 3.** General flowchart for producing host-mimicking DNA to target bacteria.The chromatogram is the data from HPLC analysis of deoxynucleosides prepared from *G. kaustophilus* chromosomes [41]. It includes 2′-deoxyadenosine (dA), 2′-deoxycytidine (dC), 2′-deoxyguanosine (dG), 2′-deoxythymidine (dT), and $N^6$-methyl-2′-deoxyadenosine ($^{6m}$dA) but not 5-methyl-2′-deoxycytidine ($^{5m}$dC) or $N^4$-methyl-2′-deoxycytidine ($^{4m}$dC).

### 3.1. A brief survey of functional RM systems

As mentioned earlier, type I–III RM systems involve DNA methylation in their functions. Therefore, the presence of methylated DNA in bacterial chromosomes indicates a type I–III RM system in the bacterium. Hence analysis of methylated DNA is an effective survey method to identify functional RM systems in target bacterium. Methylated DNA in chromosomes can be analyzed using high-performance liquid chromatography (HPLC) [15, 18, 39-45]. This method determines the presence of deoxynucleosides and methylated deoxynucleosides. Deoxynucleosides are prepared by hydrolyzing chromosomal DNA with nuclease P1 and alkaline phosphatase [39-41], are separated using reverse mode $C_{18}$-based silica columns, and are detected by ultraviolet absorption at 260 and/or 280 nm. Authentic $^{6m}$dA, $^{5m}$dC, and $^{4m}$dC are commercially available or can be prepared from methylated 2′-deoxynucleoside-5′-triphosphate by dephosphorylation using *E. coli* alkaline phosphatase [40]. Note that this analysis requires large amounts of DNA (>10 μg). Contamination with RNA, proteins, and chemicals that absorb ultraviolet radiation may also complicate accurate analysis. In some reports [18, 42, 43], deoxynucleosides are more accurately identified by combining HPLC and mass spectrometry analysis. In addition, immunochemical methods are available for analyzing methylated DNA [46-49]. Several anti-$^{5m}$C antibodies have been developed and are commercially available. Although commercially available antibodies against other methylated DNA are limited, Kong *et al.* [49] have reported successful production of rabbit polyclonal antibodies against $^{6m}$A and $^{4m}$C.

| Deoxynucleoside | Relative coefficient | |
|---|---|---|
| | Detection at 260 nm | Detection at 280 nm |
| dC | 2.34 | 1.74 |
| $^{5m}$dC | 3.51 | 1.77 |
| $^{4m}$dC | 1.77 | 1.57 |
| dA | 1.08 | 6.42 |
| $^{6m}$dA | 1.15 | 1.93 |

**Table 3.** Relative coefficients for determining deoxynucleoside molar ratios by HPLC analysis; [Relative amount of deoxynucleoside] = [Coefficient] × [Peak area on HPLC chromatogram].

Analysis of DNA using HPLC allows determination of deoxynucleoside composition and methylation frequency in chromosomes. The coefficients in Table 3 may be used for estimation. For example, HPLC analysis of *S. griseus* chromosomes revealed $^{5m}$dC but not $^{6m}$dA or $^{4m}$dC [40]. The composition ratio of $^{5m}$dC to dC was 0.7 mol%, suggesting that *S. griseus* possesses approximately one $^{5m}$C per 0.5 kb of chromosomal DNA with 67% GC content. The chromosome of *G. kaustophilus* contains $^{6m}$dA and the composition ratio to dA is 2.0 mol% [41]. This suggests that *G. kaustophilus* possesses approximately one $^{6m}$A per 0.1 kb of chromosomal DNA with 52% GC content. Although DNA methylation unrelated to RM systems have been observed, such as *E. coli* Dam and Dcm methylation [67, 68], high frequency methylations imply that the bacteria may harbor a considerable type I–III RM system. Meanwhile, the chromosomes of *S. avermitilis*, *S. coelicolor*, and *S. lividans* contain no methylated DNA (my unpublished data). This observation suggests that these bacteria harbor no type I–III RM systems. However, the possibility remains that a functional type IV system exists in these species. Potent methyl-specific restrictions have been observed in *S. avermitilis* [61], *S. coelicolor* [35], *S. bambergiensis* [62], and *S. natalensis* [65].

### 3.2. Methylation site analysis

When significant DNA methylation is observed in the target bacterium, preliminary determination of DNA methylation sites is generally required to produce host-mimicking DNA. Recent epigenetic studies have developed many methods to analyze DNA methylation [29, 30, 69-76]. Although most of these studies aimed to analyze 5-methylation of cytosine at specific sites, or differential DNA methylation in chromosomes, there are a few methods that exhaustively determine methylated consensus sites in chromosomes as follows.

In *S. griseus*, bisulfite-based analysis of a plasmid library isolated from this bacterium (Figure 4A) was used to determine the two consensus sites 5′-GAG$^{5m}$CTC-3′ and 5′-GC$^{5m}$CGGC-3′ [40]. Note that this method is not employed for methylation analysis in bacteria that cannot be transformed with exogenous plasmids, and in bacteria that have methylated nucleobases other than $^{5m}$C. For determining $^{6m}$A consensus sites in *G. kaustophilus*, chromosome digestion using methyl-sensitive restriction enzymes (Figure 4B) was used to reveal 5′-GG$^{6m}$ATC-3′ and 5′-G$^{6m}$ATCC-3′ site [41]. Methods using methyl-sensitive restriction enzymes help identify several methylation species, including $^{6m}$A, $^{5m}$C, and $^{4m}$C. However, methylation sites that can be identified by these methods are limited due to the lack of commercially available restriction enzymes. Recently, direct detection using real-time DNA sequencing has been reported [74, 75]. This method potentially enables the exhaustive determination of all methylation sites in chromosomal DNA. Although this method requires special equipments, which has limited availability, it may become one of the most promising methods for methylation analysis in the future. Also, the author has now developed a versatile immunological method for determining consensus sequences with methylated nucleobases.

### 3.3. Production of host-mimicking DNA

If the target bacterium contains no or negligible methylated DNA, methyl-free DNA should be used as host-mimicking DNA because the bacterium may harbor type IV restriction systems, as exemplified by transformation of *S. avermitilis* [61], *S. coelicolor* [35], and *S. natalensis* [65]. Methyl-free DNA can be readily produced using *E. coli* strains deficient in DNA methyltransferase genes (*dam* $^-$ *dcm* $^-$ *hsd* $^-$), such as *E. coli* IR27, ET12567, IBEC58, and HST04 (Table 4). Methyl-restrained DNA from *E. coli* GM2929 and SCS110 (*dam* $^-$ *dcm* $^-$ *hsd* $^+$) were also used for efficient transformation of *S. bambergiensis* [62] and *B. anthracis* [50], respectively. Because Hsd mediated methylation is of low frequency in *E. coli*, deficiency of this methyltion may not be essential for circumventing type IV systems.

If the target bacterium contains considerable methylated DNA, host-mimicking DNA that reconstitutes the methylation pattern of the target bacterium should be used for transformation. There are two main approaches to produce heterologous methylation of DNA. One is *in vitro* methylation using methyltransferases [53, 54, 64], such as Dam (catalyzing 5′-G$^{6m}$ATC-3′ methylation), M.TaqI (5′-TCG$^{6m}$A-3′), M.AluI (5′-AG$^{5m}$CT-3′), M.BamHI (5′-GGATC$^{4m}$C-3′), M.SssI (5′-$^{5m}$CG-3′), M.EcoRI (5′-GA$^{6m}$ATTC-3′), M.CviPI (5′-GC$^{5m}$-3′), M.HaeIII (5′-GGC$^{5m}$C-3′), M.HhaI (5′-G$^{5m}$CGC-3′), M.HpaII (5′-C$^{5m}$CGG-3′), and M.MspI (5′-$^{5m}$CCGG-3′). This approach is very simple and effective but has low cost-performance and low versatility due to the limited number of commercially available methyltransferases. In transformations of *B. cereus* [51], *B. weihenstephanensis* [51], and *H. pylori* [58], crude extracts prepared from the respective bacterium were used for DNA methylation. This method has high cost-performance and high versatility but may not be efficient because of low methyltransferase activity in crude extracts and DNA degradation by nucleases. Moreover, type I and III methylation pattern cannot be achieved by this method.

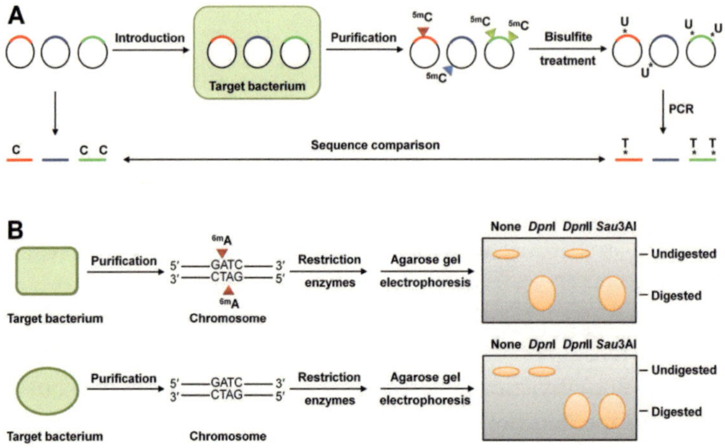


**Figure 4.** Methylation site analysis in target bacterium. (A) Bisulfite-based analysis to determine $^{5m}$C consensus sites. Bisulfite treatment converts methyl-free cytosine to uracil without affecting $^{5m}$C. Therefore, $^{5m}$C positions can be determined by comparing bisulfite-treated and -untreated DNA sequences. (B) Chromosomal digestion by methyl-sensitive restriction enzymes is used to analyze 5′-G$^{6m}$ATC-3′ methylation. The restriction enzyme DpnI cuts 5′-G$^{6m}$ATC-3′ but not 5′-GATC-3′, DpnII cuts 5′-GATC-3′ but not 5′-G$^{6m}$ATC-3′, and Sau3AI cuts 5′-GATC-3′ and 5′-G$^{6m}$ATC-3′.

Another approach is *in vivo* methylation by expressing methyltransferase genes in *E. coli* cells [38, 40, 41, 52, 55, 56]. Type II and III methylation can be reconstituted by expressing MT and M subunit genes, respectively, and type I methylation can be reconstituted by simultaneous expression of M and S subunit genes. Numerous gene sequences of methyltransferases are accumulated in the REBASE database along with their methylation sites [11]. Either plasmids or chromosomal integration can be used as expression vectors for methyltransferase genes. When the genome sequence of the target bacterium has been determined, methyltransferase genes in the genome may be used for *in vivo* methylation [40, 41, 52]. Methylation site analysis is not essential for this approach; however, functional expression of methyltransferase genes requires confirmation by HPLC analysis of recombinant *E. coli* chromosomes. A methyltransferase gene of *S. griseus*, responsible for 5′-GAG$^{5m}$CTC-3′ methylation, was found to be nonfunctional in *E. coli*. Hence, an alternative methyltransferase gene from *S. achromogenes* (*M.SacI*) was used for DNA methylation [40]. The *E. coli* host used to produce host-mimicking DNA must be a methylation-deficient strain (Table 4) because the target bacterium may have type IV systems in addition to type I–III RM systems, as exemplified by *G. kaustophilus* transformation [41]. In addition, it is desirable that the *E. coli* host is deficient in type IV system genes (*mcrA*, *mcrBC*, and *mrr*) because these may restrict heterologous methylation in *E. coli* cells. In this regard, *E. coli* strains IR27 and HST04 are appropriate for producing host-mimicking DNA through *in vivo* methylation. Although *in vivo* methylation may be more complicated than *in vitro* methylation, this approach often has excellent cost-performance, versatility, and efficiency.

A derivative of the target bacterium with methylation activity and reduced restriction activity can also be used for the production of host-mimicking DNA. In transformations of *Salmonella typhimurium* and *Staphylococcus aureus*, plasmids isolated from *E. coli* strains

http://dx.doi.org/10.5772/51691

were initially introduced and propagated in the restriction-deficient strains LB5000 [59] and RN4220 [60], respectively, and were then used for transformation of other strains. In *S. griseus* transformation, mutant HH1 that reduces restriction activity compared to the wild-type has been used [63]. This approach enables production of perfect host-mimicking DNA, although it is not easy to find a strain that is both deficient in restriction and proficient in methylation.

| Strain | Relevant genotype | Reference |
|---|---|---|
| IR21 | e14$^-$(*mcrA*$^-$) Δ*dam*::*metB* Δ(*mrr-hsdRMS-mcrBC*)114::*IS10 rpsL*104 (Str$^R$) | [41] |
| IR24 | e14$^-$(*mcrA*$^-$) Δ*dcm*::*lacZ* Δ(*mrr-hsdRMS-mcrBC*)114::*IS10 rpsL*104 (Str$^R$) | [41] |
| IR27 | e14$^-$(*mcrA*$^-$) Δ*dam*::*metB* Δ*dcm*::*lacZ* Δ(*mrr-hsdRMS-mcrBC*)114::*IS10 rpsL*104 (Str$^R$) | [40] |
| ET12567 | *dam*-13::*Tn9* (Cm$^R$) *dcm*-6 *hsdRMzjj*-202::*Tn10* (Tet$^R$) *rpsL*136 (Str$^R$) | [77] |
| IBEC58 | Δ*dam* Δ*dcm* Δ*hsdRMS* | [35] |
| HST04 | Δ(*mrr-hsdRMS-mcrBC*) Δ*mcrA dam dcm rpsL* (Str$^R$) | TB |
| JM110 | *dam dcm rpsL* (Str$^R$) | AT |
| SCS110 | *dam dcm rpsL* (Str$^R$) *endA* | AT |
| INV110 | *dam dcm* Δ(*mrr-hsdRMS-mcrBC*)102::*Tn10* (Tet$^R$) *rps*L (Str$^R$) *endA* | LT |
| GM48 | *dam*-3 *dcm*-6 | CGSC |
| GM272 | *dam*-3 *dcm*-6 *hsdS*21 | CGSC |
| GM2929 | *dam*-13::*Tn9* (Cm$^R$) *dcm*-6 *hsdR2 mcrA mcrB rpsL*136 (Str$^R$) | CGSC |

**Table 4.** *E. coli* strains deficient in genes involved in DNA methylation and/or DNA restriction.Cm$^R$: chloramphenicol resistance; Tet$^R$: tetracycline resistance; Str$^R$: streptomycin resistance; TB: Takara Bio Inc. (www.takara-bio.com); AT: Agilent Technologies Inc. (home.agilent.com); LT: Life Technologies Corporation (www.lifetechnologies.com); and CGSC: The Coli Genetic Stock Center (cgsc.biology.yale.edu).

### 3.4. Alternative methods for circumventing RM systems

In addition to host-mimicking strategies, there are some simple approaches for circumventing RM systems. One is to abolish sites recognized by RM systems. In *Clostridium difficile* transformation, five *Cdi*I sites in plasmids were abolished and used to demonstrate improved efficiency [56]. Similarly, a plasmid with three abolished *Sac*II sites was used for efficient transformation of *Bifidobacterium longum* [53]. When methyltransferase enzymes or genes are unavailable, this approach can be an effective alternative. One other approach is to reduce the restriction activity in the target bacterium temporarily by heat treatment. In *B. amyloliquefaciens* transformation, heat treatment at 46°C for 6 min increased transformation efficiency [78]. More forcible heat treatment (higher temperature and longer time) inactivates RM systems more efficiently but concurrently reduces viability of cells. Although this approach is very simple and is available for most bacteria, the heat conditions required for inactivating RM systems are not predictable and thereby may have to be determined by repeated trials.

## 4. Conclusion

In this chapter, RM systems are reviewed and some approaches to produce host-mimicking DNA are described. Analysis of chromosomal DNA using HPLC is a simple method to elucidate functional RM systems in target bacterium, and is therefore highly recommended for establishing bacterial transformation methods. When negligible DNA methylation is observed, methyl-free DNA is suitable for transformation of the bacterium. On the other hand, when significant DNA methylation is observed, a host-mimicking strategy involving methylation needs to be utilized. One weak point of this strategy is that there are no methods to exhaustively, readily, and rapidly determine methylation sites in target bacterium. When this analytical method becomes more widespread, this strategy will become a crucial technique for establishing efficient bacterial transformation methods.

## Acknowledgements

This work was supported by Grant-in-Aid for Young Scientists (B) of Japan Society for the Promotion of Science (20780080 and in part 23750083). The author would like to thank Enago (www.enago.jp) for the English language review.

## Author details

Hirokazu Suzuki*

Address all correspondence to: hirokap@xpost.plala.or.jp

Faculty of Agriculture, Kyushu University, Japan

## References

[1] Griffith, F. (1928). The Significance of Pneumococcal Types. *J. hyg. (Lond)*, 27, 113-159.

[2] Avery, O. T., MacLeod, C. M., & McCarty, M. (1944). Studies on the Chemical Nature of the Substance Inducing Transformation of Pneumococcal Types: Induction of Transformation by a Desoxyribonucleic Acid Fraction Isolated from Pneumococcus Type III. *J. exp. med.*, 79, 137-158.

[3] McCarty, M., & Avery, O. T. (1946). Studies on the Chemical Nature of the Substance Inducing Transformation of Pneumococcal Types: II. Effect of Desoxyribonuclease on the Biological Activity of the Transforming Substance. *J. exp. med.*, 83, 89-96.

[4] McCarty, M., & Avery, O. T. (1946). Studies on the Chemical Nature of the Substance Inducing Transformation of Pneumococcal types: III. An Improved Method for the Isolation of the Transforming Substance and its Application to Pneumo coccus Types II, III, and VI. *J. exp. med.*, 83, 97-104.

[5] Spizizen, J. (1958). Transformation of Biochemically Deficient Strains of Bacillus subtilis by Deoxyribonucleate. *Proc. natl. acad. sci. USA.*, 44, 1072-1078.

[6] Mandel, M., & Higa, A. (1970). Calcium-dependent Bacteriophage DNA Infection. *J. mol. biol.*, 53, 159-162.

[7] Aune, T. E., & Aachmann, F. L. (2010). Methodologies to Increase the Transformation Efficiencies and the Range of Bacteria that can be Transformed. *Appl. microbiol. biotechnol.*, 85, 1301-1313.

[8] Roberts, R. J., Belfort, M., Bestor, T., Bhagwat, A. S., Bickle, T. A., Bitinaite, J., Blumenthal, R. M., Degtyarev, S. K., Dryden, D. T. F., Dybvig, K., Firman, K., Gromova, E. S., Gumport, R. I., Halford, S. E., Hattman, S., Heitman, J., Hornby, D. P., Janulaitis, A., Jeltsch, A., Josephsen, J., Kiss, A., Klaenhammer, T. R., Kobayashi, I., Kong, H., Krüger, D. H., Lacks, S., Marinus, M. G., Miyahara, M., Morgan, R. D., Murray, N. E., Nagaraja, V., Piekarowicz, A., Pingoud, A., Raleigh, E., Rao, D. N., Reich, N., Repin, V. E., Selker, E. U., Shaw, P. C., Stein, D. C., Stoddard, B. L., Szybalski, W., Trautner, T. A., Van Etten, J. L., Vitor, J. M. B., Wilson, G. G., & Xu, S. Y. (2003). A Nomenclature for Restriction Enzymes, DNA Methyltransferases, Homing Endonucleases and their Genes. *Nucleic acids res.*, 31, 1805-1812.

[9] Arber, W., & Dussoix, D. (1962). Host Specificity of DNA Produced by Escherichia coli: I. Host Controlled Modification of Bacteriophage. *J. mol. biol.*, 5, 18-36.

[10] Roberts, R. J., Vincze, T., Posfai, J., & Macelis, D. (2003). REBASE: Restriction Enzymes and Methyltransferases. *Nucleic acids res.*, 31, 418-420.

[11] Roberts, R. J., Vincze, T., Posfai, J., & Macelis, D. (2010). REBASE-a Database for DNA Restriction and Modification: Enzymes, Genes and Genomes. *Nucleic acids res.*, 38, D 234-D236.

[12] Kobayashi, I. (2001). Behavior of Restriction-Modification Systems as Selfish Mobile Elements and their Impact on Genome Evolution. *Nucleic acids res.*, 29, 3742-3756.

[13] Snyder, L., Gold, L., & Kutter, E. (1976). A Gene of Bacteriophage T4 whose Product Prevents True Late Transcription on Cytosine-containing T4 DNA. *Proc. natl. acad. sci. USA.*, 73, 3098-3102.

[14] Moréra, S., Imberty, A., Aschke-Sonnenborn, U., Rüger, W., & Freemont, P. S. (1999). T4 Phage β-Glucosyltransferase: Substrate Binding and Proposed Catalytic Mechanism. *J. mol. biol.*, 292, 717-730.

[15] Kriaucionis, S., & Heintz, N. (2009). The Nuclear DNA Base 5-Hydroxymethylcytosine is Present in Purkinje Neurons and the Brain. *Science*, 324, 929-930.

[16] Münzel, M., Globisch, D., & Carell, T. (2011). Hydroxymethylcytosine, the Sixth Base of the Genome. *Angew. chem. int. ed.*, 50, 6460-6468.

[17] Tahiliani, M., Koh, K. P., Shen, Y., Pastor, W. A., Bandukwala, H., Brudno, Y., Agarwal, S., Iyer, L. M., Liu, D. R., Aravind, L., & Rao, A. (2009). Conversion of 5-Methylcytosine to 5-Hydroxymethylcytosine in Mammalian DNA by MLL Partner TET1. *Science*, 324, 930-935.

[18] Wu, H., & Zhang, Y. (2011). Mechanisms and Functions of Tet Protein-mediated 5-Methylcytosine Oxidation. *Genes dev.*, 25, 2436-2452.

[19] Zheng, Y., Cohen-Karni, D., Xu, D., Chin, H. G., Wilson, G., Pradhan, S., & Roberts, R. J. (2010). A Unique Family of Mrr-like Modification-dependent Restriction Endonucleases. *Nucleic acids res.*, 38, 5527-5534.

[20] Bair, C. L., & Black, L. W. (2007). A Type IV Modification Dependent Restriction Nuclease that Targets Glucosylated Hydroxymethyl Cytosine Modified DNAs. *J. mol. biol.*, 366, 768-778.

[21] Xu, S. Y., Corvaglia, A. R., Chan, S. H., Zheng, Y., & Linder, P. (2011). A Type IV Modification-dependent Restriction Enzyme SauUSI from Staphylococcus aureus subsp. aureus USA300. *Nucleic acids res.*, 39, 5597-5610.

[22] Zhou, X., He, X., Liang, J., Li, A., Xu, T., Kieser, T., Helmann, J. D., & Deng, Z. (2005). A Novel DNA Modification by sulphur. *Mol. microbiol.*, 57, 1428-1438.

[23] Wang, L. R., Chen, S., Xu, T., Taghizadeh, K., Wishnok, J. S., Zhou, X., You, D., Deng, Z., & Dedon, P. C. (2007). Phosphorothioation of DNA in Bacteria by dnd Genes. *Nat. chem. biol.*, 3, 709-710.

[24] Xu, T., Yao, F., Zhou, X., Deng, Z., & You, D. (2010). A Novel Host-specific Restriction System Associated with DNA Backbone S-Modification in Salmonella. *Nucleic acids res.*, 38, 7133-7141.

[25] Wang, L., Chen, S., Vergin, K. L., Giovannoni, S. J., Chan, S. W., De Mott, M. S. , Taghizadeh, K., Cordero, O. X., Cutler, M., Timberlake, S., Alm, E. J., Polz, M. F., Pinhassi, J., Deng, Z., & Dedon, P. C. (2011). DNA Phosphorothioation is Widespread and Quantized in Bacterial Genomes. *Proc. natl. acad. sci. USA.*, 108, 2963-2968.

[26] Liu, G., Ou, H. Y., Wang, T., Li, L., Tan, H., Zhou, X., Rajakumar, K., Deng, Z., & He, X. (2010). Cleavage of Phosphorothioated DNA and Methylated DNA by the Type IV Restriction Endonuclease ScoMcrA. *PLoS genet.*, 6, e1001253.

[27] Murray, N. E. (2000). Type I Restriction Systems: Sophisticated Molecular Machines (A Legacy of Bertani and Weigle). *Microbiol. mol. biol. rev.*, 64, 412-434.

[28] Kennaway, C. K., Obarska-Kosinska, A., White, J. H., Tuszynska, I., Cooper, L. P., Bujnicki, J. M., Trinick, J., & Dryden, D. T. F. (2009). The Structure of M.EcoKI Type I

DNA Methyltransferase with a DNA Mimic Antirestriction Protein. *Nucleic acids res.*, 37, 762-770.

[29] Ryu, J., & Rowsell, E. (2008). Quick Identification of Type I Restriction Enzyme Isoschizomers Using Newly Developed pTypeI and Reference Plasmids. *Nucleic acids res.*, 36, e81.

[30] Nagaraja, V., Stieger, M., Nager, C., Hadi, S. M., & Bickle, T. A. (1985). The Nucleotide Sequence Recognized by the Escherichia coli D Type-I Restriction and Modification Enzyme. *Nucleic acids res.*, 13, 389-399.

[31] García, L. R., & Molineux, I. J. (1999). Translocation and Specific Cleavage of Bacteriophage T7 DNA in vivo by EcoKI. *Proc. natl. acad. sci. USA.*, 96, 12430-12435.

[32] Yuan, R., Hamilton, D. L., & Burckhardt, J. (1980). DNA Translocation by the Restriction Enzyme from E. coli K. *Cell*, 20, 237-244.

[33] Dryden, D. T. F., Edwardson, J. M., & Henderson, R. M. (2011). DNA Translocation by Type III Restriction Enzymes: A Comparison of Current Models of their Operation Derived from Ensemble and Single-molecule Measurements. *Nucleic acids res.*, 39, 4525-4531.

[34] Sutherland, E., Coe, L., & Raleigh, E. A. (1992). McrBC: A Multisubunit GTP-dependent Restriction Endonuclease. *J. mol. biol.*, 225, 327-348.

[35] González-Cerón, G., Miranda-Olivares, O. J., & Servín-González, L. (2009). Characterization of the Methyl-specific Restriction System of Streptomyces coelicolor A3(2) and of the Role Played by Laterally Acquired Nucleases. *FEMS microbiol. lett.*, 301, 35-43.

[36] Waite-Rees, P. A., Keating, C. J., Moran, L. S., Slatko, B. E., Hornstra, L. J., & Benner, J. S. (1991). Characterization and Expression of the Escherichia coli Mrr Restriction System. *J. bacteriol.*, 173, 5207-5219.

[37] Mulligan, E. A., Hatchwell, E., McCorkle, S. R., & Dunn, J. J. (2010). Differential Binding of Escherichia coli McrA Protein to DNA Sequences that Contain the Dinucleotide m5CpG. *Nucleic acids res.*, 38, 1997-2005.

[38] Kurosawa, N., & Grogan, D. W. (2005). Homologous Recombination of Exogenous DNA with the Sulfolobus acidocaldarius Genome: Properties and Uses. *FEMS microbiol. lett.*, 253, 141-149.

[39] Gehrke, C. W., McCune, R. A., Gama-Sosa, M. A., Ehrlich, M., & Kuo, K. C. (1984). Quantitative Reversed-phase High-performance Liquid Chromatography of Major and Modified Nucleosides in DNA. *J. chromatogr.*, 301, 199-219.

[40] Suzuki, H., Takahashi, S., Osada, H., & Yoshida, K. (2011). Improvement of Transformation Efficiency by Strategic Circumvention of Restriction Barriers in Streptomyces griseus. *J. microbiol. biotechnol.*, 21, 675-678.

[41] Suzuki, H., & Yoshida, K. (2012). Genetic Transformation of Geobacillus kaustophilus HTA426 by Conjugative Transfer of Host-mimicking Plasmids. *J. microbiol. biotechnol.*, 22, 1279-1287.

[42] Annan, R. S., Kresbach, G. M., Giese, R. W., & Vouros, P. (1989). Trace Detection of Modified DNA Bases via Moving-belt Liquid Chromatography-Mass Spectrometry Using Electrophoretic Derivatization and Negative Chemical Ionization. *J. chromatogr.*, 465, 285-296.

[43] del Gaudio, R., Di Giaimo, R., & Geraci, G. (1997). Genome Methylation of the Marine Annelid Worm Chaetopterus variopedatus: Methylation of a CpG in an Expressed H1 Histone Gene. *FEBS lett.*, 417, 48-52.

[44] Ehrlich, M., Wilson, G. G., Kuo, K. C., & Gehrke, C. W. (1987). $N^4$-Methylcytosine as a Minor Base in Bacterial DNA. *J. bacteriol.*, 169, 939-943.

[45] Ehrlich, M., Gama-Sosa, M. A., Carreira, L. H., Ljungdahl, L. G., Kuo, K. C., & Gehrke, C. W. (1985). DNA Methylation in Thermophilic Bacteria: $N^4$-Methylcytosine, 5-Methylcytosine, and $N^6$-Methyladenine. *Nucleic acids res.*, 13, 1399-1412.

[46] Banerjee, S., & Chowdhury, R. (2006). An Orphan DNA (Cytosine-5-)-Methyltransferase in Vibrio cholerae. *Microbiology*, 152, 1055-1062.

[47] Störl, H. J., Simon, H., & Barthelmes, H. (1979). Immunochemical Detection of $N^6$-Methyladenine in DNA. *Biochim. biophys. acta.*, 564, 23-30.

[48] Lin, L. F., Posfai, J., Roberts, R. J., & Kong, H. (2001). Comparative Genomics of the Restriction-Modification Systems in Helicobacter pylori. *Proc. natl. acad. sci. USA.*, 98, 2740-2745.

[49] Kong, H., Lin, L. F., Porter, N., Stickel, S., Byrd, D., Posfai, J., & Roberts, R. J. (2000). Functional Analysis of Putative Restriction-Modification System Genes in the Helicobacter pylori J99 Genome. *Nucleic acids res.*, 28, 3216-3223.

[50] Sitaraman, R., & Leppla, S. H. (2012). Methylation-dependent DNA Restriction in Bacillus anthracis. *Gene*, 494, 44-50.

[51] Groot, M. N., Nieboer, F., & Abee, T. (2008). Enhanced Transformation Efficiency of Recalcitrant Bacillus cereus and Bacillus weihenstephanensis Isolates Upon in vitro Methylation of Plasmid DNA. *Appl. environ. microbiol.*, 74, 7817-7820.

[52] Yasui, K., Kano, Y., Tanaka, K., Watanabe, K., Shimizu-Kadota, M., Yoshikawa, H., & Suzuki, T. (2009). Improvement of Bacterial Transformation Efficiency Using Plasmid Artificial Modification. *Nucleic acids res.*, 37, e3.

[53] Kim, J. Y., Wang, Y., Park, M. S., & Ji, G. E. (2010). Improvement of Transformation Efficiency Through in vitro Methylation and SacII Site Mutation of Plasmid Vector in Bifidobacterium longum MG1. *J. microbiol. biotechnol.*, 20, 1022-1026.

[54] Chen, Q., Fischer, J. R., Benoit, V. M., Dufour, N. P., Youderian, P., & Leong, J. M. (2008). In vitro CpG Methylation Increases the Transformation Efficiency of Borrelia

burgdorferi Strains Harboring the Endogenous Linear Plasmid lp56. *J. bacteriol.*, 190, 7885-7891.

[55] Mermelstein, L. D., & Papoutsakis, E. T. (1993). In vivo Methylation in Escherichia coli by the Bacillus subtilis Phage ϕ 3T I Methyltransferase to Protect Plasmids from Restriction Upon Transformation of Clostridium acetobutylicum ATCC 824. *Appl. environ. microbiol.*, 59, 1077-1081.

[56] Purdy, D., O'Keeffe, T. A., Elmore, M., Herbert, M., McLeod, A., Bokori-Brown, M., Ostrowski, A., & Minton, N. P. (2002). Conjugative Transfer of Clostridial Shuttle Vectors from Escherichia coli to Clostridium difficile Through Circumvention of the Restriction Barrier. *Mol. microbiol.*, 46, 439-452.

[57] Tyurin, M. V., Desai, S. G., & Lynd, L. R. (2004). Electrotransformation of Clostridium thermocellum. *Appl. environ. microbiol.*, 70, 883-890.

[58] Donahue, J. P., Israel, D. A., Peek, R. M., Blaser, M. J., & Miller, G. G. (2000). Overcoming the Restriction Barrier to Plasmid Transformation of Helicobacter pylori. *Mol. microbiol.*, 37, 1066-1074.

[59] Bullas, L. R., & Ryu, J. I. (1983). Salmonella typhimurium LT2 Strains which are $r^- m^+$ for All Three Chromosomally Located Systems of DNA Restriction and Modification. *J. bacteriol.*, 156, 471-474.

[60] Schenk, S., & Laddaga, R. A. (1992). Improved Method for Electroporation of Staphylococcus aureus. *FEMS microbiol. lett.*, 94, 133-138.

[61] MacNeil, D. J. (1988). Characterization of a Unique Methyl-specific Restriction System in Streptomyces avermitilis. *J. bacteriol.*, 170, 5607-5612.

[62] Zotchev, S. B., Schrempf, H., & Hutchinson, C. R. (1995). Identification of a Methyl-specific Restriction System Mediated by a Conjugative Element from Streptomyces bambergiensis. *J. bacteriol.*, 177, 4809-4812.

[63] Yamazaki, H., Ohnishi, Y., & Horinouchi, S. (2003). Transcriptional Switch on of ssgA by A-factor, which is Essential for Spore Septum Formation in Streptomyces griseus. *J. bacteriol.*, 185, 1273-1283.

[64] Kwak, J., Jiang, H., & Kendrick, K. E. (2002). Transformation Using in vivo and in vitro Methylation in Streptomyces griseus. *FEMS microbiol. lett.*, 209, 243-248.

[65] Enríquez, L. L., Mendes, M. V., Antón, N., Tunca, S., Guerra, S. M., Martín, J. F., & Aparicio, J. F. (2006). An Efficient Gene Transfer System for the Pimaricin Producer Streptomyces natalensis. *FEMS microbiol. lett.*, 257, 312-318.

[66] Lin, L., Song, H., Ji, Y., He, Z., Pu, Y., Zhou, J., & Xu, J. (2010). Ultrasound-mediated DNA Transformation in Thermophilic Gram-positive Anaerobes. *PLoS one*, 5, e12582.

[67] Militello, K. T., Simon, R. D., Qureshi, M., Maines, R., Van Horne, M. L., Hennick, S. M., Jayakar, S. K., & Pounder, S. (2012). Conservation of Dcm-mediated Cytosine DNA Methylation in Escherichia coli. *FEMS microbiol. lett.*, 328, 78-85.

[68] Marinus, M. G., & Casadesus, J. (2009). Roles of DNA Adenine Methylation in Host-pathogen Interactions: Mismatch Repair, Transcriptional Regulation, and More. *FEMS microbiol. rev.*, 33, 488-503.

[69] Brena, R. M., Huang, T. H. M., & Plass, C. (2006). Quantitative Assessment of DNA Methylation: Potential Applications for Disease Diagnosis, Classification, and Prognosis in Clinical Settings. *J. mol. med.*, 84, 365-377.

[70] Oakeley, E. J. (1999). DNA Methylation Analysis: A Review of Current Methodologies. *Pharmacol. ther.*, 84, 389-400.

[71] Harrison, A., & Parle-McDermott, A. (2011). DNA Methylation: A Timeline of Methods and Applications. *Front genet.*, 2, 74.

[72] Fouse, S. D., Nagarajan, R. P., & Costello, J. F. (2010). Genome-scale DNA Methylation Analysis. *Epigenomics*, 2, 105-117.

[73] Sulewska, A., Niklińska, W., Kozlowski, M., Minarowski, L., Naumnik, W., Niklinski, J., Dąbrowska, K., & Chyczewski, L. (2007). Detection of DNA Methylation in Eucaryotic Cells. *Folia histochem. cytobiol.*, 45, 315-324.

[74] Eid, J., Fehr, A., Gray, J., Luong, K., Lyle, J., Otto, G., Peluso, P., Rank, D., Baybayan, P., Bettman, B., Bibillo, A., Bjornson, K., Chaudhuri, B., Christians, F., Cicero, R., Clark, S., Dalal, R., de Winter, A., Dixon, J., Foquet, M., Gaertner, A., Hardenbol, P., Heiner, C., Hester, K., Holden, D., Kearns, G., Kong, X., Kuse, R., Lacroix, Y., Lin, S., Lundquist, P., Ma, C., Marks, P., Maxham, M., Murphy, D., Park, I., Pham, T., Phillips, M., Roy, J., Sebra, R., Shen, G., Sorenson, J., Tomaney, A., Travers, K., Trulson, M., Vieceli, J., Wegener, J., Wu, D., Yang, A., Zaccarin, D., Zhao, P, Zhong, F., Korlach, J., & Turner, S. S. (2009). Real-time DNA Sequencing from Single Polymerase Molecules. *Science*, 323, 133-138.

[75] Flusberg, B. A., Webster, D., Lee, J. H., Travers, K. J., Olivares, E. C., Clark, T. A., Korlach, J., & Turner, S. W. (2010). Direct Detection of DNA Methylation During Single-molecule, Real-time Sequencing. *Nat. methods*, 7, 461-465.

[76] Bart, A., van Passel, M. W. J., van Amsterdam, K., & van der Ende, A. (2005). Direct Detection of Methylation in Genomic DNA. *Nucleic acids res.*, 33, e124.

[77] MacNeil, D. J., Gewain, K. M., Ruby, C. L., Dezeny, G., Gibbons, P. H., & MacNeil, T. (1992). Analysis of Streptomyces avermitilis Genes Required for Avermectin Biosynthesis Utilizing a Novel Integration Vector. *Gene*, 111, 61-68.

[78] Zhang, G. Q., Bao, P., Zhang, Y., Deng, A. H., Chen, N., & Wen, T. Y. (2011). Enhancing Electro-transformation Competency of Recalcitrant Bacillus amyloliquefaciens by Combining Cell-wall Weakening and Cell-membrane Fluidity Disturbing. *Anal. biochem.*, 409, 130-137.

Chapter 10

# Messenger RNA Cap Methylation in Vesicular Stomatitis Virus, a Prototype of Non-Segmented Negative-Sense RNA Virus

Jianrong Li and Yu Zhang

Additional information is available at the end of the chapter

http://dx.doi.org/10.5772/54598

## 1. Introduction

The non-segmented negative-sense (NNS) RNA viruses encompass a wide range of significant human, animal, and plant pathogens including several National Institute of Allergy and Infectious Diseases (NIAID) Category A and C biodefense pathogens. The NNS RNA viruses are classified into four families: the *Rhabdoviridae,* as exemplified by rabies virus and vesicular stomatitis virus (VSV); the *Paramyxoviridae,* as exemplified by human respiratory syncytial virus (RSV), human metapneumovirus (hMPV), human parainfluenza virus type 3 (PIV3), measles virus, mump virus, Newcastle disease virus (NDV), Nipah virus, and Hendra virus; the *Filoviridae,* as exemplified by Ebola and Marburg viruses; and the *Bornaviridae,* as exemplified by Borna disease virus. For many of these viruses, there are no effective vaccines or anti-viral drugs. RSV, hMPV, and PIV3 account for more than 70% of acute viral respiratory diseases, especially in infants, children, and the elderly [1, 2]. hPIV 1-3 have been recognized as the causative agents of croup since the late 1950's [3]. In addition, measles remains a major killer of children worldwide, despite successful vaccination programs in developed countries [4]. The most virulent strains of NDV, the viscerotropic velogenic strains (often called "exotic" NDV), are classified as High Consequence Livestock Pathogens by USDA due to their potential as agents of agricultural bioterrorism [5].

Messenger RNA modification is the essential issue in NNS RNA virus gene expression and replication. During viral RNA synthesis, NNS RNA viruses produce capped, methylated, and polyadenylated mRNAs [6-8]. Cap formation is essential for mRNA stability, efficient translation, and gene expression [9-11]. It is now firmly established that mRNA capping and methylation in NNS RNA viruses evolves in a mechanism distinct to their hosts [12-19]. Thus, mRNA cap formation is an attractive antiviral target for NNS RNA viruses. For decades, VSV has been used as a model to understand the replication and gene expression of NNS RNA viruses. Most of our understanding of mRNA modifications of NNS RNA viruses comes from studies of VSV, a prototype of the *Rhabdoviridae* family. Using VSV as a model, we will discuss (i) the unusual mechanism of mRNA capping and cap methylation; (ii) the impact of viral mRNA cap methylation in viral life cycle and viral pathogenesis; and (iii) the applications of viral mRNA cap methylation in the development of novel vaccines and broadly-active anti-viral agents.

## 2. Overview diagram of VSV mRNA synthesis and modifications

### 2.1. The structure of VSV virions

VSV virions are bullet-shaped particles 170 nm in length and 80 nm in diameter (Fig.1). Among NNS RNA viruses, VSV has the simplest RNA genome consisting of 11,161 nucleotides (nt) organized into five VSV genes encoding nucleocapsid (N), phospho- (P), matrix (M), glyco- (G), and large (L) proteins, and leader and trailer regulatory sequences arranged in the order 3'-(leader), N, P, M, G, L, (trailer)-5'[20-23]. Like all NNS RNA viruses, the genome is encapsidated with the N protein to form a nuclease-resistant helical N-RNA complex that is the functional template for mRNA synthesis as well as genomic RNA replication. The N-RNA complex is tightly associated with the viral RNA-dependent RNA polymerase (RdRp), which is comprised of the 241-kDa L protein catalytic subunit and the 29-kDa essential P protein cofactor, and results in the assembly of a viral ribonucleoprotein (RNP) complex [24, 25]. This structure contains the minimum virus encoded components of the VSV RNA synthesis machinery [26]. The RNP complex is further surrounded by the M protein which plays a crucial role in virus assembly, budding, and maintenance of the structural integrity of the virus particle [27]. The outer membrane of virion is the envelope composed of a cellular lipid bilayer. The transmembrane G protein is anchored in the viral envelope, which is essential for receptor binding and cell entry [28].

### 2.2. VSV life cycle

The overview picture of VSV life cycle is depicted in Fig.2. Upon attaching to an unknown cell receptor(s), VSV enters host cells via receptor mediated endocytosis [29]. Following low pH triggered fusion and uncoating, the RNP complex is delivered into the cytoplasm where RNA synthesis and viral replication occur [30]. During primary transcription, the input RdRp recognizes the specific signals in the N-RNA template to transcribe six discrete RNAs: a 47-nucleotide leader RNA (Le+), which is neither capped nor polyadenylated, and 5 mRNAs that are capped and methylated at the 5′ end and polyadenylated at the 3′end. These mature mRNAs are then translated by host ribosomes to yield functional viral proteins which are required for viral genome replication. During replication, the RdRP initiates at the extreme 3′ end of the genome and synthesizes a full-length complementary antigenome, which subsequently serves as template for synthesis of full-length progeny genomes. These progeny genomes can then be utilized as templates for secondary transcription, or assembled into infectious particles. Finally, viral proteins and genomic RNA are assembled into complete virus particles and the virus exits the cell by budding through the plasma membrane.

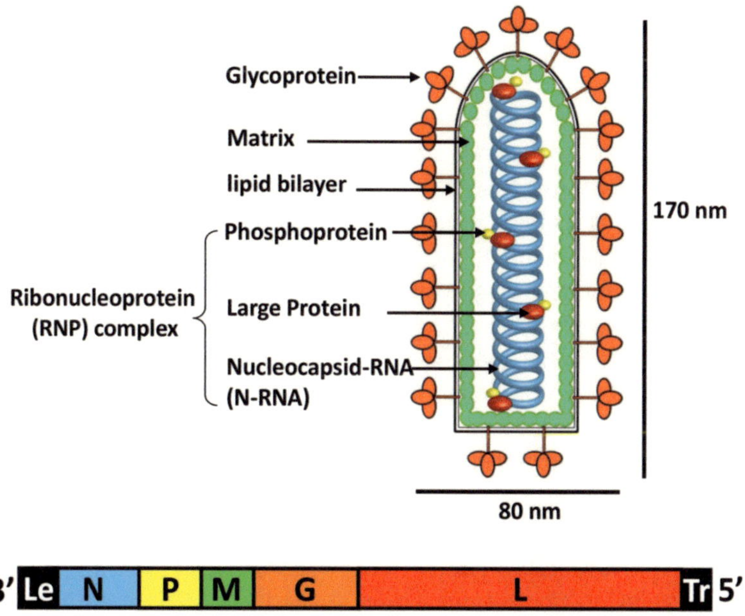


**Figure 1. VSV virion structure and genome organization.** VSV encodes five structural proteins: nucleocapsid (N), phospho- (P), matrix (M), glyco- (G), and large (L) proteins. The VSV genome is arranged in the order 3'-(leader), N, P, M, G, L, (trailer)-5'.

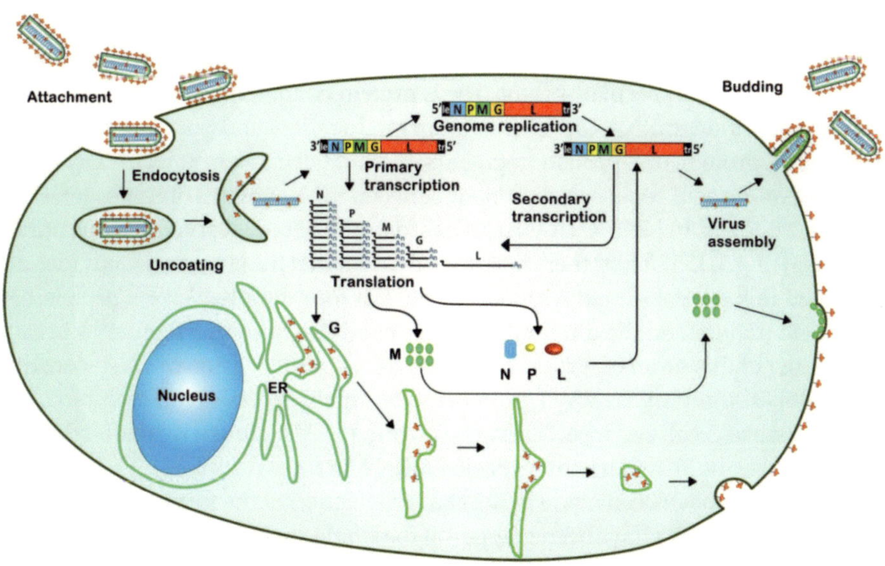


**Figure 2. Overview diagram of VSV life cycle**. Steps of virus life cycle: attachment, endocytosis, uncoating, genome replication, mRNA transcription, viral protein translation, viral assembly, and budding are shown.

### 2.3. VSV mRNA synthesis and modifications

Our current understanding of VSV mRNA synthesis and modification can be summarized as follows. In response to a specific promoter element provided by the genomic leader region, the polymerase initiates mRNA synthesis at the first gene-start sequence to synthesize N gene. The nascent mRNA is capped through an unconventional mechanism in which the GDP: polyribonucleotidyltransferase (PRNTase) of L transfers a monophosphate RNA onto a GDP acceptor through a covalent protein-RNA intermediate [12, 13, 16]. Following cap addition, VSV mRNAs are sequentially methylated at ribose 2′-O position and G-N-7 position, which is distinct from all known methylation reactions [17, 18]. Unlike traditional cap forming enzymes, the VSV capping and methylation machinery requires *cis*-acting signals in the RNA [12, 18, 31, 32]. When encountering a gene-end sequence, L polyadenylates and terminates mRNA synthesis by a programmed stuttering of the polymerase on a U7 tract [33, 34]. Termination at the end of the N gene is essential for the polymerase to initiate synthesis at the start of the next gene, to produce the P mRNA. During transcription, the RdRp complex transcribes the viral genome into five mRNAs in a sequential and gradient manner, such that 3′ proximal genes are transcribed more abundantly than 3′ distal genes [21-23]. This gradient of transcription reflects a poorly understood transcriptional attenuation event that is localized to the gene junction regions. Using this fashion, VSV produces five capped, methylated, and polyadenylated mRNAs, N, P, M, G, and L.

## 3. Large (L) polymerase protein, the multifunctional protein that modifies viral mRNA

All NNS RNA viruses encode a large (L) polymerase protein, a multifunctional protein ranging from 220-250kDa in molecular weight. The L protein contains enzymatic activities for nucleotide polymerization, mRNA cap addition, cap methylation, and polyadenylation. To date, the structure of L protein, or L protein fragments, has not been determined for any of the NNS RNA viruses. Amino acid sequence alignment between the L proteins of representative members of each family within NNS RNA viruses has identified six conserved regions numbered I to VI (CRs I–VI) (Fig.3) [35]. Thus, there is a general assent that the enzymatic activities of L protein are located in these conserved regions. For the last four decades, VSV L protein has been used a model to understand the different activities of NNS RNA virus L proteins because it is the only member of this order of viruses for which robust transcription can be reconstituted *in vitro* [6, 7, 21, 36]. In addition, the VSV L protein can be highly expressed in recombinant expression systems, such as E.coli and insect cells. The purified VSV L protein retains all the enzymatic activities that can modify short virus-specific mRNA *in trans* [12, 16, 18, 37]. In recent years, many breakthroughs have been made in the characterization of the function of VSV L protein and the enzymatic activities have been mapped at the single amino acid level (Fig.3). Within the primary sequence of L are six conserved regions shared among all NNS RNA virus L proteins. The RdRP activity has been identified in CR III and this region is also required for polyadenylation [38-40]. Consistent with this, a GDN motif is conserved in CR III of all NNS RNA virus L proteins and is functionally equivalent to the GDD polymerization motif characteristic of posi-

http://dx.doi.org/10.5772/54598

tive strand RdRPs. Mutations to the GDN motif of the VSV L protein inactivated polymerase function [40]. The mRNA capping enzyme maps to CR V [13, 16], and the capping activities of L differ from those of other viruses and their eukaryotic hosts. Specifically, an RNA:GDP PRNTase activity present within CR V transfers 5′ monophosphate RNA onto a GDP acceptor through a covalent L-pRNA intermediate [12, 13, 16]. The mRNA cap methyltransferases (MTase) map to CR VI [14, 17, 19]. Like the unconventional capping enzyme, methylation of the VSV mRNA cap structure is also unique in that mRNA cap is modified by a dual specificity MTase activity within CR VI whereby ribose 2′-O methylation precedes and facilitates subsequent guanine-N-7 (G-N-7) methylation [17, 18]. Although functions have not yet to be assigned to the other three conserved regions (CRs I, II, and IV), experiments with Sendai virus (SeV) have implicated CR I in binding P protein and CR II in binding the RNA template [41, 42].

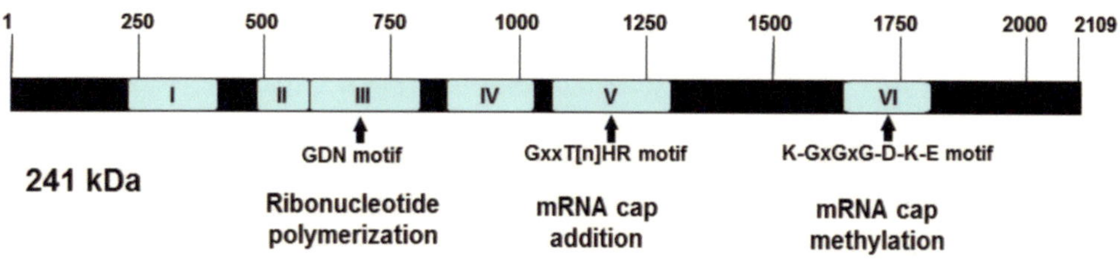


**Figure 3. Conserved regions in L proteins of NNS RNA viruses.** Six conserved regions numbered I to VI (CRs I–VI) in L protein are shown. Signature motifs for nucleotide polymerization, mRNA cap addition, and cap methylation are shown.

The location of the nucleotide polymerization, capping, and cap methylation activities within separate regions of L has led to the notion that L protein may be organized as a series of independent structural domains. Consistent with this idea, a fragment containing CRs V and VI of the SeV L protein were expressed independently and shown to retain the ability to methylate short RNAs that corresponded to the 5′ end of SeV mRNA [43]. In addition, recombinant VSV and measles virus can be recovered from infectious cDNA clones by inserting the coding sequence of green fluorescent protein between CR V and VI in L gene, suggesting that L protein folds and functions as a series of independent globular domains [44, 45]. Interestingly, mutations to a variable region between CRs V and VI (residues 1450–1481) affect mRNA cap MTase activity, feasibly suggesting that mutation to this hinge region may affect a conformational change in CR VI [46]. More recently, the molecular architecture of VSV L protein has been revealed using negative stain electron microscopy (EM) in combination with proteolytic digestion and deletion mapping [37]. It was found that VSV L protein is organized into a ring domain containing the RNA polymerase and an appendage of three globular domains containing the cap-forming activities. The capping enzyme maps to a globular domain, which is juxtaposed to the ring, and the cap methyltransferase maps to a more distal and flexibly connected globule. Interestingly, upon binding to P protein, L protein undergoes a significant structural rearrangement that may facilitate the coordination between mRNA synthesis and capping apparatus [37, 47].

# 4. An unconventional mRNA capping mechanism in VSV

## 4.1. Conventional mechanism of mRNA capping in eukaryotic cells

In eukaryotic cells, capping of mRNA is an early posttranscriptional event that is essential for subsequent processing, nuclear export, stability, and translation of mRNA [11, 48]. Cap formation is mediated by a series of enzymatic reactions (Fig.4A). First, the 5′ triphosphate end of the nascent mRNA chain (5′pppN-RNA) is hydrolyzed by an RNA triphosphatase (RTPase) to yield the diphosphate 5′ ppN-RNA. Second, an RNA guanylyltransferase (GTase) reacts with GTP to form a covalent enzyme-GMP intermediate and transfers GMP to 5′ppN-RNA via a 5′-5′ triphosphate linkage to yield 5′ GpppN-RNA. Typically, RNA GTases contain a signature Kx[D/N]G motif that functions as an active site for the capping reaction [11, 48, 49]. A lysine residue within Kx[D/N]G motif forms the enzyme-GMP covalent intermediate, prior to its transfer onto the diphosphate RNA acceptor [11, 48, 50]. This mRNA capping reaction is conserved among all eukaryotes.

Viruses are highly diverse in capping their mRNA. Many DNA viruses (such as vaccinia virus and baculovirus), double stranded RNA viruses (such as reovirus, rotavirus, and bluetongue virus), and single strand positive RNA viruses (such as West Nile virus, Fig.4B) utilize the conventional eukaryotic capping pathway [51-56]. It has been suggested that Kx[V/L/I]S motif serve as the GTase active site for reovirus and rotavirus [57]. Other viruses have evolved different mechanisms for acquiring their cap. For example, influenza virus and hantavirus furnish their mRNA with this structure by a cap-snatching mechanism, in which the viral polymerase steals host cell mRNA caps to prime viral mRNA synthesis [58, 59]. The alphaviruses, such as Sindbis, have evolved S-adenosyl-L-methionine(SAM)-dependent GTase activities that utilize distinct motifs (such as HxH motif) to transfer $7^{m}$Gp through a covalent histidine Gp intermediate to form the $7^{m}$GpppN cap [60].

## 4.2. An unconventional mRNA capping mechanism in VSV

In the early 1970′s, it was suggested that the cap structure of NNS viral mRNAs was formed by a mechanism which was unique from eukaryotic cap formation. For VSV [6], RSV [61], and spring viremia of carp virus [62], the two italicized phosphates of the 5′G*pp*p5′NpNpN triphosphate bridge have been shown to be derived from a GDP donor, rather than GMP. However, further studies on this mechanism have been seriously hampered due to the fact that the VSV capping events are tightly coupled to transcription and the capping machinery does not respond to exogenous transcripts. In 2007, this unique capping mechanism was revealed using a novel *trans* capping assay, in which a short mRNA corresponding to the first 5-nt of VSV gene start sequence was capped by a highly purified L protein in *trans* [12]. Specifically, capping of VSV mRNA was achieved by a novel polyribonucelotidyltransferase (PRNTase) which transferred a monophosphate RNA onto a GDP acceptor through a covalent L-RNA intermediate (Fig. 4C). In the first step, a GTPase associated with the VSV L protein removes the $\gamma$-phosphate group of GTP to generate GDP, an RNA acceptor. In the second step, the PRNTase activity of the L protein specifically transfers a 5′-monophosphorylated (p-) RNA moiety of pppRNA with the conserved VSV mRNA-start sequence (AACAG) to GDP to yield a GpppA capped mRNA. Interestingly, this

http://dx.doi.org/10.5772/54598

unusual VSV capping enzyme caps RNA in a sequence specific manner [12]. Specifically, VSV L protein efficiently capped pppApApCpApG (the mRNA gene start sequence), but not pppApCpGpApA (the leader RNA start sequence). In addition, the VSV L protein was not able to cap ppApApCpApG, suggesting that the L protein specifically recognizes the 5′-triphosphorylated AACAG. Further mutagenesis analysis has shown that the APuCNG (Pu, purine) sequence acts as a *cis*-acting element for the RNA capping reaction for the VSV L protein [12].

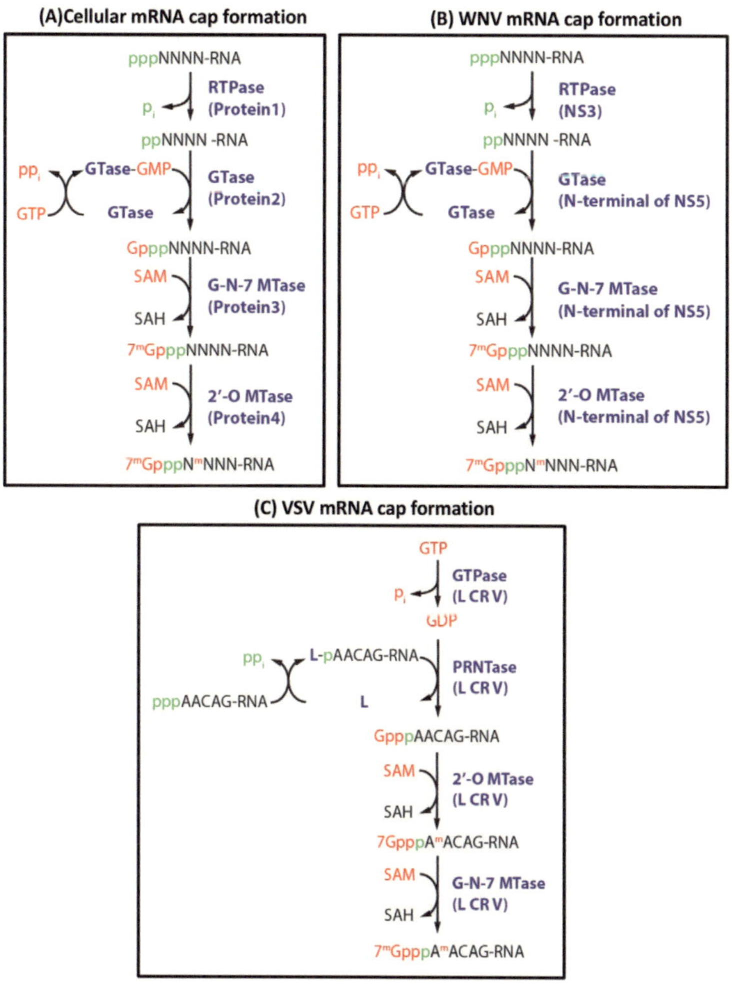


**Figure 4. Comparison of mRNA cap formation in eukaryotic cells, WNV, and VSV. (A) Cellular mRNA cap formation.** First, pppNNNN-RNA is hydrolyzed by an RNA triphosphatase (RTPase) to yield the diphosphate ppNNNN-RNA. Second, an RNA guanylyltransferase (GTase) transfers GMP to ppNNNN-RNA to yield GpppNNNN-RNA. Third, GpppNNNN-RNA is methylated by G-N-7 MTase to yield $7^{m}$GpppNNNN-RNA. Fourth, $7^{m}$GpppN-RNA is further methylated by a 2′-O MTase to yield $7^{m}$GpppN$^{m}$NNN-RNA. **(B) WNV mRNA cap formation.** First, pppNNNN-RNA is hydrolyzed by viral NS3 protein (RTPase) to yield ppNNNN-RNA. Second, viral NS5 protein (GTase) transfers GMP to ppNNNN-RNA to yield GpppNNNN-RNA. Third, GpppNNNN-RNA is methylated by N-terminus of NS5 (G-N-7 MTase) to yield $7^{m}$GpppNNNN-RNA. Fourth, $7^{m}$GpppN-RNA is further methylated by N-terminus of NS5 (2′-O MTase) to yield

$7^{m}$GpppN$^{m}$NNN-RNA. **(C) VSV mRNA cap formation.** First, a GTPase (CR V of L protein) removes the γ-phosphate group of GTP to generate GDP. Second, a polyribonucelotidyltransferase (PRNTase) (CR V of L protein) transfers a monophosphate RNA onto a GDP acceptor through a covalent L-RNA intermediate to GpppAACAG-RNA. Third, the cap structure is methylated a 2′-O MTase (CR VI of L protein) to yield GpppA$^{m}$ACAG-RNA. Fourth, GpppA$^{m}$ACAG-RNA is further methylated a G-N-7 MTase (CR VI of L protein) to yield $7^{m}$GpppA$^{m}$ACAG-RNA.

It has been a challenge to locate the active site for the novel PRNTase in the 241 kDa L protein. The only suggestive information regarding the location of the capping enzyme in L protein has come from the study of a novel inhibitor of the RSV polymerase which resulted in the synthesis of short uncapped viral RNAs *in vitro* [63]. Viral mutants resistant to this inhibitor were selected, and the resistance mutations were mapped to CR V, suggesting that CR V of L plays a role in mRNA cap formation. Sequence alignments of this region of L protein identified a total of 17 residues that were conserved among the NNS RNA viruses [16]. Guided by this information, an extensive mutagenesis analysis was performed within this region which led to the discovery of a new motif GxxT[n]HR composed of four amino acid residues (G1154A, T1157A, H1227A, and R1228A) in VSV L protein which are essential for mRNA cap formation [16]. *In vitro* RNA reconstitution assays have shown that these cap defective polymerases synthesized uncapped mRNAs that terminated prematurely. The size of these abortive transcripts ranged from 100 nt up to the full-length N mRNA, although the majority were less than 400 nt. Consistent with their inability to generate capped RNA during *in vitro* transcription reactions, G1154A, T1157A, H1227A, and R1228A were defective in *trans* capping of the 5-nt VSV gene start sequence, demonstrating that these amino acids in CR V of L protein are required for mRNA cap addition [16]. Importantly, GxxT[n]HR is highly conserved in the CR V of L proteins of all NNS RNA viruses, including Borna disease virus which replicates in nucleus. Further biochemical and mass spectrometric analyses found that H1227 in the conserved GxxT[n]HR motif of the VSV L protein is covalently linked to the 5′-monophosphate end of the RNA through a phosphoamide bond [13]. Therefore, amino acid residue H1227 is the active site of the PRNTase activity. Mutagenesis analysis also found that R1228A and R1228K mutations significantly decreased L-pRNA complex formation activities, suggesting that mutation in R1228 may affect the H1227-RNA intermediate formation [13]. Interestingly, this PRNTase activity was also found in L protein of Chandipura virus (CHPV), a rhabdovirus that is closely related to VSV [64]. Furthermore, mutations to HR motif in L protein of CHPV significantly reduced the formation of the L-pRNA covalent intermediates in the PRNTase reaction. These results demonstrate that this unconventional capping mechanism is conserved in the *Rhabdoviridae* family. Given the fact the HR motif is highly conserved in L proteins of NNS RNA viruses, it is likely that this novel capping mechanism is not only unique to rhadoviruses, but also may be utilized by other NNS RNA viruses.

## 5. An unusual mechanism of mRNA cap methylation in VSV

### 5.1. Conventional mRNA cap methylation in eukaryotic cells

In eukaryotic cells, the capped mRNA (GpppN-RNA) is typically methylated by two steps (Fig.4A) [65-68]. First, the capping guanylate is methylated by a G-N-7 methyltransferase

http://dx.doi.org/10.5772/54598

(MTase) to yield 7$^{m}$GpppN-RNA (cap 0). Second, the G-N-7 methylated cap structure can then be further methylated by a ribose-2′-O (2′-O) MTase to yield 7$^{m}$GpppN$^{m}$-RNA (cap 1). During mRNA cap methylation, S-adenosyl-L-methionine (SAM) serves as the methyl donor, and the by-product S-adenosyl-homocysteine (SAH) is the competitive inhibitor of the SAM-dependent MTase. These mRNA cap methylation reactions are conserved among all eukaryotes. In this conventional methylation reaction, G-N-7 methylation occurs prior to 2′-O methylation and the two methylase activities are carried out by two separate enzymes, each containing its own binding site for the methyl donor, SAM.

Many viruses encode their own mRNA cap methylaion machinery, the best-studied example of which is the poxvirus vaccinia virus. For vaccinia virus, the G-N-7 and 2′-O MTase activities are encoded by two separate viral proteins, D12L and VP39 [65, 68-70]. In the case of reovirus, G-N-7 and 2′-O MTases are catalyzed by two separate domains of the same viral polymerase protein [55, 71]. For VSV, G-N-7 and 2′-O MTases are accomplished by a single region (CR VI) located in the C terminus of viral polymerase protein, L (Fig.4C) [14, 17, 19]. Soon after the discovery of the dual MTase activities of VSV, the N terminus of flaviviruses polymerase protein (NS5) was found to encode both G-N-7 and 2′-O MTases (Fig.4B) [72-74]. In addition to this unusual dual MTase activity of CR VI, the order of mRNA cap methylation in VSV is unconventional in which 2′-O methylation precedes and facilitates the G-N-7 methylation [17, 18]. This is contrast to all known mRNA cap methylation reactions including flaviviruses.

### 5.2. A single MTase catalytic site in CR-VI of L protein essential for both G-N-7 and 2′-O methylation

The SAM-dependent MTase superfamily contains a series of conserved motifs (X and I to VIII) [75]. The crystal structure of several known 2′-O MTases including *E. coli* heat shock-induced methyltransferase RrmJ/FtsJ and vaccinia virus VP39 have been solved[67, 68, 70, 76]. In RrmJ, a catalytic tetrad of residues: K38, D124, K164, and E199 formed the active site of 2′-O MTase [67, 76]. Site-directed mutagenesis of RrmJ found that a catalytic triad of residues K38, D124, and K164 are essential for 2′-O MTase whereas E199 plays only a minor role in the methyltransferase reaction *in vitro*. In vaccinia virus VP39, four amino acids, K41, D138, K175, and E207, are essential for catalysis [68, 70]. By comparing the amino acid sequence of the RrmJ and VP39 with CR VI of the L protein of NNS RNA viruses, it was suggested that this region of L protein might function as a 2′-O MTase. Sequence alignments suggest that residues K1651, D1762, K1795, and E1833 of the VSV L protein correspond to a catalytic KDKE tetrad (Fig.5). In fact, this KDKE motif is conserved in CR VI of L proteins of all NNS RNA viruses with the exception of Borna disease virus. Li et al., (2005) performed an extensive mutagenesis analysis in this predicted MTase catalytic KDKE tetrad in VSV L protein [14]. Recombinant VSVs carrying individual substitutions to K1651, D1762, K1795, and E1833 were recovered from an infectious cDNA clone of VSV. Analysis of the cap structure of mRNA synthesized *in vitro* revealed that alterations to the predicted active site residues abolished both G-N-7- and ribose 2′-O MTase activities. This result demonstrated that a single KDKE tetrad in CR-VI of the VSV L protein is essential for mRNA cap G-N-7- and ribose 2′-O methylation [14]. Two models have been proposed to explain this result. One possibility is that CR VI functions as both G-N-7 and 2′-O MTases. However, this conflict the fact that all known G-N-7 and 2′-O MTases have distinct biochemistry during RNA methylation reactions. An alternative explanation is that there is a sequential model for VSV mRNA cap methylation in which the product of one MTase acts as the substrate for the second (discussed below).

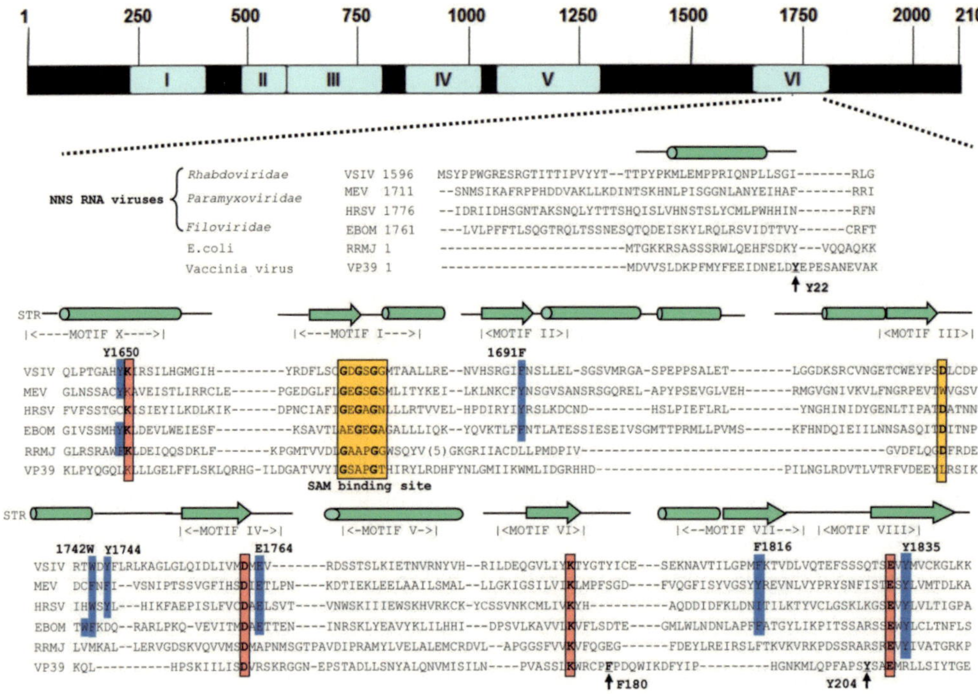


**Figure 5.** Structure-based amino acid sequence alignments of conserved domain VI of representative NNS RNA virus L proteins with known 2'-O methyltransferase, the *E. coli* RrmJ and vaccinia virus VP39. The conserved motifs (X and I to VIII) correspond to the SAM-dependent MTase superfamily. MTase catalytic site is shown by pink color. SAM binding site are shown by yellow color. Conserved aromatic residues are shown by blue color. Predicted alpha-helical regions are shown by the cylinders and the ß-sheet regions by the arrows. STR, structure of RrmJ and predicted structure for the NNS RNA viruses; EBOM, Ebola virus; VSIV, VSV Indiana type; HRSV, human respiratory syncytial virus; RRMJ, *E. coli* heat shock 2'-O MTase; VP39, vaccinia virus 2'-O MTase VP39.

http://dx.doi.org/10.5772/54598

### 5.3. A single SAM binding site in L protein essential for both G-N-7 and 2′-O methylation

The SAM-dependent MTase superfamily usually contains a G-rich motif (GxGxG) and an acidic residue (D/E) that is involved in SAM binding [75]. Sequence alignments between CR VI of NNS RNA virus L proteins and known MTases suggest that the SAM-binding residues of VSV L include G1670, G1672, G1674, G1675, and D1735 (Fig.5). Site-directed mutagenesis has been performed to define the roles of these amino acids in VSV mRNA methylation [17]. Each of these residues was individually substituted for alanine (A); or, for G4A, all four G residues were replaced with A; for G4AD, residue D1735 was also replaced with A. In addition, the flanking amino acid residues D1671 and S1673 within GDGSG motif were also substituted. Recombinant viruses were recovered from each of the *L* gene mutations. It was found that mutations to G1670, G1672, and S1673 specifically diminished G-N-7, but not 2′-O methylation, suggesting that 2′-O methylation occurs prior to G-N-7 methylation in VSV [17]. In contrast, mutants D1671, G4A, G4AD, G1675A, and D1735 were defective in both 2'-O and G-N-7 methylations. Interestingly, mutant G1674A requires a higher concentration of SAM to achieve full methylation compared with wild type VSV and methylation is more sensitive to SAH inhibition. Therefore, amino acid substitutions to the predicted SAM binding site disrupted methylation at the G-N-7 position or at both the G-N-7 and ribose 2′-O positions of the mRNA cap. However, none of these mutants are specifically defective in 2′-O methylation alone. These studies provide genetic evidence that the two methylase activities share one single SAM binding site and, in contrast to other cap methylation reactions, methylation of the G-N-7 position is not required for 2′-O methylation.

### 5.4. Mapping the potential RNA binding site that required for mRNA cap methylation

To acquire methylation, the MTase usually directly or indirectly contacts an RNA substrate. This putative substrate binding site is poorly understood in NNS RNA viruses. However, this substrate binding site has been identified in several cellular and viral mRNA 2'-O MTases [67, 68, 70, 74, 77, 78]. To achieve 2'-O methylation, the RNA substrate interacts with the cap recognition site which requires stacking between the base of the cap and aromatic rings from a MTase [76, 79, 80]. Vaccinia VP39 is one of the best characterized 2'-O MTases. In VP39, it was found that the recognition of a methylated base is achieved by stacking between two aromatic residues (Y22 and F180) and the methyl group is in contact with residue Y204 (Fig.6A) [68, 70, 79]. In addition, the carboxyl groups of residues D182 and E233 form hydrogen bonds with the NH and NH2 of the guanosine in VP39 (Fig.6A). Based on structure modeling and mutagenesis analysis, it was shown that residue F24 in West Nile virus (WNV) methylase (NS5) [81, 82] and Y29 and F173 in feline coronavirus 2'-O MTase (nsp16) [80] may play an equivalent role to residue Y22 in VP39 of vaccinia virus. The cellular cap binding protein-eukaryotic translation initiation factor 4E (eIF-4E) recognizes the cap by stacking between W56 and W102 [83]. In all known cases, aromatic residues are involved in cap binding and substrate recognition.

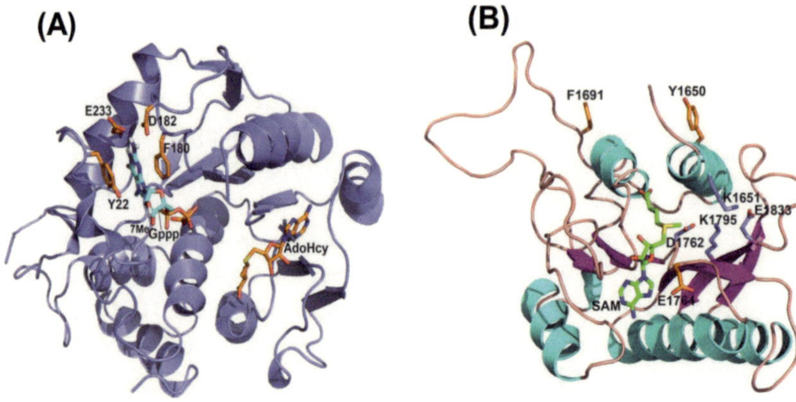


**Figure 6. The predicted structure of CR VI of VSV L protein. (A) Cap binding site of vaccinia virus 2'-O MTase, VP39**. The model was generated from the crystal structure of VP39 (PDB code: 1AV6) using PyMOL. The side chains of amino acid residues (Y22, F180, E233 and D182) involved in binding of $7^{m}$Gp cap are shown as sticks. **(B) The predicted structure of CR VI of VSV L protein**. The model was generated based on the previous predicted structure of VSV MTase (amino acid residue from 1644 to 1842 in L protein) using PyMOL software. Alpha helices are shown in blue and beta strands are shown in pink. SAM and the side chains of critical residues are shown in sticks, and the oxygen atoms and nitrogen atoms are shown in red and blue, respectively. For SAM molecule, the carbon atoms are green. For the three important amino acids (Y1650, F1691 and E1764) that may be involved in RNA substrate binding, their side-chain carbon atoms are highlighted in orange. For the predicted catalytic residues (K1651, D1762, K1795 and E1833), the carbon atoms are shown in purple.

Guided by this information, the putative RNA binding site in VSV L protein was searched through mutagenesis analysis of selected conserved residues in region VI of VSV L protein that were physiochemically similar to those involved in substrate recognition in VP39. Sequence alignment showed that there are a number of aromatic residues that are highly conserved in the MTase domain of L proteins of NNS RNA viruses (Fig. 5). Aromatic residues at positions 1650 (Y), 1691(F or Y), and 1835 (Y) are highly conserved in L proteins of NNS RNA viruses. Aromatic residues at positions 1742 (W), 1744 (Y), 1745 (F), and 1816 (F) are conserved in the L proteins of *Rhabdoviridae* and some *Paramyxoviridae* and *Filoviridae*. Therefore, these aromatic residues were selected as putative equivalents of Y22, F180, and Y204 in VP39. However, there is no amino acid precisely aligned with D182 and E233 in VP39. With the exception of two acidic amino acids in the catalytic site (K1651-D1762-K1795-E1833), position E1764 is also conserved in all L proteins. Thus, E1764 was selected as a candidate for mimicking the role of VP39 residues D182 and E233. In addition, two serine mutations at the two most conserved positions at 1693 and 1827 of VSV L protein was also examined, based on the fact that it has been shown that a serine residue was involved in RNA-protein interaction in *E. coli* 2'-O MTase, RRMJ [67, 77]. To determine the role of these amino acid residues in mRNA cap methylation, a single point mutation was introduced to an infectious clone of VSV and recombinant VSVs harboring these mutations were recovered [84]. The importance of the maintenance of the aromatic ring at amino acids Y1650 and F1691 was revealed by the observation that the substitution of Y1650 and F1691 with two other possible aromatic residues in the VSV infectious clone still produced viable recombinant viruses and produced a fully methylated mRNA cap, but alanine substitutions dramatically inhibited viral replication and completely blocked both G-N-7 and 2′-O methylation [84]. Based on the predicted structural model for the VSV MTase (amino acid residues from 1644 to 1842 in the L protein) (Fig.6B), the residues Y1650 and F1691 are located far from each other with a distance of 17.3 Å between their alpha carbon atoms. Y1650 is located in the middle of the first helix, and the F1691 is at the very C-terminal of the second helix. Perhaps, a stacking interaction with one aromatic residue causes a conformational and structural change in the VSV methylase, which results in the interaction with another aromatic residue. Changing of residue E1764 to D (maintenance of charge), Q (maintenance of size), or K (changing charge), even the very conservative change to D, dramatically inhibited both G-N-7 and 2'-O methylation [84]. The predicted structure of VSV MTase also shows that E1764, the residue adjacent to the catalytic residue D1762, is exposed to the putative SAM binding site (Fig.6B). The side chain of E1764 shows close contact to the adenyl group of SAM (3.1 Å). In addition, it was found that Y1835A was found to require a higher SAM concentration to achieve full methylation and it is more sensitive to MTase inhibitor [84].

To date, this work is the first attempt toward elucidation of the putative RNA substrate recognition site in the L protein of NNS RNA viruses, which has shed light on the possible role of several conserved aromatic amino acids, including Y1650 and F1691, in RNA binding during cap methylation. It would provide much more direct evidence for the role of these key amino acids in mediating RNA binding if the RNA binding efficiency could be measured directly. Attempts to use a gel shift assay have failed to this end [84], as the existence of multiple RNA binding sites in L protein with a size as large as 241-kDa posed a tremendous challenge in discerning the effect of single point mutation. The use of a truncated CR VI of VSV L for in vitro RNA binding assays might be a useful alternative strategy for future studies.

### 5.5. An unusual order for mRNA cap methylation in VSV

For conventional mRNA cap methylation, two separate MTases sequentially methylated the cap structure, first at the G-N-7 position and subsequently at the ribose 2′-O position [65, 66]. Analysis of the cap methylation of mRNA synthesized *in vitro* suggests that mRNA cap methylation in VSV is unusual, with methylation of ribose 2′-O occurring prior to G-N-7 methylation. First, early studies showed that at low concentrations of SAM, VSV mRNA was methylated at the 2′-O position only [85]. However, it could be chased into a doubly methylated cap structure at high SAM concentrations *in vitro*. Second, when *in vitro* mRNA synthesis was performed in the presence of MTase inhibitors such as SAH and sinefungin, G-N-7 methylation was inhibited prior to 2′-O methylation [86]. Third, a host range mutant of VSV, *hr*8, was shown to synthesize mRNA cap structures that lacked G-N-7 but were partially 2′-O-methylated [46, 87]. Finally, VSV mutants carrying mutations in the SAM binding site (such as G1670A, and G1672A) are specifically defective in G-N-7, but not 2′-O methylation [17].

This unusual order of VSV mRNA cap methylation was also biochemically demonstrated by a *trans*-methylation assay in which both ribose 2′-O and G-N-7 MTases were recapitulated by using purified recombinant L and *in vitro*-synthesized RNA [18]. It was found that VSV L modifies the 2′-O position of the cap prior to the G-N-7 position and that G-N-7 methylation is diminished by pre-2′-O methylation of the substrate RNA [18], providing compelling evidence that 2′-O methylation precedes and facilitates G-N-7 methylation. In light that both two MTase activities appear to reside in the same domain of L protein with the same SAM binding site, it is conceivable that mRNA cap and/or the SAM binding site might need to be repositioned at the end of the first methylation reaction to facilitate the second round of methylation. How this coordination happens *in vitro* is still a mystery. Bearing in mind that G-N-7 position is upstream of the ribose 2'-O position in the mRNA strand, reorientation is thus less likely to have resulted from forward movement of capped RNA through CR VI during transcription, but rather it might entail a fine spatial rearrangement. Collectively, these experiments have shown that the order of VSV mRNA cap methylation is distinct from all other known mRNA cap methylation mechanisms.

### 5.6. VSV methylases require *cis*-element in RNA

During mRNA synthesis, the VSV polymerase initiates synthesis at the first gene-start (GS) sequence (3′ UUGUCNNUAC 5′), and the nascent mRNA chain is capped and methylated, and recognizes a specific gene-end (GE) sequence (3′-AUACUUUUUUU-5′), the polymerase polyadenylates and terminates. It has been well demonstrated that the GS sequence contains a key *cis*-acting regulatory element for the initiation of mRNA synthesis [31, 32]. Specifically, the first three positions of the GS sequence have been found to be critical for mRNA synthesis. Recently, both *trans* capping assays with 5-nt oligo RNA substrates and detergent-activated virus transcription reactions pointed out the importance of positions 1, 2, 3, and 5 in mRNA cap addition, although position 5 substitutions were more tolerated [12, 31, 32]. Using a *trans* methylation assay, it was found that similar signals were required for mRNA cap methylation [18]. As expected, VSV L protein efficiently methylated a 110 nt of RNA with an authentic gene start sequence at position 2′-O. However, when the gene start sequence of this 110 nt was replaced with non-viral sequence (5′ GpppGGACGAAGAC-RNA), the efficiency of 2′-O methylation was reduced approximately 9 times. Similarly, VSV L protein efficiently methylated a pre-2′-O-methylated VSV mRNA at position G-N-7. In contrast, the efficiency of G-N-7 methylation decreased nearly 7 times when incubated with a substrate with non-VSV mRNA start RNA. Therefore, the gene start sequence of VSV mRNA contains a signal for initiation of mRNA synthesis, mRNA cap addition, and cap methylation.

### 5.7. The length of mRNA in cap methylation

In the *trans* mRNA capping assay, the VSV L protein efficiently caps the 5-nt gene start sequence [12, 16], demonstrating that a 5-nt RNA substrate is sufficient for mRNA cap addition. In order to determine the minimum length of RNA required for mRNA cap methylation, 5-,10-, 51-, and 110-nt RNAs were used as substrates for a *trans* methylation assay *in vitro* [18]. Interestingly, the 10-, 51-, and 110-nt RNAs were able to serve as substrates for both G-N-7 and ribose 2'-O methylations, whereas the 5-nt RNA was not methylated by the VSV L protein at either the G-N-7 or the ribose 2'-O position [18]. Therefore, in contrast to *trans* capping, a 5-nt substrate is not sufficient for trans methylation and likely the conserved positions 8, 9, and 10 in VSV gene start sequence are required for mRNA cap methylation. Clearly, the length of RNA required for methylation is longer than that required for capping by the VSV L protein.

### 5.8. Model for mRNA cap methylation

The process of VSV L protein-mediated cap methylation can be best summarized with the following model (Fig.7). Initially in response to a specific *cis*-acting element in the VSV gene start sequence, CR VI of L protein methylates the cap structure first at the 2'-O position to produce GpppA$^{m}$ACAG-RNA. The by-product of this reaction, SAH, is released from this reaction. Following 2'-O methylation, a second molecule of SAM binds to CR VI of L protein that may facilitate a subsequent methylation of the RNA at the G-N-7 position. Methylation at the 2'-O position favors G-N-7 methylation in the cap structure through a currently unknown mechanism. G-N-7 methlyation may be facilitated by the contact with the RNA molecule remains bound to the L protein at the end of the initial methylation at the 2'-O position. Another possibility is that CR VI of L protein exists in two different conformations. An initial conformation may favor binding of GpppRNA and SAM. Methylation of RNA at the 2'-O position perhaps induces a conformational change that facilitates the repositioning of the RNA for subsequent G-N-7 methylation, and/or favors the release of SAH as well as the binding of a subsequent molecule of SAM.

### 5.9. Comparison of mRNA cap methylation in VSV and WNV

To date, the rhabdovirus, VSV, and the flavivirus, WNV, are the two best characterized viruses that utilize a single region in the polymerase protein for both G-N-7 and 2'-O methylations. However, the mechanism of VSV mRNA methylation is distinct from that of the WNV system (Fig.4B and C). In VSV, 2'-O methylation precedes and facilitates subsequent G-N-7 methylation [17, 18]. However, WNV MTases modify the cap structure, first at the G-N-7 position and subsequently at the ribose 2'-O position [72, 73, 78]. In VSV, the G-N-7 and 2'-O MTases require similar conditions for methylation with an optimal pH at 7.0 [18]. In contrast, the G-N-7 and 2'-O MTases of WNV require an optimal pH at 6.5 and 10, respectively [72]. Both VSV and WNV MTases modify the RNA in a sequence-specific manner, but require different elements in the RNA substrate. VSV G-N-7 and 2'-O MTases require specific gene start sequences with a minimum mRNA length of 10 nucleotides [18]. In the WNV model, N-7 cap methylation requires the presence of specific nucleotides at the second and third positions and a 5' stem-loop structure within the 74-nucleotide viral RNA; in contrast, 2'-O ribose methylation requires specific nucleotides at the first and second positions, with a minimum 5' viral RNA of 20 nucleotides in length [81]. In addition, there is striking difference in the cap recognition site between the VSV and WNV MTases. For the WNV MTase, the cap recognition site is essential for 2'-O, but not G-N-7 methylation [73, 82]. Consistent with this finding, it was found that GTP and cap analogs specifically inhibited 2'-O, but not G-N-7 methylation [73, 82]. However, mutations to the putative RNA binding site in VSV L protein affected both G-N-7 and 2'-O methylations. GTP and cap analogs did not affect VSV mRNA cap methylation *in vitro*. Overall, the mechanism of VSV mRNA cap methylation is significantly different from that of WNV. Most recently, it was found that capping of flavivirus RNA is catalyzed by conventional RNA guanylyltransferase via a covalent GMP-enzyme intermediate [88]. However, VSV capping is catalyzed by a novel PRNTase [12, 13, 16, 89]. These studies suggest that VSV and perhaps other NNS RNA viruses have evolved a unique mechanism to add the cap to their mRNA and to methylate the cap structure.

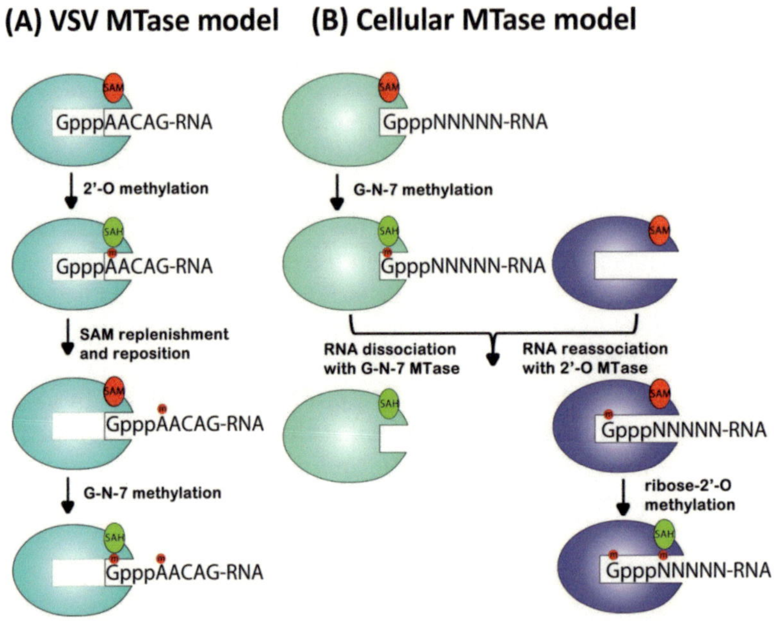


**Figure 7. Proposed model for mRNA cap methylation in VSV and eukaryotic cells. (A) VSV MTase model.** VSV mRNA cap structure is first methylated by CR VI of L protein at the 2'-O position to produce GpppA$^{m}$ACAG-RNA. The by-product, SAH, is released before the binding of a second molecule of SAM. G-N-7 methlyation may be facilitated by the contact with the RNA molecule remains bound to the polymerase at the end of the initial methylation at the 2'-O position. Or, methylation of RNA at the 2'-O position may induce a conformational change that facilitates the repositioning of the RNA for subsequent G-N-7 methylation. **(B) Cellular MTase model.** GpppNNNN-RNA is first methylated by a G-N-7 MTase to yield 7$^{m}$GpppNNNN-RNA. Following G-N-7 methylation, 7$^{m}$GpppNNNN-RNA dissociates with G-N-7 MTase, and re-associates with a separate 2'-O MTase to yield 7$^{m}$GpppN$^{m}$NNN-RNA. In this model, the two methylase activities are carried out by two separate enzymes, each containing its own SAM binding site.

### 5.10. mRNA cap methylation in other NNS RNA viruses

Limited accomplishments have been made in understanding the mechanism of mRNA cap methylation in other NNS RNA viruses, due to the lack of a robust *in vitro* mRNA synthesis for most of NNS RNA viruses, and the technical challenge of expression and purification of a functional polymerase protein or fragment. In early 1970, Colonno and Stone showed that the NDV mRNA cap structure was methylated only at G-N-7 [90]. This is distinct from the cap structures of other NNS RNA viruses which typically contain two methyl groups, at positions G-N-7 and ribose 2'-O. However, detailed characterization of the NDV methylase activities and the mechanism involved in this unique methylation is not understood. The mechanism underlying this difference and the biological significance of the lack of 2'-O MTase is not known. Sequence analysis has revealed that the proposed SAM binding region for the *Filoviridae, Rubulavirus,* and *Avulavirus* genera of the *Paramyxoviridae* contains a conserved AxGxG sequence rather than GxGxG within motif I of the SAM-dependent MTase superfamily (Fig.8). It will be interesting to determine if there is a link between this differential SAM binding sites and the lack of 2'-O methylation in NDV. Recently, it was shown that a fragment of Sendai virus L protein that includes CR VI was able to methylate short Sendai virus-specific RNA sequences *in trans* at the

G-N-7 position [43]. However, the "*trans*-methylation" assay used in their study does not allow detection of 2′-O methylation although it is known that Sendai virus encodes two MTases. More recently, recombinant Sendai virus carrying mutations in catalytic KDKE tetrad and SAM binding site were recovered from infectious clones [91, 92]. It was found that these mutations affected mRNA cap methylation. However, whether they are specifically defective in G-N-7 and/or 2′-O methylation is not known because of the assay did not have the ability to distinguish the two methyl groups. In addition, the order of methylation may be different among NNS RNA viruses. In contrast to VSV, methylation of RSV mRNA at low SAM concentrations was found at only the G-N-7 position; however, it was found to be doubly methylated at high SAM concentrations [63]. This study provided evidence that the order of mRNA cap methylation in RSV may be different with VSV. Clearly, more studies are needed to understand the mRNA cap methylation in other NNS RNA viruses.

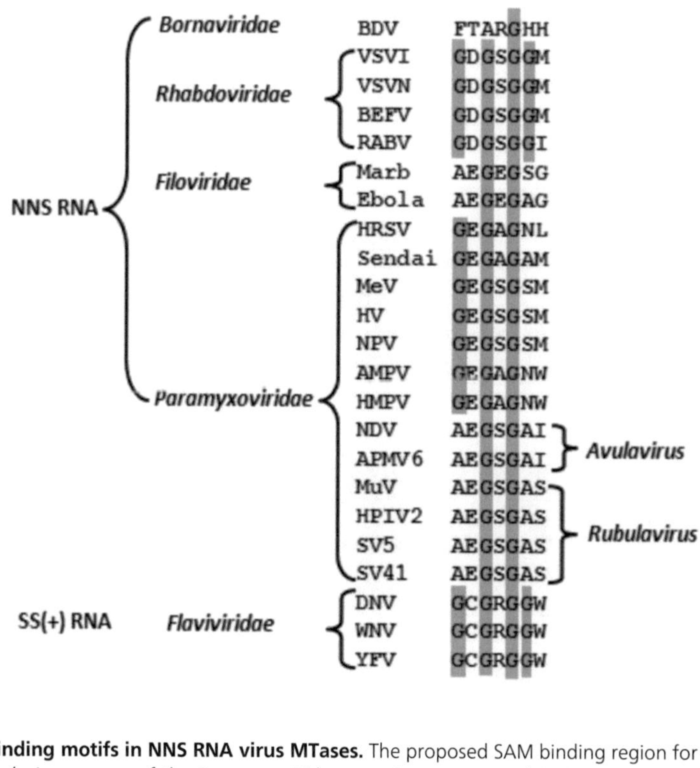


**Figure 8. SAM binding motifs in NNS RNA virus MTases.** The proposed SAM binding region for the *Filoviridae*, *Rubulavirus*, and *Avulavirus* genera of the *Paramyxoviridae* contains a conserved AxGxG sequence rather than GxGxG. NNS RNA viruses include VSVI, VSV Indiana; VSVN, VSV New Jersey; BEFV, bovine emphemeral fever virus; RABV, rabies virus; Marb, Marburg virus; MeV: measles; HV, Hendra virus; NPV, Nipah virus; AMPV, avian metapneuomovirus; HMPV, human metapneuomovirus; APMV6, avian paramyxovirus 6; MuV, mumps virus; HPIV2, human parainfluenza virus 2; SV5, simian virus 5; SV41, simian virus 41;

SS(+) RNA: single strand positive RNA viruses include DNV, dengue virus; WNV, West Nile virus; YFV, yellow fever virus.

## 6. The effects of 5′ mRNA cap addition and cap methylation on 3′ mRNA polyadenylation

VSV mRNA is capped and methylated at the 5′ end and polyadenylated at the 3′ end. Cap addition, cap methylation, and polyadenylation are carried out by three different regions (CR V, CR VI, and CR III) in L protein. During VSV mRNA synthesis, modifications of the 5′ and 3′ ends of the mRNAs are tightly coupled to transcription [21-23]. Although the detailed mechanism by which the polymerase coordinates these modification events is poorly understand, available evidence suggests there is a link between authentic 5′-end formation and 3′-end formation during VSV mRNA synthesis. Early studies demonstrated that the length of poly (A) tails on VSV mRNAs is affected by the presence of SAH, the by-product and competitive inhibitor of SAM-mediated methyltransferases [93-95]. The fact that the polymerase can synthesize full-length mRNAs *in vitro* in the absence of SAM or in the presence of SAH, suggests that transcription is not dependent on cap methylation. When *in vitro* transcription reactions are performed in the presence of SAM, the RdRp synthesizes mRNA with poly (A) tail of 100 to 200 nt in length, similar to those synthesized in VSV-infected cells. However, when VSV mRNA cap methylation was inhibited during *in vitro* transcription reactions by supplementing with 1 mM SAH, the synthesized mRNA was heterogeneous in length due to having extremely long poly (A) tails, from 700 to 2,400 nucleotides (nt) in length [93, 96]. Recent work demonstrated that SAH-induced hyperpolyadenylation also occurs in cells infected by wild-type VSV in the presence of adenosine dialdehyde (AdOX), a compound that inhibits the activity of SAH hydrolase [97]. These results indicated that chemical inhibition of VSV mRNA cap methylation by SAH resulted in hyperpolyadenylation of viral mRNA. Interestingly, this hyperpolyadenylation of VSV mRNAs has been observed in *ts*(G)16, a VSV mutant identified in 1970 based on its ability to grow at 31°C but not at 39°C [93, 98, 99]. In the absence of SAH, the mRNAs synthesized by VSV mutant *ts*(G)16 were hyperpolyadenylated at the 3′ end. Genomic sequence analysis found that the L protein of *ts*(G)16 contains two amino acid changes, C1291Y and F1488S, compared to wild type. Combined with the analysis of revertants of *ts*(G)16, it was found that F1488S, located in the variable region of L between CR V and CR VI, is responsible for the hyperpolyadenylating phenotype.

The characterization of a panel of MTase-defective VSVs may serve as a tool to understand the mechanism by which SAH or the failure to methylate the cap structure results in hyperpolyadenylation. It was found that rVSV-K1651A, a mutation in MTase active site and completely defective in G-N-7 and 2′-O methylation, synthesized excessively long poly(A) tails, similar to those produced by wild-type L in the presence of SAH [15]. Similarly, the substitution D1762E at the MTase active site, which inhibits both G-N-7 and 2′-O methylation, produces large polyadenylate in the presence or absence of SAH [97]. This data confirms the earlier work demonstrating that the inhibition of cap methylation results in large polyadenylate. In contrast, several other substitutions that inhibit cap methylation, including D1762G, D1762N, G1672P, and G1675P, did not produce hyperpolyadenylated mRNA [97].

Perhaps, K 1651A and D1762E substitutions might favor the binding of SAH at the SAM binding site in CR VI, resulting in hyperpolyadenylation without the need for supplemental SAH. Clearly, further studies are needed to understand the relationship between 5′ mRNA cap methyaltion and 3′ polyadenylation.

However, it appears clear that 5′ cap addition is required for 3′ polyadenylation, as evidenced by the polymerase mutants (G1154, T1157, H1227, and R1228) within CR V of L that inhibited cap addition also inhibit polyadenylation [15]. These cap-defective polymerases synthesized truncated transcripts that predominantly terminated within the first 500 nt of the N gene and contained short A-rich sequences at their 3′ termini. To examine how the cap-defective polymerases respond to an authentic VSV termination and re-initiation signal present at each gene junction, a 382 nt gene was inserted at the leader-*N* gene junction in the VSV genome. Using this N-RNA as the template, the cap-defective polymerases were able to synthesize full-length 382-nt transcripts that were not capped at 5′end. Interestingly, these uncapped transcripts lacked an authentic polyadenylate tail and instead contained 0 to 24 A residues [15]. In addition, the cap-defective polymerases were also unable to efficiently copy the downstream genes [15]. This finding strongly supports that 5′ mRNA cap addition and 3′ polyadenylation are mechanistically and functionally linked.

## 7. Impact of mRNA cap methylation on viral replication and gene expression

In eukaryotic cells, it is well established that G-N-7 methylation of the mRNA cap structure is essential for mRNA stability and efficient translation [11, 48, 66]. Specifically, G-N-7 methylation of the mRNA cap structure is required for recognition of the cap by the rate limiting factor for translation initiation, eIF-4E [100, 101]. The mRNA cap structures of NNS RNA viruses are typically G-N-7 and 2′-O methylated. Although the precise mechanism by which VSV mRNAs are translated is unclear, they are broadly thought to utilize a variation of the canonical cap-dependent translational pathway [102-104]. In VSV-infected cells, host mRNA translation is rapidly inhibited through the suppression of the intracellular pools of eIF-4E by a manipulation of the phosphorylation status of the 4E binding protein (4E-BP1) [104]. Nevertheless, *in vitro* experiments have shown that G-N-7 cap methylation facilitates translation of VSV proteins. MTase-defective VSV would provide a tool to study the role of mRNA cap methylation in viral protein synthesis. Ultimately, it will affect viral genome replication and gene expression since viral replication requires ongoing protein synthesis.

Based on the status of mRNA methylation, MTase-defective VSVs can be classified into three groups [14, 17, 84]. Viruses in the first group are completely defective in both G-N-7 and 2′-O methylation, including mutations in MTase active site (rVSV-K1651A, D1762A, K1795A, E1833Q, and E1833A), SAM binding site (rVSV-D1671V, G1675A, G4A, and G4AD), and putative RNA binding site (rVSV-Y1650A, F1691A, and E1764A). Viruses in the second group are specifically defective in G-N-7, but not 2′-O MTase, including mutants in SAM binding site (rVSV-G1670A, G1672A, and S1673A). Viruses in third group that require elevated SAM concentrations to permit full methylation including a mutant in SAM binding site (rVSV-G1674A) and putative RNA binding site (rVSV-Y1835A). With the exception of rVSV-G1674A and Y1835A, all MTase-defective VSVs were attenuated in cell culture as judged by diminished viral plaque size, reduced infectious viral progeny release (in single-step growth curves), and decreased levels of viral genomic RNA, mRNA, and protein synthesis. It appears that the degree of attenuation is consistent with the defects of the methylation. For example, viruses defective in both G-N-7 and 2′-O methylation had 2-5 log reductions in growth whereas viruses only defective in G-N-7 had 1-2 log declines in replication [14]. Recombinant rVSV-G1674A and Y1835A replicated as efficiently as wild type rVSV [14]. A remarkable finding is that some of the mutants in the SAM binding site (rVSV-G1675A, G4A, and G4AD) affected transcription and replication differently [17]. For these mutants, replication was enhanced 2.5- to 4-fold, and transcription decreased up to 8-fold compared with rVSV. One feature of the gene expression strategy of NNS RNA viruses is that the polymerase complex controls two distinct RNA synthetic events: genomic RNA replication and mRNA transcription [20, 105, 106]. It is possible that SAM binding influences the switch of polymerase between replicase and transcriptase. Perhaps, L protein with SAM binding favors to function as transcriptase, whereas L protein that lacks SAM binding favors replicase function.

## 8. Impact of mRNA cap methylation on viral pathogenesis *in vitro*

Although it is well studied that MTase-defective viruses were attenuated in cell culture, the impact of mRNA cap methylation on viral pathogenesis *in vitro* is poorly understood. Recently, Ma et al., (2012) examined the pathogenicity of MTase-defective VSVs in mice [107]. VSV infects a wide range of wild and domestic animals such as cattle, horses, deer, and pigs, characterized by vesicular lesions in the mouth, tongue, lips, gums, teats, and feet. Although the mouse is not the natural host of VSV, it represents an excellent small animal model to understand VSV pathogenesis because VSV causes systemic infection and fatal encephalitis [108-110]. After intranasal inoculation, VSV infects olfactory neurons in the nasal mucosa and subsequently enters the central nervous system (CNS) through the olfactory nerves. The virus is then disseminated to other areas in the brain through retrograde and possibly anterograde trans-neuronal transport, ultimately causing an acute brain infection. It was found that VSV mutants, rVSV-K1651A, D1762A, and E1833Q, which have mutations in the MTase catalytic site and are defective in both G-N-7 and 2′O methylation, were highly attenuated in mice [107]. Mice inoculated with these recombinant viruses did not show any clinical signs of VSV infection such as weight loss, ruffled fur, hyperexcitability, tremors, circling, and paralysis. Furthermore, these mutant viruses were not able to enter the brain, had dramatic defects in replication in lungs, and did not cause significant histopathological changes in lungs and brain. Recombinant rVSV-G1670A and G1672A, which have mutations in the SAM binding site and are defective in G-N-7 but not 2′-O methylation, retained low virulence in mice [107]. Mice inoculated these two recombinants exhibited weight loss of approximately 2-3 g during days 3-7 post-inoculation and showed mild illnesses such as ruffled coat for 2-3 days but recovered quickly. But, none of mice in rVSV-G1670A and G1672A had neurological symptoms. These two recombinants had moderate defects in replication in lungs and brain, and caused moderate histopathological changes in lungs. Interestingly, recombinant rVSV-G4A, which carries four mutations (G1670A, G1672A, G1674A, and G1675A) in SAM binding site and is completely defective in both G-N-7 and 2′-O methylation, exhibited an interesting pathotype [107]. Similar to VSV mutants at the MTase catalytic site, rVSV-G4A had dramatically impaired viral replication in the lungs and brain of the mice. However, the rVSV-G4A group exhibited body weight losses that were comparable to G1670A and G1672A, and clinical signs that were more severe than G1670A and G1672A. These results suggest rVSV-G4A retained low to moderate virulence despite the fact that it was attenuated for replication and or spread *in vitro*. As predicted, recombinant rVSV-G1674A, which contains a point mutation in the SAM binding site and requires elevated SAM concentrations to permit full methylation, was highly virulent to mice. These results suggest that (i) the relationship between mRNA cap methylation and viral pathogenesis is not clear cut in VSV infections; and (ii) inactivation of the predicted catalytic residues attenuates the virus to a greater extent *in vitro*, than does inactivation of the predicted SAM binding site.

## 9. 2′-O methylation and innate immunity

While it is firmly established that G-N-7 methylation is essential for mRNA stability as well as efficient translation, the role(s) of ribose 2′-O methylation have proven more elusive. Recent studies on West Nile virus (WNV) suggest that the 2′-O methylation of the 5′ cap of viral RNA functions to evade innate host antiviral responses through escape of the suppression of interferon-stimulated genes, tetratricopeptide repeats (IFIT)[111]. Specifically, mutant WNV (E218A) defective in 2′ O MTase activity was attenuated in wild-type C57BL/6 mice, but remained pathogenic in knockout mice that lacked the type I interferon (IFN) signaling pathway. In addition, a vaccinia virus mutant (J3-K175R) and mouse hepatitis virus (MHV) mutant D130A, both of which lacked 2′-O MTase activity, exhibited enhanced sensitivities to the antiviral actions of IFN mediated by IFIT proteins. Interestingly, it was also reported that 2′-O methylation of mouse and human coronavirus RNA facilitates evasion from detection by the cytoplasmic RNA sensor Mda5 [112]. Taken together, these studies suggest that 2′-O methylation of viral RNA provides a molecular signature for the discrimination of self and non-self mRNA. It is known that mRNAs of most NNS RNA viruses contain G-N-7 and 2′-O methylation. However, whether 2′-O methylation plays a similar role in all NNS RNA viruses is not known.

VSV is an excellent model to aid in the understanding the role of viral mRNA cap methylation in innate immunity. The mechanism of VSV mRNA cap methylation is unique in that 2′-O methylation precedes and facilitates the G-N-7 methylation [17, 18]. It is unknown why the order of VSV mRNA methylation is reversed compared to all known mRNA cap methylation reactions. One possibility is that the methylation of 2′-O allows VSV to successfully mimic cellular mRNA to avoid the detection by host innate immunity, which in turn promotes efficient viral replication in hosts. In fact, VSV is one of only a few viruses that replicates efficiently in a wide range of cell lines including mammalian cells, insect cells, and worms [113]. Unlike WNV, VSV that is specifically defective in G-N-7 methylation can also be successfully recovered [17]. VSV mutants defective in G-N-7 methylation or both G-N-7 and 2′-O methylations can serve as prototypes or controls to elucidate the role of methylation in innate immunity. In addition, the VSV mutant (rVSV-G4A) that was attenuated in cell culture retained low to moderate virulence, suggesting the possible role of methylation in averting the innate immune response [107]. Notably, mRNAs of NDV, an avian paramyxovirus, are not 2′-O methylated [90]. A direct comparison to determine whether 2′-O methylation of VSV has a similar biological function compared to WNV and MHV should prove very compelling.

## 10. MTase-defective viruses as live vaccine candidates

Recombinant viruses defective in MTase can be recovered from cloned full-length viral cDNA by a reverse genetics system. Viruses lacking MTase would likely be attenuated without affecting immunogenicity, since the MTase is located in L protein, which is not a neutralizing antibody target. Our group and others have identified a panel of MTase-defective VSV mutants which are attenuated in cell culture as well as in animal models [14, 17, 84, 107]. In addition, MTase-defective Sendai viruses also showed significant defects in viral growth in cell culture [91, 92]. By combining multiple substitutions within the methylation region, it should be possible to generate an attenuated virus that is genetically stable, as reversion to wild type at any single amino acid should not provide a fitness gain. Thus, ablating viral mRNA cap methylation would provide a new avenue to rationally attenuate these viruses for the development of live attenuated vaccines and exploit their use as viral vectors for vaccines, oncolytic therapy, and gene delivery. Recently, Ma et al., (2012) showed that MTase-defective VSVs were able to induce high levels of VSV-specific antibodies in mice and thus provided full protection against a virulent challenge with the VSV Indiana serotype [107]. Recombinants rVSV-K1651A, D1762A, and E1833Q which were defective in both G-N-7 and 2′-O methylation, are attractive vaccine candidates since they are not only highly attenuated but also retain high immunogenicity. Although recombinants rVSV-G1670A and G1672A retained low virulence to mice, their pathogenicity was significantly reduced compared to rVSV. The safety of using these two viruses as live vaccine candidates necessitates further investigation.

Our studies on MTase-defective VSVs also shed light on developing live vaccine candidates for other NNS RNA viruses, particularly paramyxoviruses. Within paramyxoviruses,

RSV, hMPV, and PIV3 account for the majority of respiratory diseases infants, children, and the elderly [1-3]. However, there is no vaccine available for these important viruses. Recent research found that live attenuated vaccines are the most promising vaccine candidates for paramyxoviruses [1-3]. However, it has been technically challenging to isolate a virus with low virulence while retaining high immunogenicity. Introducing mutations in the MTase may provide a novel approach to generate live attenuated viruses for these viruses. It was reported that recombinant Sendai virus carrying point mutations in the MTase catalytic site (rSeV-K1782A) and the SAM binding site (rSeV-E1805A) were attenuated in cell culture [91]. It will be of interesting to determine whether these Sendai recombinants are attenuated *in vitro.*

## 11. mRNA cap methylation as a target for anti-viral drug discovery

It appears that the entire mRNA capping and methylation machinery in NNS RNA viruses is different from that of their hosts. This difference, coupled with the fact that replication of NNS RNA viruses occurs in the cytoplasm, suggests that mRNA cap formation is an excellent target for anti-viral drug discovery. Inhibition of the viral mRNA cap formation would likely inhibit downstream events such as replication, gene expression, viral spread, and ultimately viral infection. Since the mRNA of all NNS RNA viruses contains a methylated cap structure, classes of broadly active anti-viral agents may be developed by targeting the viral cap formation. For human RSV, several compounds were shown to inhibit polymerase activity which resulted in the synthesis of short uncapped transcripts [63]. RSV mutants resistant to these inhibitors were selected and sequenced. It was found that these resistant mutants contained substitutions in CR V of L, specifically at E1269D, I1381S, and L1421F, suggesting that the mechanism of the action of these compounds is the inhibition of viral mRNA cap addition. Interestingly, these compounds showed strong antiviral activity against RSV infection in cell culture as well as in a mouse model, demonstrating that mRNA cap addition is an attractive antiviral target. It is known that SAH can inhibit viral mRNA cap methylation. Therefore, many adenosine analogues such as 3-deazaeplanocin-A are potent antiviral agents which can significantly inhibit VSV replication in cell culture [114, 115]. The mechanism of the action of these adenosine analogues is through the interference with the host enzyme SAH hydrolase that catalyzes the hydrolysis of SAH to adenosine and L-homocysteine. This reaction is reversible, and the products of this reaction are inhibitory to SAH hydrolase. Obviously, compounds that directly inhibit viral mRNA cap methylation are potent antiviral drugs. For example, sinefungin (SIN), a natural *S*-adenosyl-l-methionine analog produced by *Streptomyces griseolus*, is an inhibitor of methyltransferases. SIN is structurally related to SAM, with the exception that the methyl group that is donated from SAM is replaced by an amino group in SIN. Crystal structures of several MTases have been solved in complex with SIN, which binds to a region that overlaps the SAM binding site [116]. It was found that SIN inhibited VSV G-N-7 and 2′-O methylation with a 50% inhibitory concentration ($IC_{50}$) of 2.5 μM and 40 μM, respectively [86]. In cell culture, SIN efficiently inhibited VSV replication, gene expression, and diminished the size of viral plaques without having significant effect on cell viability. SIN was also shown to inhibit the MTases of other NNS RNA viruses such as NDV [90]. These examples demonstrate that mRNA capping and methylation is an excellent antiviral target for NNS RNA viruses. An important future direction is to develop high-throughput screening (HTS) to systemically screen compounds that can inhibit mRNA capping and/or methylation of VSV and other NNS RNA viruses. These inhibitors may be broadly active anti-viral agents against NNS RNA viruses.

## 12. Concluding remarks

In recent years, significant progress has been made in understanding the unusual mechanism of mRNA cap addition and methylation employed by VSV. First, VSV mRNA addition utilizes a novel PRNTase that transfers RNA to the GDP acceptor. Second, VSV mRNA cap methylation is catalyzed by a dual MTase that sequentially methylates the position 2′-O followed by G-N-7. Third, PRNTase and dual MTase have been mapped to single amino acid level in CR V and CR VI in the L protein, respectively. Finally, 5′ mRNA cap addition and methylation and 3′ polyadenylation are mechanistically and functionally linked. Apparently, the entire mRNA cap formation in VSV evolves a mechanism distinct to hosts. Thus, mRNA cap modification is an ideal target for vaccine and antiviral drug development. However, there are many questions need to be addressed. It is not known how polymerase coordinates nucleotide polymerization, mRNA cap addition, cap methylation, and polyadenylation. Although the general mechanism of mRNA modifications is defined, the detailed step in each reaction is still poorly understood. The GTPase required for mRNA capping has not been mapped in L protein. Besides the HR motif, it is not known which step of mRNA capping was affected by other mutations (such as T1157A and G1154A) in CR V of L protein. During mRNA cap methylation the exact mechanism by which the dual MTase methylates the 2′-O and G-N-7 is not known. The crystal structure is not known for L protein or any portion of L protein. The concept of using mRNA cap formation as antiviral target has been experimentally demonstrated, however, high-throughput screening methods toward drug discovery have not been developed. Furthermore, there is urgent need to understand the mRNA cap modification in other NNS RNA virus although it is speculated that they may also be achieved in a similar mechanism.

## Acknowledgements

Work in Dr. Jianrong Li's laboratory was supported by grants from NIH/NIAID (R01AI090060), USDA Agriculture and Food Research Initiative (2010-65119-20602), and OSU Center for Clinical and Translational Science (CCTS). Yu Zhang is a fellow of Center for RNA Biology at The Ohio State University. We thank Erin DiCaprio for critical review of this manuscript.

## Author details

Jianrong Li[1,2,3*] and Yu Zhang[1]

*Address all correspondence to: li.926@osu.edu

1 Department of Food Science and Technology, College of Food, Agricultural and Environmental Sciences, The Ohio State University, USA

http://dx.doi.org/10.5772/54598

2 Division of Environmental Health Sciences, College of Public Health, The Ohio State University, USA

3 Center for RNA Biology, The Ohio State University, Columbus, Ohio, USA

## References

[1] Collins PL, Graham BS. Viral and host factors in human respiratory syncytial virus pathogenesis. Journal of virology. 2008;82(5):2040-55.

[2] Falsey AR. Human metapneumovirus infection in adults. The Pediatric infectious disease journal. 2008;27(10 Suppl):S80-3.

[3] Sato M, Wright PF. Current status of vaccines for parainfluenza virus infections. The Pediatric infectious disease journal. 2008;27(10 Suppl):S123-5.

[4] Bloom BR. Vaccines for the Third World. Nature. 1989 Nov 9;342(6246):115-20.

[5] Alamares JG, Li J, Iorio RM. Monoclonal antibody routinely used to identify avirulent strains of Newcastle disease virus binds to an epitope at the carboxy terminus of the hemagglutinin-neuraminidase protein and recognizes individual mesogenic and velogenic strains. Journal of clinical microbiology. 2005;43(8):4229-33.

[6] Abraham G, Rhodes DP, Banerjee AK. The 5' terminal structure of the methylated mRNA synthesized *in vitro* by vesicular stomatitis virus. Cell. 1975;5:51-8.

[7] Abraham G, Rhodes DP, Banerjee AK. Novel initiation of RNA synthesis *in vitro* by vesicular stomatitis virus. Nature. 1975;255(5503):37-40.

[8] Banerjee AK, Rhodes DP. *In vitro* synthesis of RNA that contains polyadenylate by virion-associated RNA polymerase of vesicular stomatitis virus. Proceedings of the National Academy of Sciences of the United States of America. 1973;70(12):3566-70.

[9] Furuichi Y, Miura KI. A blocked structure at the 5' terminus of mRNA from cytoplasmic polyhedrosis virus. Nature. 1975;253(5490):374-5.

[10] Furuichi Y, Morgan M, Shatkin AJ, Jelinek W, Saldittgeorgieff M, Darnell JE. Methylated, blocked 5 termini in HeLa cell mRNA. Proceedings of the National Academy of Sciences of the United States of America. 1975;72(5):1904-8.

[11] Furuichi Y, Shatkin AJ. Viral and cellular mRNA capping: past and prospects. Adv Virus Res. 2000;55:135-84.

[12] Ogino T, Banerjee AK. Unconventional mechanism of mRNA capping by the RNA-dependent RNA polymerase of vesicular stomatitis virus. Mol Cell. 2007;25:85-97.

[13] Ogino T, Yadav SP, Banerjee AK. Histidine-mediated RNA transfer to GDP for unique mRNA capping by vesicular stomatitis virus RNA polymerase. Proceedings

of the National Academy of Sciences of the United States of America. 2010;107(8): 3463-8.

[14] Li J, Fontaine-Rodriguez EC, Whelan SP. Amino acid residues within conserved domain VI of the vesicular stomatitis virus large polymerase protein essential for mRNA cap methyltransferase activity. Journal of virology. 2005;79(21):13373-84.

[15] Li J, Rahmeh A, Brusic V, Whelan SPJ. Opposing Effects of Inhibiting Cap Addition and Cap Methylation on Polyadenylation during Vesicular Stomatitis Virus mRNA Synthesis. Journal of virology. 2009;83(4):1930-40.

[16] Li J, Rahmeh A, Morelli M, Whelan SP. A conserved motif in region v of the large polymerase proteins of nonsegmented negative-sense RNA viruses that is essential for mRNA capping. Journal of virology. 2008;82(2):775-84.

[17] Li JR, Wang JT, Whelan SPJ. A unique strategy for mRNA cap methylation used by vesicular stomatitis virus. Proceedings of the National Academy of Sciences of the United States of America. 2006;103(22):8493-8.

[18] Rahmeh AA, Li J, Kranzusch PJ, Whelan SPJ. Ribose 2 '-O Methylation of the Vesicular Stomatitis Virus mRNA Cap Precedes and Facilitates Subsequent Guanine-N-7 Methylation by the Large Polymerase Protein. Journal of virology. 2009;83(21): 11043-50.

[19] Grdzelishvili VZ, Smallwood S, Tower D, Hall RL, Hunt DM, Moyer SA. A single amino acid change in the L-polymerase protein of vesicular stornatitis virus completely abolishes viral mRNA cap methylation. Journal of virology. 2005;79(12): 7327-37.

[20] Whelan SPJ, Barr JN, Wertz GW. Transcription and replication of nonsegmented negative-strand RNA viruses. Biology of Negative Strand RNA Viruses: The Power of Reverse Genetics. 2004;283:61-119.

[21] Abraham G, Banerjee AK. Sequential transcription of the genes of vesicular stomatitis virus. Proceedings of the National Academy of Sciences of the United States of America. 1976;73(5):1504-8.

[22] Ball LA. Transcriptional mapping of vesicular stomatitis virus in vivo. Journal of virology. 1977;21(1):411-4.

[23] Ball LA, White CN. Order of transcription of genes of vesicular stomatitis virus. Proceedings of the National Academy of Sciences of the United States of America. 1976;73(2):442-6.

[24] Emerson SU, Wagner RR. Dissociation and reconstitution of the transcriptase and template activities of vesicular stomatitis B and T virions. Journal of virology. 1972;10(2):297-309.

[25] Emerson SU, Yu YH. Both NS and L proteins are required for *in vitro* RNA synthesis by vesicular stomatitis virus. Journal of virology. 1975;15(6):1348-56.

[26] Szilagyi JF, Uryvayev L. Isolation of an infectious ribonucleoprotein from vesicular stomatitis virus containing an active RNA transcriptase. Journal of virology. 1973;11(2):279-86.

[27] Gaudin Y, Barge A, Ebel C, Ruigrok RW. Aggregation of VSV M protein is reversible and mediated by nucleation sites: implications for viral assembly. Virology. 1995;206(1):28-37.

[28] Hammond C, Helenius A. Folding of VSV G protein: sequential interaction with BiP and calnexin. Science. 1994;266(5184):456-8.

[29] Matlin KS, Reggio H, Helenius A, Simons K. Pathway of vesicular stomatitis virus entry leading to infection. Journal of molecular biology. 1982;156(3):609-31.

[30] Follett EA, Pringle CR, Wunner WH, Skehel JJ. Virus replication in enucleate cells: vesicular stomatitis virus and influenza virus. Journal of virology. 1974;13(2):394-9.

[31] Stillman EA, Whitt MA. Transcript initiation and 5 '-end modifications are separable events during vesicular stomatitis virus transcription. Journal of virology. 1999;73(9): 7199-209.

[32] Wang JT, McElvain LE, Whelan SPJ. Vesicular stomatitis virus mRNA capping machinery requires specific cis-acting signals in the RNA. Journal of virology. 2007;81(20):11499-506.

[33] Barr JN, Whelan SP, Wertz GW. cis-Acting signals involved in termination of vesicular stomatitis virus mRNA synthesis include the conserved AUAC and the U7 signal for polyadenylation. Journal of virology. 1997;71(11):8718-25.

[34] Hwang LN, Englund N, Pattnaik AK. Polyadenylation of vesicular stomatitis virus mRNA dictates efficient transcription termination at the intercistronic gene junctions. Journal of virology. 1998;72(3):1805-13.

[35] Poch O, Blumberg BM, Bougueleret L, Tordo N. Sequence comparison of five polymerases (L proteins) of unsegmented negative-strand RNA viruses: theoretical assignment of functional domains. Journal of General Virology. 1990;71:1153-62.

[36] Baltimore D, Huang AS, Stampfer M. Ribonucleic acid synthesis of vesicular stomatitis virus, II. An RNA polymerase in the virion. Proceedings of the National Academy of Sciences of the United States of America. 1970;66(2):572-6.

[37] Rahmeh AA, Schenk AD, Danek EI, Kranzusch PJ, Liang B, Walz T, et al. Molecular architecture of the vesicular stomatitis virus RNA polymerase. Proceedings of the National Academy of Sciences of the United States of America. 2010;107(46):20075-80.

[38] Chattopadhyay A, Raha T, Shaila MS. Effect of single amino acid mutations in the conserved GDNQ motif of L protein of Rinderpest virus on RNA synthesis *in vitro* and in vivo. Virus research. 2004;99(2):139-45.

[39] Smallwood S, Hovel T, Neubert WJ, Moyer SA. Different substitutions at conserved amino acids in domains II and III in the Sendai L RNA polymerase protein inactivate viral RNA synthesis. Virology. 2002;304(1):135-45.

[40] Sleat DE, Banerjee AK. Transcriptional activity and mutational analysis of recombinant vesicular stomatitis virus RNA polymerase. Journal of virology. 1993;67(3): 1334-9.

[41] Chandrika R, Horikami SM, Smallwood S, Moyer SA. Mutations in conserved domain I of the Sendai virus L polymerase protein uncouple transcription and replication. Virology. 1995;213(2):352-63.

[42] Smallwood S, Easson CD, Feller JA, Horikami SM, Moyer SA. Mutations in conserved domain II of the large (L) subunit of the Sendai virus RNA polymerase abolish RNA synthesis. Virology. 1999;262(2):375-83.

[43] Ogino T, Kobayashi M, Iwama M, Mizumoto K. Sendai virus RNA-dependent RNA polymerase L protein catalyzes cap methylation of virus-specific mRNA. Journal of Biological Chemistry. 2005;280(6):4429-35.

[44] Duprex WP, Collins FM, Rima BK. Modulating the function of the measles virus RNA-dependent RNA polymerase by insertion of green fluorescent protein into the open reading frame. Journal of virology. 2002;76(14):7322-8.

[45] Ruedas JB, Perrault J. Insertion of enhanced green fluorescent protein in a hinge region of vesicular stomatitis virus L polymerase protein creates a temperature-sensitive virus that displays no virion-associated polymerase activity *in vitro*. Journal of virology. 2009;83(23):12241-52.

[46] Grdzelishvili VZ, Smallwood S, Tower D, Hall RL, Hunt DM, Moyer SA. Identification of a new region in the vesicular stomatitis virus L polymerase protein which is essential for mRNA cap methylation. Virology. 2006;350(2):394-405.

[47] Rahmeh AA, Morin B, Schenk AD, Liang B, Heinrich BS, Brusic V, et al. Critical phosphoprotein elements that regulate polymerase architecture and function in vesicular stomatitis virus. Proceedings of the National Academy of Sciences of the United States of America. 2012;109(36):14628-33.

[48] Shuman S. Structure, mechanism, and evolution of the mRNA capping apparatus. Progress in Nucleic Acid Research and Molecular Biology. 2001;66:1-40.

[49] Mizumoto K, Kaziro Y. Messenger RNA capping enzymes from eukaryotic cells. Progress in Nucleic Acid Research and Molecular Biology. 1987;34:1-28.

[50] Venkatesan S, Moss B. Eukaryotic mRNA capping enzyme-guanylate covalent intermediate. Proceedings of the National Academy of Sciences of the United States of America. 1982;79(2):340-4.

[51] Sutton G, Grimes JM, Stuart DI, Roy P. Bluetongue virus VP4 is an RNA-capping assembly line. Nature Structural & Molecular Biology. 2007;14(5):449-51.

[52] Shuman S, Hurwitz J. Mechanism of mRNA capping by vaccinia virus guanylyltransferase: characterization of an enzyme--guanylate intermediate. Proceedings of the National Academy of Sciences of the United States of America. 1981;78(1):187-91.

[53] Cleveland DR, Zarbl H, Millward S. Reovirus guanylyltransferase is L2 gene product lambda 2. Journal of virology. 1986;60(1):307-11.

[54] Furuichi Y, Muthukrishnan S, Tomasz J, Shatkin AJ. Mechanism of formation of reovirus mRNA 5'-terminal blocked and methylated sequence, m7GpppGmpC. Journal of Biological Chemistry. 1976;251(16):5043-53.

[55] Reinisch KM, Nibert M, Harrison SC. Structure of the reovirus core at 3.6 angstrom resolution. Nature. 2000;404(6781):960-7.

[56] Henderson BR, Saeedi BJ, Campagnola G, Geiss BJ. Analysis of RNA binding by the dengue virus NS5 RNA capping enzyme. PloS one. 2011;6(10):e25795.

[57] Luongo CL, Reinisch KM, Harrison SC, Nibert ML. Identification of the guanylyltransferase region and active site in reovirus mRNA capping protein lambda2. The Journal of biological chemistry. 2000;275(4):2804-10.

[58] Dias A, Bouvier D, Crepin T, McCarthy AA, Hart DJ, Baudin F, et al. The cap-snatching endonuclease of influenza virus polymerase resides in the PA subunit. Nature. 2009;458(7240):914-8.

[59] Mir MA, Duran WA, Hjelle BL, Ye C, Panganiban AT. Storage of cellular 5' mRNA caps in P bodies for viral cap-snatching. Proceedings of the National Academy of Sciences of the United States of America. 2008;105(49):19294-9.

[60] Ahola T, Kaariainen L. Reaction in alphavirus mRNA capping: formation of a covalent complex of nonstructural protein nsP1 with 7-methyl-GMP. Proceedings of the National Academy of Sciences of the United States of America. 1995;92:507-11.

[61] Barik S. The structure of the 5' terminal cap of the respiratory syncytial virus mRNA. Journal of General Virology. 1993;74:485-90.

[62] Gupta KC, Roy P. Alternate capping mechanisms for transcription of spring viremia of carp virus: evidence for independent mRNA initiation. Journal of virology. 1980;33(1):292-303.

[63] Liuzzi M, Mason SW, Cartier M, Lawetz C, McCollum RS, Dansereau N, et al. Inhibitors of respiratory syncytial virus replication target cotranscriptional mRNA guanylylation by viral RNA-dependent RNA polymerase. Journal of virology. 2005;79(20): 13105-15.

[64] Ogino T, Banerjee AK. The HR motif in the RNA-dependent RNA polymerase L protein of Chandipura virus is required for unconventional mRNA-capping activity. Journal of General Virology. 2010;91:1311-4.

[65] Cong P, Shuman S. Methyltransferase and subunit association domains of vaccinia virus mRNA capping enzyme. The Journal of biological chemistry. 1992;267:16424-9.

[66] Fabrega C, Hausmann S, Shen V, Shuman S, Lima CD. Structure and mechanism of mRNA cap (guanine-N7) methyltransferase. Molecular Cell. 2004;13(1):77-89.

[67] Hager J, Staker BL, Bugl H, Jakob U. Active site in RrmJ, a heat shock-induced methyltransferase. Journal of Biological Chemistry. 2002;277(44):41978-86.

[68] Hodel AE, Quiocho FA, Gershon PD. VP39 - an mRNA cap-specific 2'-O-methyltransferase. In: X.D. Cheng RMB, editor. S-adenosylmethionine-dependent methyltransferase:structures and functions: World Scientific Publishing; 1999. p. 255-82.

[69] De lPM, Kyrieleis OJP, Cusack S. Structural insights into the mechanism and evolution of the vaccinia virus mRNA cap N7 methyl-transferase. EMBO J. 2007;26:4913-25.

[70] Hodel AE, Gershon PD, Shi XN, Quiocho FA. The 1.85 angstrom structure of vaccinia protein VP39: A bifunctional enzyme that participates in the modification of both mRNA ends. Cell. 1996;85(2):247-56.

[71] Luongo CL, Contreras CM, Farsetta DL, Nibert ML. Binding site for S-adenosyl-L-methionine in a central region of mammalian reovirus lambda2 protein. Evidence for activities in mRNA cap methylation. The Journal of biological chemistry. 1998;273(37):23773-80.

[72] Ray D, Shah A, Tilgner M, Guo Y, Zhao Y, Dong H, et al. West nile virus 5'-cap structure is formed by sequential guanine N-7 and ribose 2'-O methylations by nonstructural protein 5. Journal of virology. 2006;80:8362-70.

[73] Dong H, Ren S, Zhang B, Zhou Y, Puig-Basagoiti F, Li H, et al. West nile virus methyltransferase catalyzes two methylations of the viral RNA cap through a substrate-repositioning mechanism. Journal of virology. 2008;82(9):4295-307.

[74] Egloff M-P, Decroly E, Malet H, Selisko B, Benarroch D, Ferron F, et al. Structural and Functional Analysis of Methylation and 5'-RNA Sequence Requirements of Short Capped RNAs by the Methyltransferase Domain of Dengue Virus NS5. J Mol Biol. 2007;372:723-36.

[75] Martin JL, McMillan FM. SAM (dependent) I AM: the S-adenosylmethionine-dependent methyltransferase fold. Curr Opin Struct Biol. 2002;12:783-93.

[76] Bugl H, Fauman EB, Staker BL, Zheng FH, Kushner SR, Saper MA, et al. RNA methylation under heat shock control. Molecular Cell. 2000;6(2):349-60.

[77] Hager J, Staker BL, Jakob U. Substrate binding analysis of the 23S rRNA methyltransferase RrmJ. Journal of Bacteriology. 2004;186(19):6634-42.

[78] Zhou Y, Ray D, Zhao Y, Dong H, Ren S, Li Z, et al. Structure and function of flavivirus NS5 methyltransferase. Journal of virology. 2007;81:3891-903.

[79] Hu G, Gershon PD, Hodel AE, Quiocho FA. mRNA cap recognition: dominant role of enhanced stacking interactions between methylated bases and protein aromatic

side chains. Proceedings of the National Academy of Sciences of the United States of America. 1999;96(13):7149-54.

[80] Decroly E, Imbert I, Coutard B, Bouvet M, Selisko B, Alvarez K, et al. Coronavirus nonstructural protein 16 is a cap-0 binding enzyme possessing (nucleoside-2'O)-methyltransferase activity. Journal of virology. 2008;82(16):8071-84.

[81] Dong H, Ray D, Ren S, Zhang B, Puig-Basagoiti F, Takagi Y, et al. Distinct RNA elements confer specificity to flavivirus RNA cap methylation events. Journal of virology. 2007;81:4412-21.

[82] Dong H, Ren S, Li H, Shi P-Y. Separate molecules of West Nile virus methyltransferase can independently catalyze the N7 and 2'-O methylations of viral RNA cap. Virology. 2008;377:1-6.

[83] Marcotrigiano J, Gingras AC, Sonenberg N, Burley SK. Cocrystal structure of the messenger RNA 5' cap-binding protein (eIF4E) bound to 7-methyl-GDP. Cell. 1997;89(6):951-61.

[84] Zhang X, Wei Y, Ma Y, Hu S, Li J. Identification of aromatic amino acid residues in conserved region VI of the large polymerase of vesicular stomatitis virus is essential for both guanine-N-7 and ribose 2'-O methyltransferases. Virology. 2010;408(2): 241-52.

[85] Testa D, Banerjee AK. Two methyltransferase activities in the purified virions of vesicular stomatitis virus. Journal of virology. 1977;24(3):786-93.

[86] Li J, Chorba JS, Whelan SP. Vesicular stomatitis viruses resistant to the methylase inhibitor sinefungin upregulate RNA synthesis and reveal mutations that affect mRNA cap methylation. Journal of virology. 2007;81(8):4104-15.

[87] Horikami SM, Moyer SA. Host range mutants of vesicular stomatitis virus defective in *in vitro* RNA methylation. Proceedings of the National Academy of Sciences of the United States of America-Biological Sciences. 1982;79(24):7694-8.

[88] Issur M, Geiss BJ, Bougie I, Picard-Jean F, Despins S, Mayette J, et al. The flavivirus NS5 protein is a true RNA guanylyltransferase that catalyzes a two-step reaction to form the RNA cap structure. RNA. 2009;15:2340-50.

[89] Koonin EV, Moss B. Viruses know more than one way to don a cap. Proceedings of the National Academy of Sciences of the United States of America. 2010;107(8): 3283-4.

[90] Colonno RJ, Stone HO. Newcastle disease virus mRNA lacks 2'-O-methylated nucleotides. Nature. 1976 1976;261(5561):611-4. PubMed PMID: WOS:A1976BU52600052.

[91] Murphy AM, Grdzelishvili VZ. Identification of sendai virus L protein amino acid residues affecting viral mRNA cap methylation. Journal of virology. 2009;83(4): 1669-81.

[92] Murphy AM, Moerdyk-Schauwecker M, Mushegian A, Grdzelishvili VZ. Sequence-function analysis of the Sendai virus L protein domain VI. Virology. 2010;405(2): 370-82.

[93] Hunt DM. Vesicular stomatitis virus mutant with altered polyadenylic acid polymerase activity *in vitro*. Journal of virology. 1983;46(3):788-99.

[94] Hunt DM. Effect of analogues of S-adenosylmethionine on *in vitro* polyadenylation by vesicular stomatitis virus. The Journal of general virology. 1989;70 ( Pt 3):535-42.

[95] Hunt DM, Mehta R, Hutchinson KL. The L protein of vesicular stomatitis virus modulates the response of the polyadenylic acid polymerase to S-adenosylhomocysteine. The Journal of general virology. 1988;69 ( Pt 10):2555-61.

[96] Rose JK, Lodish HF, Brock ML. Giant heterogeneous polyadenylic acid on vesicular stomatitis virus mRNA synthesized *in vitro* in the presence of S-adenosylhomocysteine. Journal of virology. 1977;21(2):683-93.

[97] Galloway SE, Wertz GW. S-adenosyl homocysteine-induced hyperpolyadenylation of vesicular stomatitis virus mRNA requires the methyltransferase activity of L protein. Journal of virology. 2008;82(24):12280-90.

[98] Hunt DM, Hutchinson KL. Amino acid changes in the L polymerase protein of vesicular stomatitis virus which confer aberrant polyadenylation and temperature-sensitive phenotypes. Virology. 1993;193(2):786-93.

[99] Hunt DM, Smith EF, Buckley DW. Aberrant polyadenylation by a vesicular stomatitis virus mutant is due to an altered L protein. Journal of virology. 1984;52(2):515-21.

[100] Muthukrishnan S, Both GW, Furuichi Y, Shatkin AJ. 5'-Terminal 7-methylguanosine in eukaryotic mRNA is required for translation. Nature. 1975;255(5503):33-7.

[101] Muthukrishnan S, Moss B, Cooper JA, Maxwell ES. Influence of 5'-terminal cap structure on the initiation of translation of vaccinia virus mRNA. The Journal of biological chemistry. 1978;253(5):1710-5.

[102] Lodish HF, Porter M. Translational control of protein synthesis after infection by vesicular stomatitis virus. Journal of virology. 1980;36(3):719-33.

[103] Lodish HF, Porter M. Vesicular stomatitis virus mRNA and inhibition of translation of cellular mRNA--is there a P function in vesicular stomatitis virus? Journal of virology. 1981;38(2):504-17.

[104] Connor JH, Lyles DS. Vesicular stomatitis virus infection alters the eIF4F translation initiation complex and causes dephosphorylation of the eIF4E binding protein 4E-BP1. Journal of virology. 2002;76(20):10177-87.

[105] Qanungo KR, Shaji D, Mathur M, Banerjee AK. Two RNA polymerase complexes from vesicular stomatitis virus-infected cells that carry out transcription and replication of genome RNA. Proceedings of the National Academy of Sciences of the United States of America. 2004;101(16):5952-7.

[106] Whelan SPJ, Wertz GW. Transcription and replication initiate at separate sites on the vesicular stomatitis virus genome. Proceedings of the National Academy of Sciences of the United States of America. 2002;99(14):9178-83.

[107] Ma Y WY, Divers E, Whelan SPJ, Li J. , editor The impact of mRNA cap methylation status on the pathogenesis of vesicular stomatitis virus in vivo. American Soceity for Virology; 2011; Minneapolis, Minnesota, USA.

[108] Sabin AB, Olitsky PK. Influence of Host Factors on Neuroinvasiveness of Vesicular Stomatitis Virus : Iii. Effect of Age and Pathway of Infection on the Character and Localization of Lesions in the Central Nervous System. The Journal of experimental medicine. 1938;67(2):201-28.

[109] Sabin AB, Olitsky PK. Influence of Host Factors on Neuroinvasiveness of Vesicular Stomatitis Virus : Ii. Effect of Age on the Invasion of the Peripheral and Central Nervous Systems by Virus Injected into the Leg Muscles or the Eye. The Journal of experimental medicine. 1937;66(1):35-57.

[110] Sabin AB, Olitsky PK. Influence of Host Factors on Neuroinvasiveness of Vesicular Stomatitis Virus : I. Effect of Age on the Invasion of the Brain by Virus Instilled in the Nose. The Journal of experimental medicine. 1937;66(1):15-34.

[111] Daffis S, Szretter KJ, Schriewer J, Li J, Youn S, Errett J, et al. 2'-O methylation of the viral mRNA cap evades host restriction by IFIT family members. Nature. 2010;468(7322):452-6.

[112] Zust R, Cervantes-Barragan L, Habjan M, Maier R, Neuman BW, Ziebuhr J, et al. Ribose 2'-O-methylation provides a molecular signature for the distinction of self and non-self mRNA dependent on the RNA sensor Mda5. Nature immunology. 2011;12(2):137-43.

[113] Wilkins C, Dishongh R, Moore SC, Whitt MA, Chow M, Machaca K. RNA interference is an antiviral defence mechanism in Caenorhabditis elegans. Nature. 2005;436(7053):1044-7.

[114] De Clercq E. Antivirals and antiviral strategies. Nature Reviews Microbiology. 2004;2(9):704-20.

[115] de Clercq E, Montgomery JA. Broad-spectrum antiviral activity of the carbocyclic analog of 3-deazaadenosine. Antiviral research. 1983;3(1):17-24.

[116] Schluckebier G, Zhong P, Stewart KD, Kavanaugh TJ, Abad-Zapatero C. The 2.2 A structure of the rRNA methyltransferase ErmC' and its complexes with cofactor and cofactor analogs: implications for the reaction mechanism. Journal of molecular biology. 1999;289(2):277-91.

Chapter 11

# The Methylation of Metals and Metalloids in Aquatic Systems

Robert P. Mason

Additional information is available at the end of the chapter

http://dx.doi.org/10.5772/51774

## 1. Introduction

This chapter will focus on the formation processes and fate of the more common methylated metals and metalloids in the aquatic environment, focusing on both the ocean and freshwater ecosystems. In addition to the formation of the methylated compounds, the biotic and abiotic degradation of these compounds in the natural environment will also be discussed. The formation pathways and the microbes responsible for environmental methylation of different elements will be examined in detail with the focus on the organometallic or organic metalloid compounds of Hg, As, Sb and Se. Methylated compounds of other metal(loids)s will also be discussed. Such compounds are defined here as those in which the attachment of the organic moiety to the metal/metalloid ion is directly through a carbon-metal bound. Most of these bonds are covalent, especially for the metals and metalloids which have filled d and f orbitals [1]. There is an ever growing field of organometallic chemistry related to the use of manufactured transition metal compounds as catalysts or in organic production synthesis, or for other uses (e.g. alkylated Pb and butylated Sn compounds). These compounds will not be discussed in detail.

Most of the compounds that will be discussed contain one or more methyl group attached to the metal or metalloid atom (Table 1). Methylated halogens are formed in the environment but their formation and fate will not be included in this chapter. Methylation of transition metals does not occur under environmental conditions. In terms of the Periodic Table this chapter will focus on Groups 12-16, but will not directly discuss the major elements of Groups 14-16 (C, N, O, Si, P and S). Organometallic compounds with other alkyl groups (ethylated, butylated or phenyl-metal compounds) in the environment are mostly added as a result of human activity [1]. Most of these methylated compounds are formed biotically in the environment by microorganisms but abiotic pathways of methylation by methyl donor reactions within the aquatic system will also be discussed. Methylation within cells is a fundamental biochemical process and can be carried out by a number of biochemical pathways. It appears, however, that the mechanisms of methylation of metals and metalloids are carried out by one of three pathways, involving either: S-adenosylmethionine, methylcobalamin or N-methyltetrahydrofolate (Figure 1) [1].

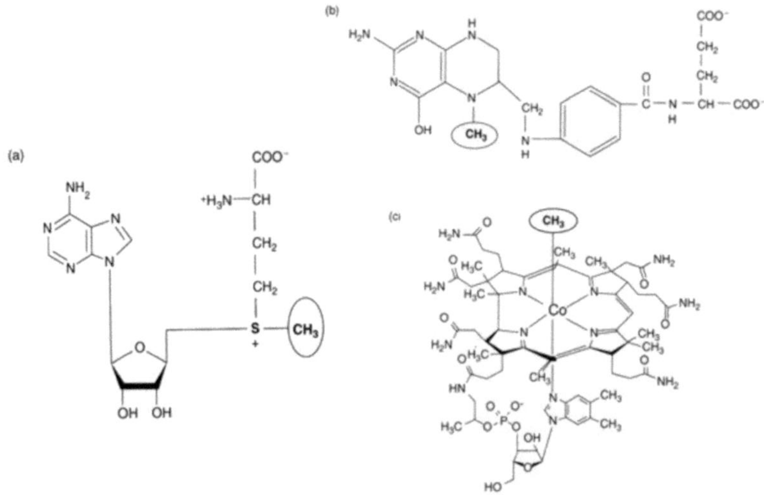

**Figure 1.** The primary methylating enzymes for metals and metalloids in organisms: a) SAM, b) tetrahydrofolate and c) methylcobalamin.

For example, methylation of Hg by sulfate-reducing and iron-reducing bacteria [2, 3] involves methylcobalamin, or related Co-containing enzymes. As ionic Hg ($Hg^{II}$) is the form that is methylated, methylation requires a methyl *carbanion* ($CH_3^-$), with methylation via a $SN_2$ reaction, and this process is not possible via the other methylation pathways. In contrast, the methyl group given up by S-adenosylmethionine (SAM) and N-methyltetrahydrofolate is a *carbocation* ($CH_3^+$). Thus there are fundamental differences in the potential methylating biochemicals and the pathways by which they react with metals and metalloids. For example, the so-called "Challenger" pathway of methylation of As by SAM requires that initially the $As^V$ is reduced to $As^{III}$ and then methylated [4, 5]. The methylated product is oxidized to the $As^V$ state during the methylation step and must be further reduced before addition of more methyl groups. Methylation of Se appears to follow a similar mechanism. In contrast, the methylation of Sn and other cations is thought to involve mainly the cobalamin pathway, in a similar fashion to Hg, with these elements being methylated while in their most oxidized form. There is no concrete evidence for the methylation of reduced Hg ($Hg^I$ or $Hg^0$) in the environment [2]. This is probably a result of the unstable nature of $Hg^I$ in the environment and the chemical nature of $Hg^0$. As a dissolved gas in most environmental aquatic systems it is not accumulated to any significant degree by microorganisms [6], or other organisms, unless it is oxidized upon uptake. So, therefore while $Hg^0$

could likely be methylated by SAM, methylation of $Hg^{II}$ by other pathways appears to be more efficient.

| Element | Methylated species | Element | Methylated species |
|---|---|---|---|
| As | $(CH_3)_4As_2$, $(CH_3)_3As$,$(CH_3)_3AsO$, $(CH_3)_2AsH$, $CH_3AsH_2$, $CH_3AsO(OH)_2$, $CH_3AsO(OH)$ | Sb | $(CH_3)_3Sb$,$(CH_3)_3SbO$, $(CH_3)_2SbH$, $CH_3SbH_2$ |
| Cd | $(CH_3)_2Cd$, $CH_3Cd^+$ | Hg | $(CH_3)_2Hg$, $CH_3Hg^+$, $CH_3HgH$ |
| Bi | $(CH_3)_3Bi$, $(CH_3)_2BiH$, $CH_3BiH_2$, $(CH_3)_2B^+$, $CH_3Bi^{2+}$ | Se | $(CH_3)_2Se_2$, $(CH_3)_2Se$, $(CH_3)_2SeS$, $(CH_3)_2SeH$ |
| Ge | $(CH_3)_3GeH$, $(CH_3)_2GeH_2$, $CH_3GeH_3$, $(CH_3)_2Ge^{2+}$, $CH_3Ge^{3+}$ | Sn | $(CH_3)_4Sn$,$(CH_3)_3AsH$, $(CH_3)_2SnH_2$,$CH_3SnH_3$ |
| Te | $(CH_3)_2Te$, | Tl | $(CH_3)_2Te^+$ |
| Pb | $(CH_3)_4Pb$, $(CH_3)_3PbH$ | | |

**Table 1.** Known forms of the various methylated compounds in the environment, including those that are formed by hydride generation but could exist as hydrides in the environment. Table compiled from [7-9].

Therefore, the various pathways of methylation are entirely distinct and which pathway dominates is a function of the differences in the speciation and oxidation state of the metal and metalloid in aquatic systems. For example, there is some evidence for the methylation of As and other metalloids in anoxic sediments via the cobalamin pathway [5, 10, 11]. In contrast to metal cations, the metalloids are present in environmental solutions mostly as an oxyanion of a weak acid, and therefore their form depends on pH. It has been proposed that Hg is taken up as a neutral Hg-sulfide complex via passive diffusion prior to methylation by sulfate-reducing bacteria (SRB), which are thought to be the most important methylating organisms [12]. However, there is also the potential for active transport of metals, especially through their uptake via channels designed for major ion transport, such as the channels for phosphate assimilation, or for the acquisition of required metals, such as Fe and Zn, or when combined with low molecular weight thiols [13].

Arsenic is a compound that appears to be methylated by organisms to reduce its toxicity [14]. In low phosphate environments, concentrations of arsenate can rival those of phosphate and given their similar chemistry, organisms can take up $As^V$ inadvertently. Methylation appears to be a way to detoxify the As and allow for its secretion into the environment. This is more prevalent in marine waters where As concentrations are higher, as discussed further below. In contrast, methylation of Hg and other metals enhances their toxicity [15]. However, most of the methylated Se compounds are derived from the decomposition of larger organic Se biochemicals such as selenoproteins [16]. Throughout the chapter such contrasts will be illustrated.

In summary, this chapter will specifically consider the methylation of elements in Groups 12-16 of the periodic table in aquatic systems, with a focus of those present as minor or trace elements. Most of these elements, especially those lower in the periodic table (i.e. higher atomic mass) form covalent bonds with carbon because of the shielding of the nuclear charge that occurs due to the presence of electrons in filled d and f orbitals. For the metals in Group 12, the tendency to form methylated compounds increases down the group. However, for Groups 15 and 16, the metalloids As and Se are methylated more readily than the elements below them in the periodic table, as in these cases the ionic character increases with atomic number. These and other differences within groups result in both similarities and differences in the methylation of the elements and in their stability, fate and transport in the environment, and their ability to biomagnify in aquatic food chains. Before discussing the processes whereby the metal(loids) are is methylated in the environment, it is useful to discuss briefly the distribution and fate of these elements in marine and freshwater environments.

## 2. The Distribution of Methylated Species in the Ocean and in Freshwaters

Representative vertical profiles in the North Pacific Ocean for the metal(loid)s discussed in this chapter are shown in Figure 2 [17]. Many of the elements that form methylated species in marine systems (e.g. As, Se, Sb, Ge) exist as oxyanions, and in a number of oxidation states [14, 18-20]. The reduced form of the element is often present because the methylation pathway involves reduction prior to methylation (the so-called Challenger mechanism), as discussed further below, or because of biological or photochemical reduction within organisms or the water column. In addition to be found as methylated compounds, many metalloids are incorporated into larger metalloid-containing species, such as arsenobetaine and selenoproteins [21, 22]. For example, As is found as $As^{III}$, $As^{V}$, mono-, di- and tri-methyl arsenic in marine waters (Figure 3a), and as arsenobetaine, arsenosugars and other As-containing carbohydrates in organisms. In the open ocean water column, methylation of As is mostly by phytoplankton as this is a detoxification/elimination mechanism. Arsenic ($As^{V}$) is taken up inadvertently by microorganisms in low phosphate waters (both exist as polyprotic acids with similar pKa's) and these relatively high concentrations of As can interfere with phosphate biochemistry within the cells.

The methylation of Hg, and other cations (e.g. Sn, Pb), does not involve oxidative methylation and therefore the reduced form of these metals, if present, is due to reductive processes that are not directly related to methylation. For Hg, however, the reduced form, elemental Hg ($Hg^{0}$) can be formed through the demethylation of $CH_3Hg$ and its subsequent reduction [23, 24]. The presence of the reduced forms of the elements in ocean surface waters, such as $Hg^{0}$ and $As^{III}$ is contrary to what is expected based on thermodynamic equilibrium calculations, and this further suggests their formation through microbial processes. However, reduction of Hg can be abiotic as well [25], as its redox couple is such that photochemical reduction is possible in surface waters.

As an example of the distribution of the metalloids in the ocean, profiles of the various species of As and Sb are shown in Figure 3a-c for the North Pacific Ocean. Methylated As and Sb species are present in the surface waters where phytoplankton activity occurs and the concentrations at depth are low or below detection, depending on the stability of the methylated form. In estuarine environments and freshwaters, $As^{III}$ and the methylated forms can be a larger fraction of the total dissolved As [20, 26]. The distribution and speciation of Sb is similar to that of As in the ocean water column [14]. The dominant oxidation state is +V, but with the presence of the +III oxidation state in the upper waters and the presence of methylated species, making up about 10% of the total dissolved Sb. The ancillary parameters shown in Figure 4 for the upper Pacific Ocean [27] give some indication of the physical factors influencing the distribution of the metalloids. The density profile shows an area of rapid changing density which coincides with rapid changes in temperature and salinity, which occurs closer to the surface in the northern latitudes. This stratification separates the more productive surface ocean, where most primary production occurs, from the deeper colder waters where microbial activity is much lower. Therefore, most of the microbial methylation of the metalloids occurs in the upper waters of the ocean, overall within the top 1000 m, and if driven mostly by phytoplankton, within the top 100 m.

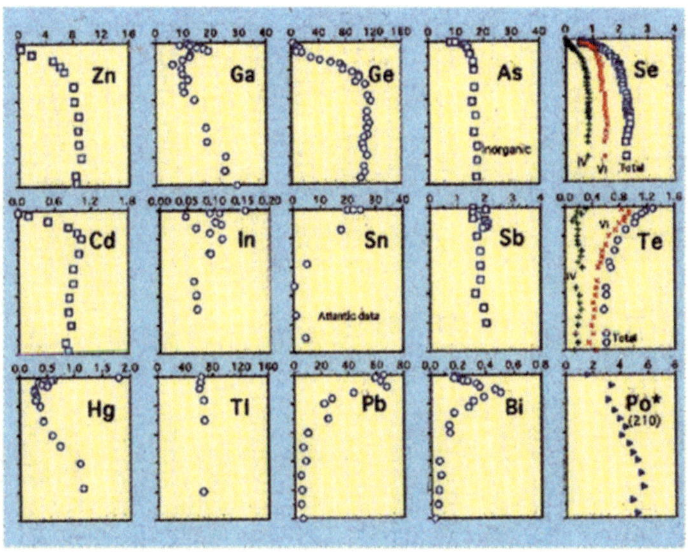


**Figure 2.** Vertical profiles of the total metal concentration in open North Pacific Ocean water as compiled by Nozaki 1997. The y-axis is the depth from the surface to 5 km. symbols represent the concentration range: squares for nmol/kg circles for pmol/kg and filled triangle for mBq/kg. Figure reprinted with permission from the American Geophysical Union (AGU).

For Se, methylated Se compounds are found in natural waters, as well as both the oxidized and reduced inorganic forms (Figure 3d). The two main inorganic redox states are found but their concentrations are somewhat depleted in the surface waters (Figure 3d), likely due to their uptake and incorporation into biota [14]. Selenium is an essential element although only required at low concentrations. The distribution of organic Se ($Se^{-II}$) suggests its persistence through the water column, either due to its continual formation and release from microbes and/or from organic matter dissolution, or due to its stability. Volatile methylated

Se compounds can be formed (analogs to methylated sulfide species, i.e. the suite of compounds: $(CH_3)_2S_ySe_Z$; y=z=0-2; y+z=1 or 2)) in the surface ocean through the decomposition of larger Se-containing biomolecules [28, 29]. The evasion of these compounds could also result in depletion of Se from surface waters [28, 30]. The cycling of Se in the upper ocean is not well understood and needs further study [14].

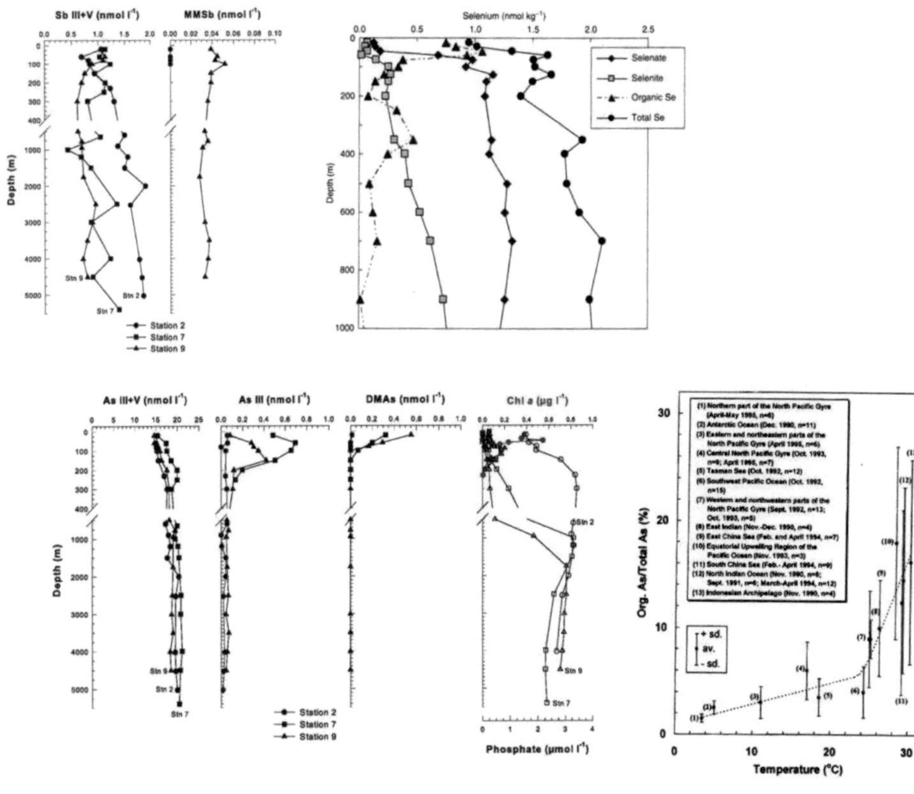


**Figure 3.** a) Arsenic speciation and distribution in the North Pacific Ocean. Taken from Cutter and Cutter (2006); b) relationship between the relative amount of organic As compounds in seawater and the water temperature. Taken from Santosa et al., 1997; c) Antimony speciation and distribution in the North Pacific Ocean. Taken from Cutter and Cutter (2006); d) Selenium speciation and distribution in the North Pacific Ocean. Taken from Cutter (2010). e) Speciation of germanium in the North Pacific Ocean. Taken from Cutter (2010). Figures a) and c) reprinted with permission from AGU; b) with permission from Wiley; c) and e) with permission from Elsevier

Tessier et al. [31] developed methods for the simultaneous measurement of a number of volatile metal(loid) species in various estuaries in France. They were able to detect the methylated Se species, a variety of Sn compounds, as well as $Hg^0$. Many of the compounds were found at low concentrations (e.g. $(CH_3)_2Se_2$, $(CH_3)_2SSe$, $(C_4H_9)_xSn(CH_3)_{4-x}$ (x=1-3), $(CH_3)_4Sn$ and $(CH_3)_2Hg$) and the dominant species for each element was $Hg^0$, $(CH_3)_2Se$ and $(C_4H_9)_3SnCH_3$.The concentration of $(CH_3)_2Se$ was higher in spring, suggesting production in conjunction with phytoplankton activity. For Sn and Hg, concentrations of volatile compounds were in the sub-pM range while concentrations were in the pM range for $(CH_3)_2Se$. In each case, there was some evidence of a gradient across the estuary that is likely related to water mixing and changes in ecosystem productivity.

Germanium (Ge) is a most unusual element in that its ocean distribution is dominated by its methylated forms (Figure 3e). Germanium is found as the mono- and dimethylated species with the monomethyl species being the dominant form throughout the water column [14]. It has a conservative distribution which indicates its high stability and little is known about its formation mechanisms [32]. There is also little information on the ocean distribution of tin (Sn) (Figure 2) [33]. Much of the focus of study of this element has been due to its use as antifouling agents (e.g. tetrabutyltin) and these compounds will not be discussed in detail. In the surface ocean its concentration is higher than at depth, showing that it is scavenged from the ocean by sinking particles. Bismuth is also higher in surface waters and has a deep water scavenged profile (Figure 2) [33].

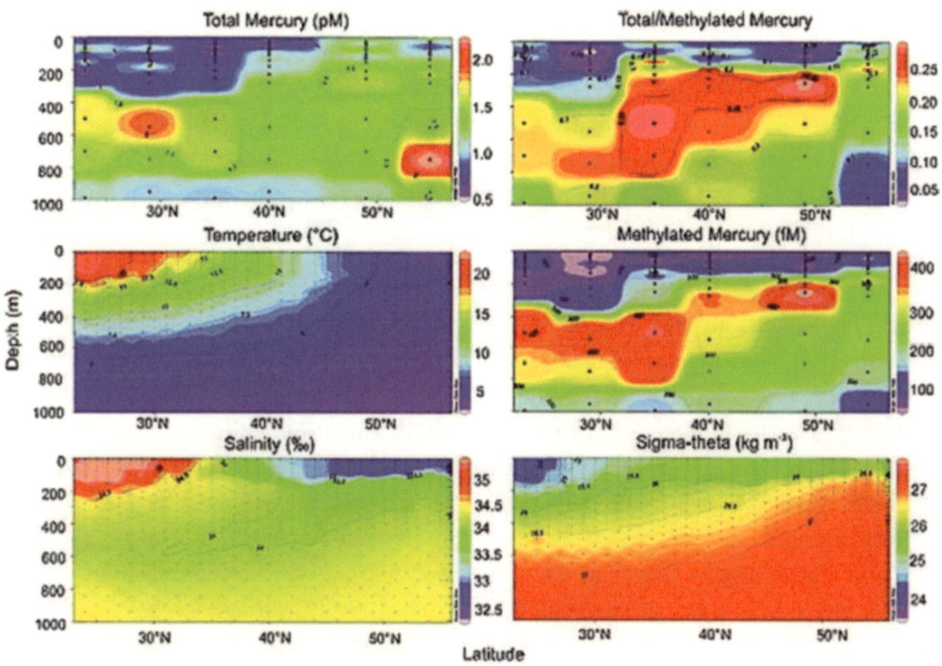


**Figure 4.** Distributions of total mercury, total methylated mercury (sum of mono and dimethylmercury), and their ratio, temperature, salinity and sigma-theta (a measure of water density) for a transect sampling waters at latitude 152°W in the North Pacific. Taken from Sunderland et al. (2009). Figure reprinted with permssion from AGU.

In the late 1980's, methylated Hg compounds were detected in the water column of the remote ocean [25] and in lakes, and it was shown that the formation of $CH_3Hg$ was relatively ubiquitous in aquatic systems [34]. In ocean waters, and in some freshwater systems, dimethylmercury ($(CH_3)_2Hg$) has been measured and its presence is mostly found in the water column, although there is some evidence for $(CH_3)_2Hg$ in sediment porewaters

[35]. The relative importance of different bacteria in the production of $CH_3Hg$ and $(CH_3)_2Hg$ in these diverse natural aquatic environments is not clearly understood, although it has been a topic of recent investigation. The distribution of Hg in the North Pacific Ocean is shown in Fig 4 [27]. As can be seen, the distribution of methylated Hg is different from that of As, Sb and the other metalloids as the concentration is low in the surface waters, and maximal in the mid-depth waters. This study and a number of other investigations [25, 27, 36-38] have concluded that the profiles are best explained by formation of methylated Hg in conjunction with the decomposition of organic matter that sinks from the surface ocean, and that the formation is microbially-mediated. Studies in the Arctic Ocean have shown that in situ methylation occurs in the water column in this region [39], further confirming this pathway. This contrasts lakes where most of the methylation is thought to occur in the sediments [2].

Overall, given the limited data for some elements it is difficult to examine in detail the locations and processes of formation of many of the metal(loid)s in marine systems. In summary, the metal(loid)s show the following distributions (Figure 2): a) distributions with lower surface ocean concentrations, reflecting uptake in the surface ocean, either into plankton and the food web or by abiotic particles, and release at depth; or b) higher surface water concentrations, reflecting either the dominance of atmospheric inputs (e.g. Pb) or the strong scavenging of the element from deep waters by particles. Overall, however, their distributions are modified to a degree by the formation of methylated or reduced species and the stability and fate of these compounds relative to the more oxidized forms.

Studies of many of the metal(loid)s are also limited for freshwater environments. Mercury has been the most studied and the factors controlling Hg methylation in sediments in the Florida Everglades is summarized in Fig 5a [2]. Across the Everglades there is a strong organic matter and sulfate gradient that drives the activity of the SRB's (sulfate reduction rate (SRR) in the figure). The product of sulfate reduction, sulfide, complexes Hg and reduces its bioavailability to the methylating organisms, as discussed further below. The bioavailable fraction is represented in Figure 5a as $HgS^0$, the neutral complex concentration. The maximum in methylation rate and the highest fraction as $CH_3Hg$ in sediments (%MeHg in the figure) is found at the right combination of bioavailability and bacterial activity, at low sulfide but sufficient sulfate concentrations [2, 40]. Similar results have been found for estuarine and coastal sediments [41-44], as shown in Figure 5b. Higher sulfide levels in coastal sediments result in a strong hindrance of methylation at concentrations above 0.1 mM sulfide in sediment porewaters [2, 42]. This is shown in Figure 5. In the estuarine sediments, lower methylation rates and %$CH_3Hg$ are found at depth as sulfide levels increase. The highest fractional conversion of Hg to $CH_3Hg$ occurs in low organic matter, shelf sediments where microbial activity is lower but Hg is much more bioavailable [41-44]. Studies in lakes show comparable data, and also suggest that there is the potential for methylation within the water column of seasonally or permanently stratified lakes where oxygen is depleted and sulfide is present [45]. In these environments, the highest methylation is within the redox interface, which is consistent with the discussion of methylated Hg formation in the ocean and in sediments, although truly anoxic conditions are not found in the ocean water column.

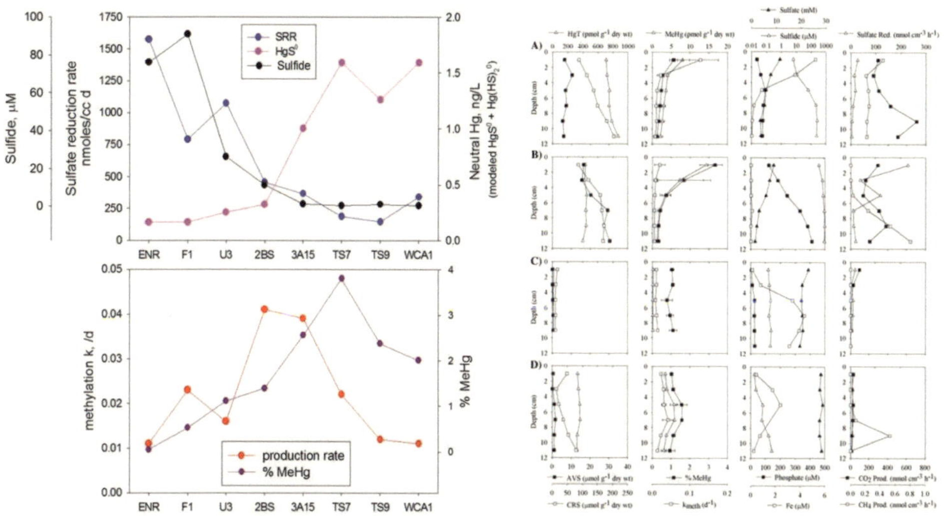


**Figure 5.** a) Changes in the concentration of various parameters including the concentration of bioavailable Hg ($HgS^0$) as well as the methylation rate for sites across the eutrophication gradient in the Florida Everglades. Taken from Benoit et al. (2003); b) The vertical distribution of parameters, including mercury speciation (total (HgT) and methyl-mercury (MeHg)), and also the rates of microbial processes (mercury methylation ($k_{meth}$), sulfate reduction, $CO_2$ and methane production). The sediment reduced sulfide content is indicated by the concentration of labile reduced sulfide (AVS) and pyrite (CRS). The four sample locations include sites in the Chesapeake Bay (A and B) and sites on the shelf (C and D). Taken from Hollweg et al. (2009). Figure a) reprinted with permission of the American Chemical Society (ACS), b) with permission from Elsevier.

Arsenic speciation and methylation in freshwater ecosystems has also received attention and this has been driven mostly by studies in As contaminated environments. Methylation processes are similar to that found in the ocean with most of the methylated species being confined to the surface waters and levels in deeper waters depending on a variety of conditions [46-50]. Both seasonally and permanently stratified lakes have been examined and while high levels of the inorganic forms of As are found in anoxic waters, this is not the case for the methylated species. A study in the hydrothermal environment at Yellowstone National Park, USA found that there were volatile As compounds emitted in locations with high aqueous As (up to 50 μM levels) [51]. Concentrations of volatile As in surface waters were from <1 to 2.5 μM. Species identified were $(CH_3)_2AsCl$, $(CH_3)_3As$, $(CH_3)_2AsCCH_3$ and $(CH_3)_2AsCl_2$. There are also some reports of volatile As compounds in some marine environments [52]. Studies of the other methylated metal(loid)s in freshwater environments are very limited, with some examination of the formation pathways and speciation of Sb and Se [53-55]. Aspects of the factors influencing formation will be discussed further below. Overall, there is a need for further research on the methylation of metal(loid)s besides As and Hg in aquatic systems.

## 3. Biotic Transformations

Of the species that exist in solution as cations, Hg is the element that is methylated to the highest extent, and has been the most studied, primarily as a result of concerns of the human and environmental impact of the accumulation of $CH_3Hg$ in fish, and their consumption [56]. The results of these extensive studies can be extrapolated to other cations that are methylated, but more study is also required to investigate their fate and how they are methylated and bioaccumulated. In terms of the oxyanions, As has received the most attention and again this is driven by concerns over toxicity and the fact that methylation reduces the toxicity of As relative to reduced inorganic As. Methylated compounds of both As and Se can also be formed by the decomposition of larger biochemicals produced in microbes and larger organisms. These pathways will also be discussed in addition to the discussion of the direct methylation pathways.

### 3.1. The biotic methylation of mercury

Acute exposure incidents in Japan and elsewhere in the 1960's provided the first evidence that inorganic Hg could be converted into the more toxic and bioaccumulative $CH_3Hg$ [15, 56]. Methylation of Hg in sediments by the resident microorganisms was subsequently demonstrated and many of the early studies examining the role of microbes in methylation were in coastal and estuarine sediments [34]. Selective microbial inhibition studies indicated that methylation was primarily mediated by SRB's [57, 58] but recent studies suggest that phylogenetically similar microbes (e.g. Fe-reducers in the genera *Geobacter*) can also methylate Hg [3, 59]. Additionally, there has been recent demonstration of methylation being related to the activity of methanogens in lake periphyton [60] and it is possible that further examination of different environments may lead to further understanding of the Hg methylation process. The site, or more likely sites, of methylation within cells has not been clearly identified and not all SRB's methylate Hg, and even organisms from the same genus has different abilities to methylate Hg [2]. While initial studies suggested that methylation was associated with the Acetyl-CoA pathway and cobalamin in one estuarine organism (*Desulfovibrio desulfuricans* LS) [61-63], this link does not hold across a variety of organisms, as organisms without this pathway methylate Hg, and *vice versa* [64, 65]. For SRB's, both complete and incomplete organic carbon oxidizers are methylators of Hg. Recent studies have also shown differences in the rate of methylation in biofilms compared to free living SRB in culture [66]. It was shown that the gene expression, and in particular the activity of the Acetyl-CoA pathway, was different for the same organism when growing under these different conditions and that the expression of the pathway coincided with the increased methylation in the biofilms. These results appear to confirm the notion that methylation is accidental and not a detoxifying mechanism in these organisms.

In a number of ecosystems, $CH_3Hg$ production has been shown to be strongly related to Hg interactions with sulfide, e.g. [2, 43, 44, 67]. Neutrally charged dissolved Hg-S species (HOHgSH and $Hg(SH)_2$) are believed to be much more bioavailable to sulfate-reducing bacteria [12, 68] than charged complexes. They have a relatively high $K_{ow}$ and dominate at low environmental sulfide concentrations. At higher sulfide, negatively charged Hg-S species and Hg polysulfide species dominate [69]. Therefore, methylation is most prevalent in environments where sulfate reduction is high, but sulfide accumulation is low (Figure 5) [2]. These locations are often the upper layers of sediments, as inputs of fresh organic matter and oxygen diffusion into sediments result in high rates of Fe and sulfate reduction in regions of relatively low sulfide content. Other complexes of Hg are potentially bioavailable and complexes with small organic ligands can have a relatively high $K_{ow}$ [70]. This is demonstrated by the fact that a bacterial culture of *Geobacter sulfurreducens* can methylate $Hg^{II}$ when present in the medium as a cysteine complex at a much faster rate than as either sulfide or chloride complexes [71, 72]. Most studies therefore highlight the importance of speciation in determining the rate of methylation in sediments and freshwater systems but the role and activity of the methylating bacteria cannot be ignored. It has been well demonstrated that speciation affects the uptake and methylation of inorganic Hg and the same impact is probable on the rate of demethylation of $CH_3Hg$, and on the uptake and methylation of other cations.

The discussion above about methylation in sediments and freshwater systems does not explain the sources and sinks for $CH_3Hg$ in the open ocean. A recent examination of the sources and sinks for $CH_3Hg$ and $(CH_3)_2Hg$ (hereafter represented as $\sum CH_3Hg$) to the ocean [25] suggest that external sources (riverine inputs and coastal sources and atmospheric deposition) are insufficient to account for the $\sum CH_3Hg$ sinks in the ocean, which include accumulation into biota and removal by fisheries, photochemical and biological degradation into inorganic Hg, and net removal to the deep ocean and deep sea sediments. This indicates that production within the ocean water column is important. While both $CH_3Hg$ and $(CH_3)_2Hg$ are broadly distributed throughout the ocean water column, they have observed concentrations are difficult to explain without *in situ* production [25]. Initial studies in the equatorial Pacific Ocean suggested sub-thermocline maxima in both $CH_3Hg$ and $(CH_3)_2Hg$ [38, 73-75] have been confirmed by more recent studies in the North and South Atlantic and Pacific Oceans, the Mediterranean Sea, the Southern Ocean and other locations [27, 36, 37, 76-80]. Figure 4 is representative of a typical profile for the upper ocean. These vertical distributions are most consistent with *in situ* formation of $\sum CH_3Hg$ in association with the decomposition of organic matter. The link to organic carbon degradations is demonstrated, for example, by the relationship between the amount of $\sum CH_3Hg$ and the extent of organic carbon remineralization [27], and correlations between $\sum CH_3Hg$ and apparent oxygen utilization, another measure of carbon degradation [36-38, 75, 78]. The $\sum CH_3Hg$ distribution across studies suggests that the transition regions (the base of the euphotic zone), and subsurface waters where particulate organic matter is being degraded, are locations of enhanced net methylation of Hg. However, there is still little concrete information about the microbes responsible for Hg methylation and for the primary factors driving the relative magnitude of this process across ocean basins.

### 3.2. The biotic methylation of arsenic and antimony

The methylation of As (Figure 6) is thought to be a detoxifying mechanism for bacteria and phytoplankton [5], especially those in the marine environment where the concentration of As is relatively high compared to the required nutrient phosphate, as both exist in solution as oxyanions. However, the first indication of As methylation was the demonstration of the release of volatile As-containing compounds from wallpaper in the 1800's in Europe, from the use of As-containing pigments in their coloration [4, 5]. It was further realized that mold and damp enhanced their formation and therefore a biological role for the production of these volatile compounds was concluded, mostly based on work done by an Italian physician, Gosio. This early work was followed by Challenger and his colleagues in the early 20th century, who developed the original mechanism for As methylation that still bears his name [4].

It is now known that methylation of As and other metalloids is carried out by a wide variety of fungi, yeasts and bacteria, and eukaryotes [4, 21, 81]. Methylation of As is the most prevalent of the elements in Group 15 occurring in microbes, algae, plants and animals while methylation of Sb is more restricted to eukaryotic and prokaryotic microorganisms. It is thought that As is mainly taken up by phytoplankton through phosphate uptake channels. It is however also possible that the methylated As species are formed during the degradation of As biochemicals during degradation of cellular material [4]. Inorganic As is present in environmental waters as an oxyacid in both oxidation states: arsenic acid (arsenate) $AsO(OH)_3$ or $H_3AsO_4$ ($pK_{a1}$ = 2.2; $pK_{a2}$ = 7.0; $pK_{a3}$ = 11.5) and arsenous acid (arsenite) $As(OH)_3$ ($pK_{a1}$ = 9.3). The pKa's of arsenic acid are very similar to those of phosphate (respectively, 2.1, 7.2 and 12.4) and therefore the speciation of $As^V$ and phosphate in most environmental waters is analogous. At the typical pH of environmental waters, the major species will be $H_2AsO_4^{-}$ and $HAsO_4^{2-}$. It generally appears that phosphate uptake is active and in conjunction with $Na^+$ co-transport and therefore a similar mechanism is likely for As. In open ocean surface waters, phosphate concentrations are often very low (<0.5 μM) and As concentrations are typically around 10-20 nM [14, 20]. Therefore, given this relatively small difference in concentration, inadvertent uptake of As is possible [21]. The methylated forms of As can be released from the cells into the environment or they can be incorporated into larger molecules and their toxicity reduced as a result.

The Challenger mechanism of As, and other metalloid, methylation involves a series of reductive methylation steps where the addition of the methyl group is via a carbocation addition reaction (Figure 6). The details of the mechanism are relatively well known although some aspects of the biochemistry within the cell are not entirely elucidated. It is thought that cellular thiols, such as glutathione, are involved in the reduction steps and that S-adenosylmethionine (SAM) is the main methylating agent. The reduction is linked to glutathione oxidation and is enzymatically controlled. Arsenite and related methyltransferase enzymes are associated with the methylation step [4, 8]. The products are the simple reduced methylated species ($(CH_3)_xAsO(OH)_{3-x}$, x=1-3) as well as oxidized forms, such as trimethylarsine oxide ($(CH_3)_3AsO^-$). Volatile forms are also produced by some organisms (Table 1), and these are the methylated As hydrides, such as ($(CH_3)_xAsH_{3-x}$; x = 1-3) [9]. In marine algae, As is found in a variety of organic compounds, such as arsenosugars and As-containing carbohydrates, with the most common compound being arsenobetaine (trimethylarsinio acetate) ($(CH_3)_3AsCH_2COO^-$) [21]. It is thought that these products are formed from further reactions of the methylated derivatives and that they are ultimately generated by processes similar to that invoked in the Challenger mechanism. The methylated species are also found in measurable concentrations in many environmental waters, both freshwater and marine, as discussed above, and their presence has mostly been correlated with phytoplankton activity although their production via bacteria present in conjunction with the algae is also possible. It is suggested that these compounds are actively exported by the phytoplankton.

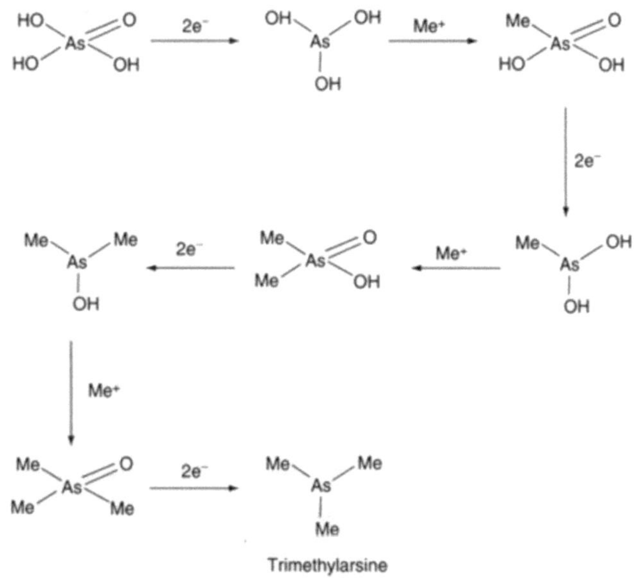


**Figure 6.** Representation of the steps involved in the methylation of arsenic via the Challenger process. Figure taken from Feldman (2003) and used with permission from Wiley.

Based on the $pK_a$ values, it is evident that the reduced form of As is present as an undissociated acid at physiological pH's and in most environmental solutions, and therefore that there is the possibility of its loss via passive diffusion from the cells into the surrounding media. There are a number of instances where measurements in the environment have shown that the concentration of reduced inorganic As is greater than that of $As^V$, and release of $As^{III}$ after microbial reduction is the most likely explanation [16]. There have been a number of As reductases indentified in microbes and these processes appear to be separate from the methylation pathways, and therefore involve different reductants, such as thioredoxin and glutaredoxin [4]. Similar to other metal reductases, the operons are attached to plasmids in bacteria.

Antimony (Sb) has a similar chemistry to As and therefore it is expected to behave in a similar manner to As in terms of uptake and methylation [7]. Its compounds have been widely used in industry, medicine, as a poison, and as cosmetics. The methylated forms, $(CH_3)_xSb_{3-x}$ (x = 1-3), are well-known (Table 1), as are many other organo-Sb compounds, and many have been synthesized for industrial purposes. Volatile Sb compounds were suggested as a possible cause for Sudden Infant Death Syndrome, as Sb compounds were used as flame retardants in mattresses, and this lead to the examination of the mechanisms of their formation [4, 7]. A number of fungi and bacteria have been identified that can methylate Sb, and methylation is much higher in the presence of $Sb^{III}$ and it is apparent that many organisms are not able to reduce and methylate $Sb^{V}$ [54]. Therefore, the methylation of Sb may be less ubiquitous than that of As, and there appears to be complex interactions if both As and Sb are present in the same culture in terms of relative methylation [4, 7]. Overall, little is known of the speciation and form of Sb in natural waters, and the formula is given either as $Sb(OH)_5$ or $HSb(OH)_6$, which dissociates in water to form the anion, $Sb(OH)_6$ - ($pK_{a1}$ =2.2). There is evidence from measurements in seawater and in the presence of marine algae that reduction to $Sb^{III}$ occurs and that the monomethylated form exists in environmental waters [54]. It is also present in freshwaters, and evidence for its formation in environments such as landfills [56]. Overall, however, it appears that $Sb^{V}$ is the major form in environmental solutions. The presence of volatile Sb compounds in landfill gases and other methanogenic environments confirms that methylation of Sb is microbially mediated [4, 82].

Most studies have invoked the Challenger mechanism to explain the methylation of As and other metalloids by SAM in the environment, especially in oxic waters but there is some speculation that the pathway of methylation may be different for anaerobic organisms. In this case, it has been suggested that methylation may involve cobalamin and therefore involve a different mechanism whereby a carbanion or a radical from methylcobalamin is added to $As^{III}$ in the presence of mediating enzymes [4, 7]. Methanogenic Achaea, for example, were shown to methylate a variety of metalloids of Groups 15 and 16 (As, Se, Sb, Te, and Bi) [10]. The mechanism was attributed to side reactions with methylcobalamin. Additionally, it was demonstrated that methylation of As(V) did not occur and that methylation of As(III) did not involve oxidation, and was therefore similar in process to the methylation of Hg whereby the methyl group is added as a carbanion rather than a carbocation. While Weufel et al. [10] were able to demonstrate the formation of higher methylated compounds, another study [11] suggested that the reaction pathway produces only monomethylated forms, which contrasts the environment where higher methylated forms are often more abundant. In addition to methylation of As, cobalamin has also been shown to methylate Sb [11].

Studies have also focused on the methylation of As and other metalloids in sediments [83]. Laboratory incubation of marine sediments have produced volatile arsines ($(CH_3)_xAsH_{3-x}$; x=0-3) and other methylated compounds ($(CH_3)_xAsO(OH)_{3-x}$; x=1-3). In other experiments, incubation of sediments showed the production of both methylated As and Sb species [84]. It appeared that the dimethylated species dominated for both metalloids. Also, the initial rate of formation of the methylated species was faster for As than for Sb. After the completion of the experiment (76 days) all methylated forms of As and Sb were found distributed through the sediment column (0-12 cm) and in the overlying water. While the experiment lasted 76 days, in many instances the peak in concentration occurred relatively early in the experiment suggesting demethylation was occurring in the latter parts of the experiment.

Also, in most cases the porewater concentrations were similar or lower than those of the overlying water.

The relative concentration of the various compounds changed over the course of the incubations in both these experiments [83, 84] and these changes are likely related to the changing microbial community with time and the sequential nature of the methylation processes, as well as demethylation. Field sampling of sediment porewater confirmed the presence of these compounds in the environment, but also showed that these compounds were a small fraction (<1%) of the total As. Another study of estuarine porewaters also found the presence of methylated As, but again these were a relative small fraction of the total (<4%) [85]. This contrasts the oxic water column where higher relative amounts occur (Figure 3). Results with lake sediments [86] were similar as these studies also suggested that anaerobic bacteria (Fe, Mn or sulfate-reducing bacteria) were mostly responsible for the transformations found. Overall, these studies suggest that methylation of As and other metalloids can occur in sediments and that anaerobic bacteria are responsible for the methylation, contrasting the formation mechanisms in the oxic environment. Overall, the links and interactions between the various pathways are complex, and it is difficult to distinguish the relative importance of the various processes in As methylation in sediments and other environments.

### 3.3. The biotic formation of methylated selenium compounds

Selenium, an element in Group 16, has important and complex organometallic chemistry, and is readily methylated. In organisms, Se has a large number of biochemical roles as it is incorporated into a number of enzymes [52]. The methylation of Se was first investigated by Challenger and since these early studies it has been shown that Se has an extensive biochemistry and that compounds, such as selenoproteins are important constituents of organisms as they act as anti-oxidants and have other roles in the cellular machinery [16, 81, 87]. Compounds such as selenomethionine and Se-adenosylselenomethionine (SeSAM), are found in cells, where Se has replaced S, as could be expected as these elements are from the same group of the periodic table. The methylating ability of SeSAM has been shown to be greater than that of SAM [7].

It has been suggested that $CH_3SeH$ and the cation $CH_3Se^+$ are some of the compounds responsible for the toxicity of Se. Additionally, analogs to the methylated S-containing compounds $(CH_3)_2S$ (DMS) and $(CH_3)_2S_2$ have been identified ($(CH_3)_2Se$, $(CH_3)_2SSe$ and $(CH_3)_2Se_2$) [7]. It appears likely that these compounds are the degradation products produced by certain microorganisms that exist in ocean waters, being formed from the decomposition of 3-dimethyl-selenopropionate ($(CH_3)_2Se^+CH_2CH_2COO^-$) (Figure 7) [7]. Similar processes likely account for their formation in terrestrial waters and other environments. The importance of this pathway was confirmed by growing a freshwater green algae on selenate in the absence of sulfate and showing the formation of the volatile methylated species [53]. This production was reduced when sulfate was added to the medium. Another study also demonstrated the release of volatile methylated Se compounds from green algae. This study also showed the potential for As to inhibit the formation of the Se compounds

[55]. Overall, the formation of methylated Se compounds is relatively ubiquitous as they are apparently produced by both bacteria and algae.

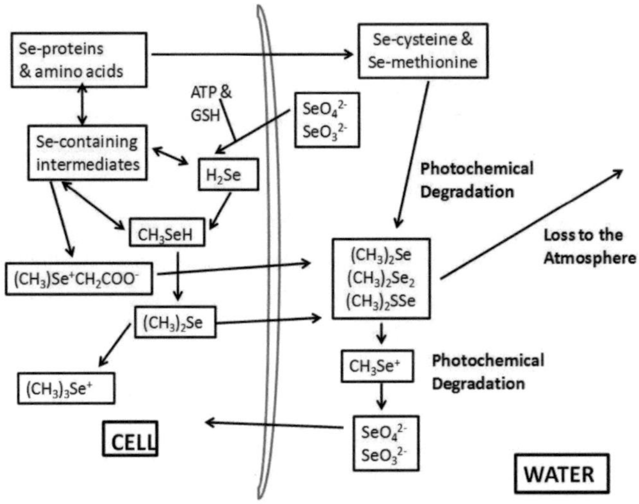


**Figure 7.** Pathways for the formation and decomposition of methylated selenium compounds in the environment

However, direct methylation is also possible. In freshwater environments, γ-Proteobacteria, such as *Pseudomonas* spp. have been identified as Se methylators. Additionally, a gene encoding for the bacterial thiopurine methyltransferase has been shown to methylate selenite and (methyl)selenocysteine into dimethylselenide and dimethyldiselenide [88]. One potential pathway of formation that interlinks the Se and Hg cycles relates to the potential for $CH_3Hg$, present in the cell as a thiol complex (represented here as $CH_3HgR$), to bind to Se-containing amino acids or thiols (represented here as SeR). It is proposed that two CH3HgSeR react to form $(CH_3Hg)_2Se$ and $R_2Se$, and then $(CH_3Hg)_2Se$ decomposes to $(CH_3)_2Hg$ and HgSe [89]. A similar pathway was proposed many years ago involving $(CH_3Hg)_2S$ for the formation of $(CH_3)_2Hg$, which was purportedly formed in sediments [90]. Demethylation of $(CH_3)_2Se$ is found in anoxic sediments and it is speculated that methanogens are using this compound for growth in an analogous fashion to their utilization of DMS. In summary, it is likely that in sediments and other low oxygen/anoxic environments, direct methylation is occurring while in the water column the production of the methylated Se compounds results from decomposition of Se-containing biomolecules.

### 3.4. The biotic formation of other methylated compounds

A number of metal(loid)s not yet discussed are known to form organometallic compounds although there is little information on the formation, stability and toxicity of many of them, or on how they are formed in aquatic systems. In Group 12, Zn does not form any stable small methylated compounds in aquatic systems. In contrast, Cd, above Hg in the periodic table, has been isolated from the environment as methylated compounds [9], although

$(CH_3)_2Cd$ is relatively unstable in water. There have been few studies of organic Cd compounds in the environment in contrast to the inorganic chemistry of Cd that has been well-studied. Initial evidence for the formation of $CH_3Cd^+$ was by bacterial cultures isolated from polar waters [91], and these same cultures also produced methylated Pb and Hg compounds. In the environment, evidence suggests that the peak concentration of these methylated species coincided with that of chlorophyll a, suggesting a microbial role in the formation of these compounds in polar waters. These studies of the formation of methylated Cd compounds in ocean waters require more confirmation. It is known that Cd can be abiotically methylated by methylcobalamin so this represents the potential biotic methylation pathway in aquatic systems [7].

For the other Group 13 elements, there is little evidence for the formation of methylated compounds except for Tl. This is a potentially toxic and bioaccumulative metal and the chemistry of inorganic Tl has received some attention [7]. It appears that $Tl^I$ is oxidized and methylated at the same time (i.e. likely via the Challenger mechanism) producing a mono-, di- or trimethylated product of, respectively, +2, +1 and 0 charge. This process occurs under anaerobic conditions with little evidence of aerobic methylation [82]. None of these compounds are highly stable but there is some initial evidence for the presence of these compounds at low pM concentrations in the Atlantic Ocean, mostly as $(CH_3)_2Tl^+$ [92], and ranging up to nearly 50% of the total Tl, and present throughout the water column. The profile of the methylated species correlated with chlorophyll a in the upper waters, suggesting its microbial production. These authors also found methylation to occur in an anaerobic lake sediment [92]. There is no evidence for methylated In and Ga complexes in the environment.

Alkylation of Group 14 elements occurs for Sn and Pb and Ge. Alkyl Pb and Sn compounds have been widely produced for use in industrial and other applications, but these will not be discussed here. Studies have shown that a variety of microbes can methylate Sn [8]. For Ge, the mono-, di-, tri- and tetramethylated compounds have been found in the environment. In the ocean, $Ge^{IV}$ has its highest concentrations in deep ocean waters with depleted concentrations in surface waters (Figure 3e) ([82] and references therein). For much of the ocean, the dominant form is monomethylated ($CH_3Ge^{3+}$), and its distribution suggests it is relatively stable. The other methylated Ge species ($(CH_3)_2Ge^{2+}$ and $(CH_3)_3Ge^+$) occur in seawater at somewhat lower concentrations (Figure 3e). It is apparent that methylated Ge compounds can be produced under anaerobic conditions and that these species are not produced in oxic waters in the presence of algae. These compounds can also be made in the laboratory through reactions with $CH_3I$ and methylcobalamin, suggesting that this is the pathway for methylation in the environment, although it has also been suggested that these compounds are formed via the Challenger mechanism [7].

Besides As and Sb, bismuth (Bi) is found under some conditions as methylated compounds, although the methylation is restricted to prokaryotes [5, 82]. As the compounds of Bi are used in industrial and pharmaceutical applications, such as Pepto-Bismol, its presence in sewage treatment plants, and in municipal waste deposits, and the loss of volatile forms of Bi from these environments is not surprising [9]. Bismuth, in contrast to As and Sb, exists in environmental media as a +3 ion rather than as an oxyanion. It also can be found in the mono-, di- and tri- methylated form, and $(CH_3)_3Bi$ is non-polar while the other forms are ions, which exist as complexes in solution (Table 1). The trimethylated form is less stable than its As and Sb analogs. For example, methylated Bi compounds are produced by methanogens in culture [7]. The hydride ($BiH_3$) has also been isolated from bacterial cultures (Table 1). In the biotic formation of methylated Bi compounds, it is possible that the methyl group is donated by methylcobalamin, which is consistent with its form in solution as ionic complexes [5, 82]. This contrasts the methylation of As and Sb. However, there is little detailed information available about the exact nature of the methylation process for Bi.

There is evidence for the formation of organo-Te compounds and the mechanisms for their formation appear to be similar to the mechanisms for the formation of organic Se-containing compounds [82], which is also in Group 16 of the periodic table. Certain bacteria have been shown to methylate Te and form dimethylated compounds, and there is a complex interaction between the ability of these organisms to methylate and the Se concentration [8]. This suggests that Se and Te, which are electronically similar, behave similarly in this regard. Both exist in solution as oxyacids although the pKa's of the selenic and selenous acid are much lower than the corresponding values for telluric and tellurous acid [93]. There has been some suggestion that Po can be methylated but the conditions under which this occurred suggests that these compounds are unlikely in natural environments [7]. The mechanism of methylation is not known and as Po exists in various oxidation states, there are a number of potential methylation pathways. More research is needed to examine in more detail the methylation and cycling of Po and the other less-studied heavy metals and metalloids.

## 4. Microbially-Mediated Decomposition of Methylated Compounds

The pathways for the decomposition of organometal(loid)s often occur in a stepwise fashion with the removal of successive methyl (or other alkyl) groups from the central metal(loid) atom. Examples include the decomposition of $(CH_3)_2Hg$ to $CH_3Hg^+$ to $Hg^{II}/Hg^0$ and $(CH_3)_4Sn$ or $(CH_3)_4Pb$ to the tri, di and monomethyl forms. Microbial demethylation is likely to be a detoxifying mechanism in many cases, but there is also evidence that some microbes can use the low molecular weight methyl compounds as a carbon source. Both of these pathways will be highlighted with specific examples. For most of the metal(loid)s, the degradation pathways are less studied than the methylation reactions. The one exception is the demethylation of $CH_3Hg$ using the *mer* operon [23] (Figure 8). This pathway can decompose other alkyl as well as phenyl Hg compounds.

A number of microbes appear to be important in the demethylation of $CH_3Hg$ although the mechanisms are not as well understood in many environments [23, 24]. In uncontaminated environments, the major products appear to be Hg and $CO_2$ and therefore this pathway has been termed *oxidative demethylation*, in contrast to *reductive demethylation*, where $CH_4$ is the major carbon product [24]. The mechanism of oxidative demethylation may be analogous to monomethylamine degradation by methanogens or acetate oxidation by SRB's. Reductive demethylation appears to be prevalent in more contaminated environments and at high $CH_3Hg$ and Hg concentrations it has been shown that a series of inducible genes can be activated (the *mer* operon) that can aid in detoxification of $CH_3Hg$ via demethylation (the *mer B* gene which encodes for organomercury lyase), and reduction of $Hg^{II}$ to $Hg^0$ (the *mer A* gene which produces mercury reductase) (Figure 8). The *mer B* gene can decompose a variety of organomercury compounds. There is also a regulatory gene (*mer R*), as well as transport genes and their transport proteins in the cell membrane [23]. The overall operon is contained on a plasmid and is readily transferred between bacteria in the environment. However, while membrane $Hg^{II}$ transport proteins are present in bacteria with the *mer* operon, they are absent in SRB and therefore are not involved in the transport of Hg associated with methylation.

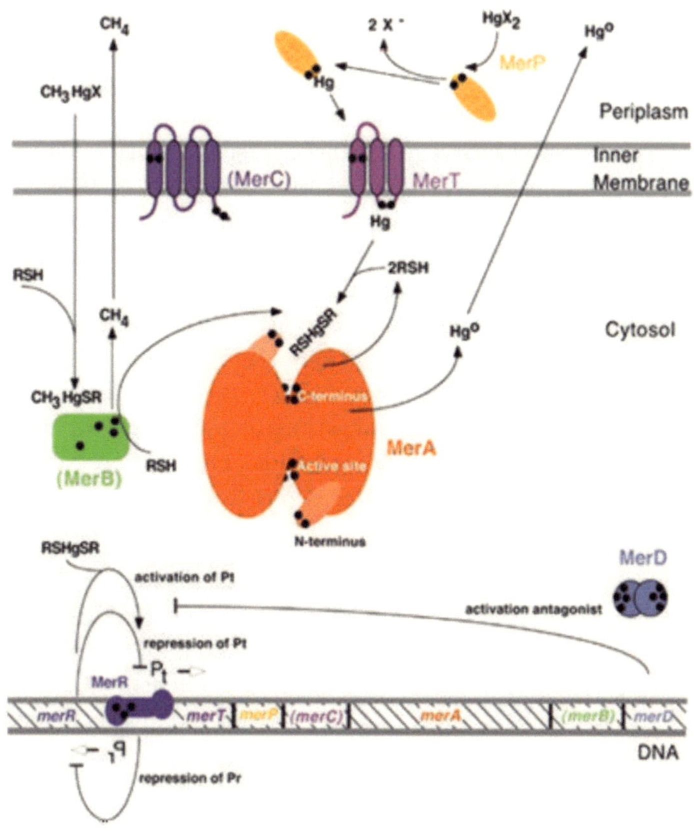


**Figure 8.** Representation of the *mer* operon and the processes whereby mercury species are transformed. Taken from Barkay et al. (2003) and used with permission from Elsevier.

However, while methane and $Hg^0$ are the primary products of *mer*-mediated Hg demethylation, $CO_2$ has also been observed as a major demethylation product in many studies [24, 94, 95] and this oxidative demethylation is not considered an active detoxification pathway. A variety of aerobes and anaerobes have been implicated in carrying out oxidative demethylation which has been observed in freshwater, estuarine and alkaline-hypersaline sediments

[24, 94, 96]. However, the identity of the organisms responsible for oxidative demethylation in the environment remains poorly understood and no specific organism has been isolated. One study confirmed the ability of two sulfate reducing bacterial strains and one methanogen strain to demethylate mercury in pure culture [97]. The authors however argued that the $CO_2$ seen in these studies resulted from oxidation of methane released from $CH_3Hg$ after cleavage via organomercurial lyase and was actually a secondary product and not the primary product of demethylation. However, this view is not universally accepted based on other their studies under both aerobic and anaerobic conditions [24]. Overall, the relative importance of *mer*-mediated versus oxidative demethylation is poorly understood. In systems that are not highly contaminated, oxidative demethylation appears to dominate, under both aerobic and anaerobic conditions. The Hg concentrations that would cause a switch from one pathway to the other are only loosely defined. The end-product of oxidative demethylation has been presumed to be Hg(II), but that has not been confirmed in most studies.

Studies in freshwater and marine sediments [24, 42, 67, 94, 98] however confirm that the rate of demethylation is rapid, and that the rate constant for this process is higher than that of methylation, and that demethylation occurs across the redox gradient. Many of these studies have used stable isotope approaches, where isotopically-labelled inorganic Hg, and $CH_3Hg$ made using a different isotope of Hg, are spiked into sediments or water and the transformations of each followed under the same conditions. Another approach is to use radiolabelled Hg and $^{14}C$-labeled $CH_3Hg$ but these approaches cannot be done at the trace levels of the stable isotope method. There is an obvious advantage of simultaneously examining both of the reactions in the same experiment. These studies [42, 67, 98] have shown overall that the fraction of Hg as $CH_3Hg$ in sediments is often closely related to the ratio of the rate constants, which suggests that both reactions are pseudo first order and that the system reaches steady state relatively rapidly. Given that demethylation rate constants on the order of 10 $d^{-1}$ have been measured in some sediment, the time to steady state is a few days.

Biodegradation studies of other methylated compounds are limited but these are likely to occur in sediments and reduced environments [82, 99]. One study examining the degradation of methylated As compounds in a lake showed that the decomposition occurred in the presence of suspended particulate but not in filtered water, implicating microbial processes in the decomposition. Degradation occurred in the dark under anaerobic conditions. Studies of alkylated Sn compounds have similarly shown their degradation in the sediment and it is likely that anaerobic microbes can demethylate most of the commonly found methylated metal(loid)s in the environment.

## 5. Abiotic Formation and Degradation Pathways in Aquatic Systems

A variety of methyl donors exist in environmental solutions and these have the potential to methylate the metal(loid)s discussed here. Pathways include the following primary mechanisms: 1) cross-methylation i.e. transfer of a methyl group from one metal(loid) compound to another e.g. $(CH_3)_4Pb + Hg^{II} \rightarrow (CH_3)_3Pb^+ + CH_3Hg^+$; and 2) methylation by other methyl-containing compounds such as methyliodide ($CH_3I$). For example, experiments examining the potential for the abiotic methylation of $As^{III}$ by $CH_3I$ found that the reaction proceeded, but only at very high pH's (>10), above those typically found in the environment [100]. Monomethylarsenic was the only product formed. This study therefore suggests that abiotic formation of methylated As is not likely in the environment. Other studies have shown that $CH_3I$ can methylate Pb, Sn and Ge [8], and there are also studies showing the methylation of $Hg^0$ by $CH_3I$, but not with $Hg^{II}$ [101]. Again, these studies do not suggest that these reactions are important in the environment. For example, the rate of formation of $CH_3Hg$ from $Hg^0$ in the presence of $CH_3I$, given typical environmental concentrations of these species, is insufficient to account for any substantial portion of the $CH_3Hg$ found in natural waters. For Hg, the same conclusion is reached in terms of methyl transfer reactions between methylated tin compounds and $Hg^{II}$, even though it appeared that the presence of Cl and high pH, which would be found in seawater, enhanced the reaction rate [101]. Overall, the results of a number of studies over time [52, 101-104] lead to the conclusion that abiotic formation of $CH_3Hg$ in the environment by these pathways is not important.

There have been a number of studies that have shown the potential for the transfer of a methyl group from an organic compound to $Hg^{II}$, and the formation of $CH_3Hg$ in environmental waters [102, 104, 105], including precipitation [106]. However, most of these experiments have been conducted at unrealistic concentrations of both Hg and the organic compound, as well as having a ratio of Hg/organic matter much greater than found in the environment. Additionally, the reactions are often done at low pH or high temperature. Clearly, these experiments show that $CH_3Hg$ can be manufactured abiotically, which is no surprise, but the results of these studies have little environmental relevance. For example, in the laboratory, $CH_3Hg$ is routinely manufactured through the reaction with cobalamin. This does not however suggest that this is occurring abiotically in the environment.

In terms of abiotic decomposition, the stability of organometal(loid)s in water is related to the polarity of the metal carbon bond with more polarity enhancing hydrolysis and decomposition [107]. However, while many organometal(loid)s may be thermodynamically unstable, they are often kinetically stable and are not degraded abiotically as readily as may be expected. For example, $CH_3Hg$ which is less stable in water at low pH but the reaction is kinetically hindered [108]. Photochemical processes however can enhance the degradation rate. This is an important loss process for methylated Hg. Dimethylmercury is much less stable to photochemical degradation than $CH_3Hg$ [109]. In the ocean, the rate of $CH_3Hg$ photodecomposition varies, with some studies showing relative rapid rates of degradation, while others have shown little degradation [110-112]. It is likely that complexation to $Cl^-$or NOM in seawater impacts this rate, but these effects have been little studied compared to in freshwater systems [111, 113, 114]. The degradation of $CH_3Hg$ in freshwater has received more study and photochemical oxidants and UV radiation are important in driving the degradation [114-117] with various reactive oxygen species implicated in the reactions [113, 118]. For the methylated Se compounds, it is likely that oxidation occurs in the presence of light, especially UV radiation, as has been found for methylated S compounds (e.g. $(CH_3)_2S$) [29, 119].

A photochemical degradation study will tetraethyllead showed that first order decrease of the reactant with the subsequent buildup and decay of the intermediates [120]. The final product was $Pb^{II}$. It is likely that tetramethyllead would be degraded in a similar fashion. For Se, photodecomposition of selenoamino acids can produce significant amounts of volatile selenium species in both light and dark conditions in the laboratory, with $(CH_3)_2SSe$ and $(CH_3)_2Se_2$ being the major products, with small amounts of $(CH_3)_2Se$ being formed [29]. Inorganic selenium oxyanions did not produce any volatile products. It was hypothesized that formation of $H_2O_2$ under the experimental conditions initiated the decomposition reactions. Overall, it is likely that multi-methylated species can be photochemically decomposed by the stepwise removal of methyl groups. This is discussed above and is true for the decomposition of $(CH_3)_2Hg$.

## 6. Conclusion

The methylation of metal(loid)s in the environment is important to the fate and transport of many of the elements in Groups 12-16 of the periodic table. This is true for elements besides those that have received the most attention (Hg, As and Se). Much of the research done on these three elements can be extrapolated to the other elements based on knowledge about the chemistry of the elements in environmental waters and the uptake and fate of the elements within cells. While there is still more research needed to fully understand the methylation, demethylation and fate and transport of Hg, As and Se, this is even more necessary for the other metal(loid)s discussed in this chapter.

## Acknowledgements

Acknowledgements The support of NSF and NIH, especially grant P42 ES007373 from NIEHS, is acknowledged for support of studies and work cited and in supporting the chapter prepartion. The contents of this chapter are solely the responsibility of the author and do not represent the official views of NIH.

## Author details

Robert P. Mason*

Address all correspondence to: robert.mason@uconn.edu

Departments of Marine Sciences and Chemistry, University of Connecticut, USA

## References

[1] Craig. (2003). *Organometallic Compunds in the Environment*, John Wiley and Sons, Chichester, 22.

[2] Benoit, J. M., Gilmour, C. C., Heyes, A., Mason, R. P., & Miller, C. L. (2003). Geochemical and biological controls over methylmercury production and degradation in aquatic ecosystems. *Biogeochemistry of Environmentally Important Trace Elements*, ACS Symposium Series #, book editors are Cai, Y and Braids, OC, 835, 262-297.

[3] Kerin, E. J., Gilmour, C. C., Roden, E., Suzuki, M. T., Coates, J. D., & Mason, R. P. (2006). Mercury methylation by dissimilatory iron-reducing bacteria. *Applied and Environmental Microbiology*, 72(12), 7919-7921.

[4] Bentley, R., & Chasteen, T. G. (2002). Microbial methylation of metalloids: Arsenic, antimony, and bismuth. *Microbiology and Molecular Biology Reviews*, 66(2), 250.

[5] Sun, H. (2010). *Biological Chemistry of Arsenic, Antimony and Bismuth*, Hoboken, Wiley.

[6] Mason, R. P., Reinfelder, J. R., & Morel, F. M. M. (1996). Uptake, toxicity and trophic transfer of mercury in a coastal diatom. *Environ Sci. Technol*, 30(6), 1835-1845.

[7] Thayer, J. S. (2002). Biological methylation of less-studied elements. *Applied Organometallic Chemistry*, 16(12), 677-691.

[8] Dopp, E., Hartmann, L. M., Florea-M, A., Rettenmeier, A. W., & Hirner, A. V. (2004). Environmental distribution, analysis andtoxicity of organo metal(loid) compounds. *Critical Reviews in Toxicology*, 34(3), 301-333.

[9] Feldman, J. (2003). Volatilization of metals from a landfill site. In Biogeochemistry of Environmentally Important Trace Elements. Cai, Y.; Braids, O. C., Eds. ACS Series: Washington, DC, 128-140.

[10] Wuerfel, O., Thomas, F., Schulte, M. S., Hensel, R., & Diaz-Bone, R. A. (2012). Mechanism of multi-metal(loid) methylation and hydride generation by methylcobalamin and cob(I)balmain: a side reaction of methanogenesis. *Applied Organometallic Chemistry*, 26(2), 94-101.

[11] Wehmeier, S., Raab, A., & Feldmann, J. (2004). Investigations into the role of methylcobalamin and glutathione for the methylation of antimony using isotopically enriched antimony(V). *Applied Organometallic Chemistry*, 18(12), 631-639.

[12] Benoit, J. M., Gilmour, C. C., & Mason, R. P. (2001). Aspects of bioavailability of mercury for methylation in pure cultures of *Desulfobulbus propionicus* (1pr3). *Applied and Environmental Microbiology*, 67(1), 51-58.

[13] Morel, F., Milligan, A. J., & Saito, M. A. (2004). Marine Bioinorganic chemistry: The role of trace metals in the oceanic cycles of major nutrients. In The Oceans and Marine Geochemistry in Holland, HD and Turekian, KK (Exec Eds) *Treatise on Geochemistry* Elderfield, H., Ed. Elsevier Pergamon: Amsterdam , 6

[14] Cutter, G. A. (2010). Metalloids and oxyanions. *Marine Chemistry and Geochemistry*, Steele, J. H.; Thorpe, S. A.; Turekian, K. K., Eds. Elsevier: Amsterdam, 64-71.

[15] Clarkson, T. (1994). The toxicology of mercury and its compounds its compounds. In Mercury. *Mercury Pollution: Integration and Synthesis*, Synthesis Watras CJ and Huckabee, JW (Eds), Lewis Publishers, 631-641.

[16] Stolz, J. E., Basu, P., Santini, J. M., & Oremland, R. S. (2006). Arsenic and selenium in microbial metabolism. *Annual Review of Microbiology*, 60, 107-130.

[17] Nozaki, Y. (2010). Elemental distribution: An overview. Steele, J. H.; Thorpe, S. A.; Turekian, K. K., Eds. Elsevier: Amsterdam. *Marine Chemistry and Geochemistry*, 7-12.

[18] Cutter, G. A., & Cutter, L. S. (1998). Metalloids in the high latitude north Atlantic Ocean: Sources and internal cycling. *Marine Chemistry*, 61(1-2), 25-36.

[19] Cutter, G. A., & Cutter, L. S. (2001). Sources and cycling of selenium in the western and equatorial Atlantic Ocean. *Deep-Sea Research Part Ii-Topical Studies in Oceanography*, 48(13), 2917-2931.

[20] Cutter, G. A., & Cutter, L. S. (2006). The Biogeochemistry of arsenic and antimony in the North Pacific Ocean. *Geochemistry Geophysics Geosystems*, 7, Art # Q05M08.

[21] Edmonds, J. S., & Francesconi, K. A. (2003). Organoarsenic compounds in the marine environment. *Organometallic Compounds in the Environment*, Craig, P. J., Ed. Wiley: Chichester, 195-222.

[22] Craig, P. J., & Maher, W. A. (2003). Orgnaoselenium compounds in the environment. *Organometallic Compounds in the Environment*, Craig, P. J., Ed. wiley: Chichester, 391-398.

[23] Barkay, T., Miller, S. M., & Summers, A. O. (2003). Bacterial mercury resistance from atoms to ecosystems. *Fems Microbiology Reviews*, 27(2-3), 355-84.

[24] Marvin Di, Pasquale. M., Agee, J., Mc Gowan, C., Oremland, R. S., Thomas, M., Krabbenhoft, D., & Gilmour, C. C. (2000). Methyl-mercury degradation pathways: A comparison among three mercury-impacted ecosystems. *Environmental Science & Technology*, 34(23), 4908-4916.

[25] Mason, R. P., Choi, A. L., Fitzgerald, W. F., Hammerschmidt, C. H., Lamborg, C. H., Soerensen, A. L., & Sunderland, E. M. (2012). Mercury biogeochemical cycling in the ocean and policy implications. *Environmental Research.*

[26] Nice, A. J., Lung, W. S., & Riedel, G. F. (2008). Modeling arsenic in the Patuxent Estuary. *Environmental Science & Technology*, 42(13), 4804-4810.

[27] Sunderland, E. M., Krabbenhoft, D. P., Moreau, J. W., Strode, S. A., & Landing, W. M. (2009). Mercury sources, distribution, and bioavailability in the North Pacific Ocean: Insights from data and models. *Global Biogeochemical Cycles*, 23, Art # GB2010.

[28] Amouroux, D., Liss, P. S., Tessier, E., Hamren-Larsson, M., & Donard, O. F. X. (2001). Role of oceans as biogenic sources of selenium. *Earth and Planetary Science Letters*, 189(3-4), 227-283.

[29] Amouroux, D., Pecheyran, C., & Donard, O. F. X. (2000). Formation of volatile selenium species in synthetic seawater under light and dark experimental conditions. *Applied Organometallic Chemistry*, 14(5), 236-244.

[30] Amouroux, D., & Donard, O. F. X. (1997). Evasion of selenium to the atmosphere via biomethylation processes in the Gironde estuary, France. *Marine Chemistry*, 58(1-2), 173-188.

[31] Tessier, E., Amouroux, D., & Donard, O. F. X. (2003). Biogenic volatilization of trace elements from European estuaries. *Biogeochemistry of Environmentally Important Trace Elements*, Cai, Y.; Braids, O. C., Eds, 835, 151-165.

[32] Santosa, S. J., Wada, S., Mokudai, H., & Tanaka, S. (1997). The contrasting behaviour of arsenic and germanium species in seawater. *Applied Organometallic Chemistry*, 11(5), 403-414.

[33] Orians, K. J., & Merrin, C. L. (2010). Refractory metals. *Marine Chemsitry and Geochemistry*, Steele, J. H.; Thorpe, S. A.; Turekian, K. K., Eds. Elsevier: Amsterdam, 52-63.

[34] Fitzgerald, W., & Lamborg, C. H. (2005). Geochemsitry of mercury in the environment. *Environmental Geochemistry*, Holland HD and Turekian, KK (Eds), Elsevier: Amsterdam, 9, 107-147.

[35] Mason, R. P., & Benoit, J. M. (2003). Organomercury compounds in the environment. *Organometallic Compounds in the Environment*, Second ed.; Craig, P. J., Ed. John Wiley and Sons: Chichester, 57-99.

[36] Heimburger, L. E., Cossa, D., Marty, J. C., Migon, C., Averty, B., Dufour, A., & Ras, J. (2010). Methyl mercury distributions in relation to the presence of nano- and picophytoplankton in an oceanic water column (Ligurian Sea, North-western Mediterranean). *Geochimica Et Cosmochimica Acta*, 74(19), 5549-5559.

[37] Cossa, D., Heimburger, L. E., Lannuzel, D., Rintoul, S. R., Butler, E. C. V., Bowie, A. R., Averty, B., Watson, R. J., & Remenyi, T. (2011). Mercury in the Southern Ocean. *Geochimica Et Cosmochimica Acta*, 75(14), 4037-4052.

[38] Mason, R. P., & Fitzgerald, W. F. (1993). The distribution and biogeochemical cycling of mercury in the equatorial Pacific-Ocean. *Deep-Sea Research Part I-Oceanographic Research Papers*, 40(9), 1897-1924.

[39] Lehnherr, I., St. Louis, V. L., Hintelmann, H., & Kirk, J. L. (2009). Production and cycling of methylated ercury species in Arctic marine waters. Paper presented at 9th International Conference on Mercury As a Global Polutant, China. *Nature Geoscience*, 4(5), 298-302.

[40] Gilmour, C. C., Riedel, G. S., Ederington, M. C., Bell, J. T., Benoit, J. M., Gill, G. A., & Stordal, M. C. (1998). Methylmercury concentrations and production rates across a trophic gradient in the northern Everglades. *Biogeochemistry*, 40(2-3), 327-345.

[41] Hollweg, T. A., Gilmour, C. C., & Mason, R. P. (2009). Methylmercury production in sediments of Chesapeake Bay and the mid-Atlantic continental margin. *Marine Chemistry*, 86-101.

[42] Hollweg, T. A., Gilmour, C. C., & Mason, R. P. (2010). Mercury and methylmercury cycling in sediments of the mid-Atlantic continental shelf and slope. *Limnology and Oceanography*, 55(6), 2703-2722.

[43] Hammerschmidt, C. R., & Fitzgerald, W. F. (2004). Geochemical controls on the production and distribution of methylmercury in near-shore marine sediments. *Environmental Science & Technology*, 38(5), 1487-1495.

[44] Sunderland, E. M., Gobas, F., Branfireun, B. A., & Heyes, A. (2006). Environmental controls on the speciation and distribution of mercury in coastal sediments. *Marine Chemistry*, 102, 111-123.

[45] Chen, C. Y., Driscoll, C. T., & Kamman, N. C. (2012). Mercury hotspots in freshwater ecosystems. *Mercury in the Environment*, Bank, M. S., Ed. University of California Press: Berkeley and Los Angeles, 143-166.

[46] Sohrin, Y., Matsui, M., Kawashima, M., Hojo, M., & Hasegawa, H. (1997). Arsenic biogeochemistry affected by eutrophication in Lake Biwa, Japan. *Environmental Science & Technology*, 31(10), 2712-2720.

[47] Hasegawa, H. (1997). The behavior of trivalent and pentavalent methylarsenicals in Lake Biwa. *Applied Organometallic Chemistry*, 11(4), 305-312.

[48] Aurillo, A. C., Mason, R. P., & Hemond, H. F. (1994). Speciation and fate of arsenic in 3 lakes of The Aberjona Watershed. *Environmental Science & Technology*, 28(4), 577-585.

[49] Rahman, M. A., & Hasegawa, H. Arsenic in freshwater systems: Influence of eutrophication on occurrence, distribution, speciation, and bioaccumulation. *Applied Geochemistry*, 27(1), 304-314.

[50] Mc Knight-Whitford, A., Chen, B. W., Naranmandura, H., Zhu, C., & Le , X. C. New Method and Detection of High Concentrations of Monomethylarsonous Acid Detected in Contaminated Groundwater. *Environmental Science & Technology*, 44(15), 5875-5880.

[51] Planer-Friedrich, B, Lehr, C, Matschullat, J, Merkel, B. J, Nordstrom, D. K, & Sandstrom, M. W. (2006). Speciation of volatile arsenic at geothermal features in Yellowstone National Park. *Geochimica Et Cosmochimica Acta*, 70(10), 2480-2491.

[52] Weber, J. H. (1999). Volatile hydride and methyl compounds of selected elements formed in the marine environment. *Marine Chemistry*, 65(1-2), 67, 75.

[53] Neumann, P. M., De Souza, M. P., Pickering, I. J., & Terry, N. (2003). Rapid microalgal metabolism of selenate to volatile dimethylselenide. *Plant Cell and Environment*, 26(6), 897-905.

[54] Andrewes, P., Cullen, W. R., Feldmann, J., Koch, I., Polishchuk, E., & Reimer, E. (1998). The production of methylated organoantimony compounds by Scopulariopsis brevicaulis. *Applied Organometallic Chemistry*, 12(12), 827-842.

[55] Oyamada, N., Takahashi, G., & Ishizaki, M. (1991). Methylation of inorganic selenium-compounds by fresh-water green-algae, *Ankistrodesmus* sp *chlorella-vulgaris* and *Selenastrum* sp. *Eisei Kagaku-Japanese Journal of Toxicology and Environmental Health*, 37(2), 83-88.

[56] Clarkson, T. W. (1990). Human health risks from methylmercury in fish. *Environ. Toxicol. Chem.*, 9, 821-823.

[57] Compeau, G., & Bartha, R. (1985). Sulfate-reducing bacteria: principal methylators of mercury in anoxic estuarine sediment. *Appl. Environ. Microbiol.*, 50, 498-502.

[58] Gilmour, C. C, Henry, E. A, & Mitchell, R. (1992). Sulfate stimulation of mercury methylation in freshwater sediments. *Environ. Sci. Technol*, 26, 2281-2287.

[59] Fleming, E. J., Mack, E. E., Green, P. G., & Nelson, D. C. (2006). Mercury methylation from unexpected sources: Molybdate-inhibited freshwater sediments and an iron-reducing bacterium. *Applied and Environmental Microbiology*, 72, 457-464.

[60] Hamelin, S., Amyot, M., Barkay, T., Wang, Y. P., & Planas, D. (2011). Methanogens: Principal methylators of mercury in lake periphyton. *Environ. Sci. Technol.*, 18, 7693-7700.

[61] Choi, S. C., Chase, T., & Bartha, R. (1994). Metabolic Pathways Leading to Mercury Methylation in *Desulfovibrio-desulfuricans* LS. *Applied and Environmental Microbiology*, 60(11), 4072-4077.

[62] Choi, S. C., & Bartha, R. (1993). Cobalamin-mediated mercury methylation by Desulfovibrio desulfuricans LS. *Applied and Environmental Microbiology*, 60(11), 290-295.

[63] Choi, S. C., Chase, J. R., , T., & Bartha, R. (1994). Enzymatic catalysis of mercury methylation by Desulfovibrio desulfuricans LS. *Applied and Environmental Microbiology*, 60(11), 1342-1346.

[64] Ekstrom, E. B., & Morel, F. M. M. (2008). Cobalt limitation of growth and mercury methylation in sulfate-reducing bacteria. *Environmental Science & Technology*, 42(1), 93-99.

[65] Ekstrom, E. B., Morel, F. M. M., & Benoit, J. M. (2003). Mercury methylation independent of the acetyl-coenzyme a pathway in sulfate-reducing bacteria. *Applied and Environmental Microbiology*, 69(9), 5414 -5422.

[66] Lin, C. C., & Jay, J. A. (2007). Mercury methylation by planktonic and biofilm cultures of Desulfovibrio desulfuricans. *Environmental Science & Technology*, 41(19), 6691-6697.

[67] Heyes, A., Mason, R. P., Kim, E. H., & Sunderland, E. (2006). Mercury methylation in estuaries: Insights from using measuring rates using stable mercury isotopes. *Marine Chemistry*, 102(1-2), 134-147.

[68] Benoit, J. M., Gilmour, C. C., & Mason, R. P. (2001). The influence of sulfide on solid phase mercury bioavailability for methylation by pure cultures of *Desulfobulbus propionicus* (1pr3). *Environmental Science & Technology*, 35(1), 127-132.

[69] Jay, J. A, Morel, F. M. M, & Hemond, H. F. (2000). Mercury speciation in the presence of polysulfides. *Environmental Science & Technology*, 34(11), 2196-2200.

[70] Mason, R. P. (2000). The bioaccumulation of mercury, methylmercury and other toxic trace metals into pelagic and benthic organisms. *Coastal and Estuarine risk Assessment*, Newman, M. C., Hale, R.C., Ed. CRC Press: Boca Raton, 127-149.

[71] Schaefer, J. K., & Morel, F. M. M. (2009). High methylation rates of mercury bound to cysteine by *Geobacter sulfurreducens*. *Nature Geoscience*, 2(2), 123-126.

[72] Schaefer, J. K., Rocks, S. S., Zheng, W., Liang, L. Y., Gu, B. H., & Morel, F. M. M. (2012). Active transport, substrate specificity, and methylation of Hg(II) in anaerobic bacteria. *Proceedings of the National Academy of Sciences of the United States of America*, 108(21), 8714-8719.

[73] Mason, R. P., & Fitzgerald, W. F. (1991). Mercury speciation in open ocean waters. *Water Air and Soil Pollution*, 56, 779-789.

[74] Kim, J. P., & Fitzgerald, W. F. (1988). Gaseous mercury profiles in the tropical Pacific Ocean. *Geophysical Research Letter*, 15, 40-43.

[75] Mason, R. P., & Fitzgerald, W. F. (1990). Alkylmercury species in the equatorial Pacific. *Nature*, 347, 457-459.

[76] Hammerschmidt, C. H., & Bowman, K. L. (2012). Vertical methylmercury distribution in the subtropical North Pacific Ocean. *Marine Chemistry*, 132, 77-82.

[77] Mason, R. P., Rolfhus, K. R., & Fitzgerald, W. F. (1998). Mercury in the North Atlantic. *Marine Chemistry*, 61, 37-53.

[78] Mason, R. P., & Sullivan, K. A. (1999). The distribution and speciation of mercury in the South and equatorial Atlantic. *Deep-Sea Research Part Ii-Topical Studies in Oceanography*, 46(5), 937.

[79] Horvat, M., Kotnik, J., Logar, J. M., Fajon, V., Zvonaric, T., & Pirrone, N. (2003). Speciation of mercury in surface and deep-sea waters in the Mediterranean Sea. *Atmos. Environ.*, 37(1), S 93-S108.

[80] Lamborg, C. H., Hammerschmidt, C. R., Saito, M., Goepfert, T. R., & Lam, P. J. (2009). Mercury methylation in the gyre and Benguela upwelling regions of the tropical

South Atlantic Ocean. In 9th International Conference on Mercury As a Global Polutant China

[81] Plant, J., Kinniburgh, D. G., Smedley, P. L., & Fordyce, F. M. (2005). Arsenic and Selenium. *Environmental Geochemistry*, Holland HD and Turekian, KK (Eds). Elsevier: Amsterdam, 9, 17-65.

[82] Feldman, J. (2003). Other organometallic compounds in the environment. *Organometallic Compounds in the Environment*, Craig, P., Ed. John Wiley and Sons: Chichester, 353-390.

[83] Reimer, K. J. (1989). The methylation of arsenic in marine sediments. *Applied Organometallic Chemistry*, 3, 475-490.

[84] Duester, L., Vink, J. P. M., & Hirner, A. V. (2008). Methylantimony and-arsenic species in sediment pore water tested with the sediment and fauna incubation experiment. *Environ. Sci. Technol.*, 42, 5866-5871.

[85] Ebdon, L., Walton, A. P., Millward, g. E., & Whitfield, M. (1987). Methylated arsenic species in estuarine porewaters. *Applied Organometallic Chemistry*, 1, 427-433.

[86] Bright, D. A., Brock, S., Cullen, W. R., Hewitt, G. M., Jafaar, J., & Reimer, K. J. (1994). Methylation of arsenic by anaerobic microbial consortia isolated from lake sediment. *Applied Organometallic Chemistry*, 8(4), 415-422.

[87] Stolz, J. F., & Oremland, R. S. (1999). Bacterial respiration of arsenic and selenium. *Fems Microbiology Reviews*, 615(627), 61-27.

[88] Ranjard, L., Nazaret, S., & Cournoyer, B. (2003). Freshwater bacteria can methylate selenium through the thiopurine methyltransferase pathway. *Appl. Environ. Microbiol.*, 69, 3784-3790.

[89] Khan, M. A. K., & Wang, F. Y. (2009). Mercury-selenium compounds and their toxicological significance: Toward a molecular understanding of the mercury-selenium antagonism. *Environmental Toxicology and Chemistry*, 28, 1567-1577.

[90] Craig, P. J., & P. D. B. (1978). The role of hydrogen sulfide in the transport of mercury. *Nature*, 275, 635-637.

[91] Pongratz, R., & Heumann, K. G. (1999). Production of methylated mercury, lead and cadmium by marine bacteria as a significant source of atmospheric heavy metals in polar regions. *Chemosphere*, 14(6), 89.

[92] Schedlbauer, O. F., & Heumann, K. G. (2000). Biomethylation of thallium by bacteria and first determination of biogenic dimethylthallium in the ocean. *Applied Organometallic Chemistry*, 330-340.

[93] Perrin, D. D. (1982). Ionization Constants for Inorganic Acids and Bases in Aqueous Solution. Pergammon Press: Oxford.

[94] Oremland, R. S., Culbertson, C. W., & Winfrey, M. R. (1991). Methylmercury decomposition in sediments and bacterial cultures: Involvement of methanogens and sulfate reducers in oxidative demthylation. *Appl. Environ. Microbiol.*, 57, 130-137.

[95] Oremland, R. S., Miller, L. G., Dowdle, P., Connel, T., & Barkay, T. (1995). Methylmercury oxidative degradation potentials in contaminated and pristine sediments of the Carson River, Nevada. *Appl. Environ. Microbiol.*, 61, 2745-2753.

[96] Marvin-Dipasquale, M., & Oremland, R. (1998). Bacterial methylmercury degradation in Florida Everglades peat sediment. *Environ. Sci. Technol.*, 32, 2556-2563.

[97] Pak, K. R., & Bartha, R. (1998). Mercury methylation and demethylation in Anoxic Lake sediments and by strictly anaerobic bacteria. *Applied and Environmental Microbiology*, 64, 1013-1017.

[98] Kim, E. H., Mason, R. P., Porter, E. T., & Soulen, H. L. (2006). The impact of resuspension on sediment mercury dynamics, and methylmercury production and fate: A mesocosm study. *Marine Chemistry*, 102(3-4), 300-315.

[99] Craig, P. J. (1986). Organomercury compounds in the environment. Organometallic Compounds in the Environment. Craig, P. J., Ed. Longman Essex.

[100] Chen, B. W., Wang, T., He, B., Yuan, C. G., Gao, E. L., & Jiang, G. B. (2006). Simulate methylation reaction of arsenic(III) with methyl iodide in an aquatic system. *Applied Organometallic Chemistry*, 20(11), 747-753.

[101] Celo, V., Lean, D. R. S., & Scott, S. L. (2006). Abiotic methylation of mercury in the aquatic environment. *Science of the Total Environment*, 368(1), 126-137.

[102] Weber, J. (1993). Review of possible paths for abiotic methylation of mercury(II) in the aquatic environment. *Chemosphere*, 26, 2063-2077.

[103] Weber, J., Evans, R., Jones, S., & Hines, M. (1998). Conversion of mercury (II) into mercury (0), monomethylmercury cation, and dimethylmercury in saltmarsh sediment slurries. *Chemosphere*, 36, 1669-1687.

[104] Weber, J., Reisinger, K., & Stoeppler, M. (1985). Methylation of mercury (II) by fulvic acid. *Environ. Technol.*, 6, 203-208.

[105] Yin, Y. G., Chen, B. W., Mao, Y. X., Wang, T., Liu, J. F., Cai, Y., & Jiang, G. B. (2010). Possible alkylation of inorganic Hg(II) by photochemical processes in the environment. *Chemosphere*, 88(1), 8-16.

[106] Hammerschmidt, C. R., Lamborg, C. H., & Fitzgerald, W. F. (2007). Aqueous phase methylation as a potential source of methylmercury in wet deposition. *Atmospheric Environment*, 41(8), 1663-1668.

[107] Craig, P. J., & Maher, W. A. (2003). Organoselenium compounds in the environment. *Organometallic Compounds in the Environment*, Craig, P., Ed. John Wiley and Sons: Chichester, 391-398.

[108] Stumm, W., & Morgan, J. J. (1996). Aquatic Chemistry. John Wiley and Sons: New York.

[109] Mason, R. P., Lawson, N. M., & Sheu, G. R. (2001). Mercury in the Atlantic Ocean: factors controlling air-sea exchange of mercury and its distribution in the upper waters. *Deep-Sea Research Part Ii-Topical Studies in Oceanography*, 48(13), 2829.

[110] Whalin, L., Kim, E. H., & Mason, R. (2007). Factors influencing the oxidation, reduction, methylation and demethylation of mercury species in coastal waters. *Marine Chemistry*, 107(3), 278-294.

[111] Black, , F. J., Poulin, B. A., & Flegal, A. R. (2012). Factors controlling the degradation of monomethylmercury in surface waters. *Geochimica et Cosmochimica Acta*, 84, 492-507.

[112] Suda, I., Suda, M., & Hirayama, K. (1993). Degradation of methyl and ethyl mercury by singlet oxygen generated from sea water exposed to sunlight or ultraviolet light. *Arch. Toxicol.*, 67, 365-368.

[113] Zhang, T., & Hsu-Kim, H. (2010). Photolytic degradation of methylmercury enhanced by binding to natural organic ligands. *Nature Geoscience*, 3(7), 473-476.

[114] Hammerschmidt, C. R., & Fitzgerald, W. F. (2010). Iron-mediated photochemical decomposition of methylmercury in an arctic Alaskan lake. *Environ Sci Technol*, 44, 6138-6143.

[115] Gardfeldt, K., Sommar, J., Stromberg, D., & Feng, X. B. (2001). Oxidation of atomic mercury by hydroxyl radicals and photoinduced decomposition of methylmercury in the aqueous phase. *Atmospheric Environment*, 35(17), 3039-3047.

[116] Inoko, M. (1981). Studies on the photochemical decomposition of organomercurials--methylmercury(II) chloride. *Environmental Pollution B*, 2, 3-10.

[117] Sellers, P., Kelly, C. A., Rudd, J. W. M., & Mac Hutchon, A. R. (1996). Photodegradation of methylmercury in lakes. *Nature*, 380, 694-697.

[118] Chen, J, Pehkonen, S. O, & Lin, C.-J. (2003). Degradation of monomethylmercury chloride by hydroxyl radicals in simulated natural waters. *Water Research*, 37, 2496-2504.

[119] Yang, G. P., Li, C. X., Qi, J. L., Hu, L. G., & Hou, H. J. (2007). Photochemical oxidation of dimethylsulfide in seawater. *Acta Oceanologica Sinica*, 26, 34-42.

[120] Yoshinaga, J. (2003). Organolead compounds in the environment. Craig, P. J., Ed. Chichester. *Organometallic Compounds in the Environment*, 151-194.